Tutorials in Differential Diagnosis

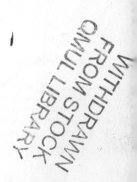

For Churchill Livingstone

Publisher: Laurence Hunter
Editorial Co-ordination: Editorial Resources Unit
   Copy Editor: Jennifer Bew
   Indexer: J. Roderick Gibb
Production Controller: Lesley W. Small
Design: Design Resources Unit
Sales Promotion Executive: Marion Pollock

Tutorials in Differential Diagnosis

Eric R Beck BSc MB BS FRCP
Consultant Physician,
Whittington Hospital, London;
Honorary Senior Clinical Lecturer in Medicine,
University College and Middlesex School of
Medicine, London

John L Francis MSc MB BS FRCP
Consultant Physician,
Staffordshire General Infirmary, Stafford

Robert L Souhami BSc MD FRCP
Kathleen Ferrier Professor of Clinical Oncology;
Consultant Physician, University College
and Middlesex School of Medicine, London

THIRD EDITION

CHURCHILL LIVINGSTONE
EDINBURGH LONDON MADRID MELBOURNE NEW YORK AND TOKYO 1992

CHURCHILL LIVINGSTONE
Medical Division of Longman Group UK Limited

Distributed in the United States of America by Churchill
Livingstone Inc., 650 Avenue of the Americas, New York,
N.Y. 10011, and by associated companies, branches and,
representatives throughout the world.

First edition 1974 (Pitman Publishing Ltd)
Second edition 1982
    Reprinted 1987 (Churchill Livingstone)
    Reprinted 1986
Third edition 1992
    Reprinted 1994
    Reprinted 1995

ISBN 0 443 04472 4

British Library Cataloguing Publication Data
A catalogue record for this book is available from the
British Library.

Library of Congress Cataloguing in Publication Data
Beck, Eric R.
    Tutorials in differential diagnosis/Eric R.Beck, John L.
Francis, Robert L. Souhami. — 3rd ed.
        p.   cm.
        Previous American ed. has title: Tutorials in differential
diagnosis. c 1974
        Includes index.
        1. Diagnosis, Differential. I. Francis, John L. II. Souhami,
Robert L. III. Beck, Eric R. Differential diagnosis. IV. Title.
        [DNLM: 1. Diagnosis, Differential. WB 141 B393t]
RC71.5.B37 1992
616.07'5-dc20
DNLM/DLC
for Library of Congress
91-29308
CIP

The
publisher's
policy is to use
**paper manufactured
from sustainable forests**

Produced by Longman Singapore Publishers (Pte) Ltd.
Printed in Singapore

Preface

In the course of our experience of undergraduate and postgraduate teaching, we have noticed that although many students have a wide theoretical knowledge they often lack the ability to apply this to individual clinical problems. Symptoms and signs are the raw material of medicine: this is how doctors are confronted by patients on their first day in the wards as a student and for the rest of their professional life. While patients present with symptoms, most textbooks are written in the form of descriptions of diseases. This book attempts to give a symptom rather than a disease-orientated approach. It is intended for students, for postgraduates studying for higher examinations, and for all those who wish to refresh themselves on common problems in internal medicine.

Each chapter discusses a common symptom or sign. It attempts to relate this to normal and abnormal function so as to give a basis for understanding. The clinical features which are important in the differential diagnosis are emphasized and there is a discussion of those investigations which will help to establish the diagnosis. Subjects have been selected which are either important in the day-to-day practice of general medicine, or which are poorly understood by students and postgraduates. At the end of each chapter there is an illustrative case history with questions. This is followed by a detailed discussion of the case. These problems serve as a challenge to the reader's diagnostic ability and as a test of comprehension of the chapter. They will be of value to those taking the MRCP(UK) examinations which contain this type of case problem.

Since the second edition in 1982, HIV infection and AIDS have become important health problems. Like syphilis in the past, these disorders must now be considered in the differential diagnosis of disease affecting many systems of the body.

Diagnostic methods continue to increase in sophistication and power, while at the same time becoming progressively less invasive. The newer imaging techniques in particular have revolutionised the approach to many diagnostic problems.

It has, therefore, been necessary to make considerable changes in this third edition so that these new and exciting developments can be given due weight and their incorporation into diagnostic protocols clearly demonstrated.

E R Beck
J L Francis
R L Souhami

London and Stafford, 1992

Contents

1. Palpitations

Patients and doctors often differ in their understanding of medical terms. Doctors usually use the term palpitations to mean a feeling of the heart thumping inside the chest. Patients may also use it to describe a feeling of breathlessness, especially when excited, a feeling of fright and panic, and pain in the chest, usually over the heart .

Awareness of the heart's action does not only occur when it is beating rapidly, although paroxysmal tachycardia is one of the commonest causes of palpitations. A slow heartbeat of excessive force, as may occur paroxysmally from a phaeochromocytoma producing noradrenaline, can also give rise to this complaint. Similarly, a patient may become aware of irregularity of the heartbeat as with atrial fibrillation or ectopic beats.

Palpitations may be due to a primary cardiac disorder, whether acute or chronic, or to a condition elsewhere in the body which is having a secondary effect on the heart.

With the increasing use of cardiac monitoring, especially after myocardial infarction, it is found that patients may have a wide variety of transient arrhythmias. Some of these, if ignored, can have dangerous consequences. However, 'palpitations' occurring during intensive care in the coronary unit will not usually present any diagnostic problem and will not therefore be discussed further.

HISTORY AND EXAMINATION

The first point is to ask what the patient means by his symptom of palpitations. Here it may be useful to ask him to tap out what he feels is his heart rhythm. One must decide whether the patient is aware of the palpitations all the time or whether they occur only in clear-cut attacks. If the patient is vague about the length of time he has had the symptom this suggests a sinus tachycardia or established atrial fibrillation. If he can clearly remember the abrupt onset of one or more episodes then it is likely to be some form of paroxysmal tachycardia. Occasionally the patient may be aware of an equally abrupt termination, though usually an episode fades away. He may even have learnt, or have been taught, simple tricks which

terminate the attacks. For example swallowing ice, pressure on the eyeballs or carotid sinus massage, by causing reflex stimulation of the vagus may end paroxysms of supraventricular tachycardia. Polyuria is another feature of paroxysmal tachycardia that should be sought, as the patient may hesitate to volunteer the information thinking it irrelevant. This may come on within a few minutes of the onset of the tachycardia and consists of passing large amounts of dilute urine. It is related to a raised left atrial pressure stimulating the release of the hormone atrial naturetic peptide (ANP) and is confined to those with otherwise normal hearts.

Cardiac neurosis

Precipitating factors obviously are an important point in the history. The patient with an anxiety state may notice a rapid pulse at times of stress, or may only be aware of it when totally unoccupied apart from introspection. In such a situation his discovery that the heart is beating rapidly may in turn give rise to anxiety that something is wrong with it and so create a vicious circle. It is, of course, normal for the heart to accelerate on exercise, but undue acceleration or failure to decelerate on stopping the exercise is another feature of anxiety or cardiac neurosis (effort syndrome). It is also a feature of lack of physical fitness. The sleeping pulse rate will be normal. The condition was first described amongst army recruits in the First World War who often had systolic murmurs of innocent origin. They had been allowed to worry about their health as a result of their physicians' failure to recognize that their hearts were normal. The term 'effort syndrome' is applied more widely nowadays to patients with psychosomatic symptoms which are referred to the cardiovascular system and may often suggest cardiac disease. The heart will usually be entirely normal although occasionally the patient may indeed have mild rheumatic or ischaemic heart disease. The symptoms and ensuing disability, however, are out of all proportion to the underlying lesion.

This diagnosis can only be made by a carefully taken and interpreted history. The patient often has a past history of depression or anxiety or of phobic symptoms. Sometimes his symptoms will afford a protection from the situation he seeks to avoid (as in warfare). The content of dreams or nightmares may be a useful clue. In addition to palpitations there is often the complaint of chest pain after effort. This is a dull ache, often associated with tenderness in the left infra-mammary region, rather than the retrosternal pain of cardiac ischaemia. It may persist for hours or days. Breathlessness, characteristically described as inability to take a satisfactory breath in, is often manifested by the patient taking deep sighs. He is usually unable to hold his breath for 30 seconds as a normal person can. Some authorities attach significance to the absence of a period of apnoea following forced hyperventilation in these patients. Headaches, described as pressure on top of the head or a tight band, excessive sweating in the 'emotional' areas of palms and axillae, and coarse tremor are all common features. This condition has deliberately been discussed first because a positive diagnosis should be made, and not arrived at by exclusion of other causes.

Provoking factors

The effect of exercise on an irregular pulse can be of value in differentiating multiple extrasystoles from atrial fibrillation. The patient may either have noticed, or he can be exercised to show, that extrasystoles tend to disappear, whereas the irregular ventricular response to atrial fibrillation becomes more pronounced. Sometimes a relationship between extrasystoles and heavy smoking or coffee drinking may be established. Patients with phaeochromocytomas which discharge adrenaline or noradrenaline paroxysmally may, in addition to palpitations, notice sweating, pallor and headache. Certain bending, twisting, or rolling movements of the trunk, or, rarely, deep palpitation of the abdomen, may also provoke such an attack.

Associated features

Other symptoms may either suggest underlying organic heart disease or indicate that there is some non-cardiac cause. If true angina occurs during an attack of palpitations it is likely that the fall in cardiac output resulting from the arrhythmia is the cause. The coronary circulation will probably be already impaired due either to a low cardiac output, as in mitral or aortic stenosis, or to extensive atherosclerosis of the coronary arteries.

Patients may have symptoms suggestive of anaemia or thyrotoxicosis, and it should be remembered that in the elderly, thyrotoxicosis may present with cardiac symptoms alone. Another manifestation of a change in cardiac rhythm in the elderly may be dizziness or fainting due to the accompanying fall in cardiac output (see Ch. 19). If palpitations are accompanied by episodes of diarrhoea, flushing, and wheezing, the possibility of carcinoid syndrome due to an argentaffinoma must be considered.

Finally, an ever-increasing number of drugs given for non-cardiac conditions may affect the heart. Sympathomimetic drugs such as those used in the treatment of asthma may cause marked tachycardia. Psychotropic drugs such as the phenothiazines (e.g. chlorpromazine) increase electrical excitability and have been incriminated as a cause of ventricular fibrillation (similarly, they may render the treatment of epilepsy more difficult). The combination of a sympathomimetic drug, such as a bronchodilator, and a monoamine oxidase inhibitor in the treatment of depression, may give rise to hypertensive crises in which palpitations may occur. Cardiac drugs may be the cause of the palpitations, but because the patient may have been taking them for many years this may be overlooked. The introduction of a potent diuretic may precipitate digoxin toxicity as a result of hypokalaemia even though the digoxin dosage is unaltered. Digoxin must be remembered not only as a cause of bradycardia, pulsus bigeminus (coupled ectopic beats) and heart block, but also sometimes as a cause of atrial tachycardia often with varying degrees of block.

DIFFERENTIATION OF TACHYCARDIA

Although most patients with palpitations will have an electrocardiogram performed, in many cases its chief value will be to reassure the patient that there is no serious cardiac disease present. In sinus tachycardia the history and examination of other systems will often point to the cause.

Table 1.1 The causes of tachycardia

A. Sinus tachycardia

Fever
Anaemia
Anxiety
Menopause
Thyrotoxicosis
Phaeochromocytoma
Carcinoid syndrome
Drugs – sympathomimetics, atropine
Porphyria

B. Paroxysmal tachycardia

1. *Supraventricular* – (narrow complex)
a) Atrial and nodal, including Wolff–Parkinson–White syndrome
b) Atrial flutter
c) Atrial fibrillation

2. *Ventricular* – (Broad complex)
a) Ventricular tachycardia
b) Ventricular fibrillation

In patients suspected of attacks of paroxysmal tachycardia, it is self-evident that most will be learned by seeing a patient during an attack. Between attacks, the heart and ECG may be completely normal. One exception to this, where the diagnosis is best made between attacks, is the Wolff–Parkinson–White syndrome (WPW). Here there is a characteristic ECG pattern of apparent shortening of the PR interval caused by a delta wave on the upstroke of the R wave (Fig. 1.1). The electrical impulse originating in the atria bypasses the atrioventricular node (which momentarily delays the normal impulse). This pre-excitation occurs through an alternative conduction pathway called the bundle of Kent and fuses with that passing normally through the AV node. Patients with WPW are prone to attacks of paroxysmal atrial tachycardia during which the ECG does not show the characteristic delta waves and apparent PR shortening. This is a re-entrant tachycardia initiated by an atrial extrasystole occurring prematurely and being conducted normally through the AV node but not through the bundle of Kent, which is still refractory from the previous normal beat. By the time the impulse has traversed the AV node however, the bundle of Kent has recovered and permits retrograde conduction to the atria and thence through the AV node again, initiating a

tachycardia. Atrial fibrillation, which is a less commonly associated arrhythmia, may occur and is then often more rapid than when due to other causes, since the normal delay created by the AV node is bypassed. A very small number of patients have an associated congenital cardiac lesion (e.g. Ebstein's anomaly). Even in a normal heart, sudden death can occur.

A similar mechanism, without the ECG characteristics of WPW, gives rise to the AV re-entrant paroxysmal supraventricular tachycardia which is a common and usually benign arrhythmia without underlying cause.

Clinically indistinguishable atrial and nodal tachycardias may arise due to other mechanisms causing enhanced automaticity to foci other than the usual sinoatrial (SA node). Not only is there more likely to be underlying disease or an iatrogenic cause (digoxin toxicity) but their treatment differs from that of re-entrant tachycardia.

When paroxysmal atrial tachycardia, which is regular and constant, arises from a nodal source, the atria may contract simultaneously with the ventricles. Because the AV valves will be closed the right atrial contraction wave is reflected into the jugular vein and may be seen as a giant ('cannon') wave.

Paroxysmal atrial flutter or fibrillation will usually be easy to recognize on the ECG. In the former there is

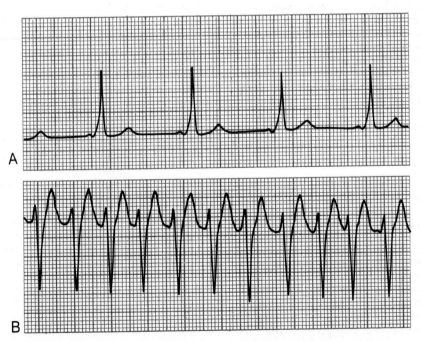

Fig 1.1 A. Standard lead I of a patient with Wolff–Parkinson–White syndrome. Note the short PR interval and the slurred upstroke of the R wave
B. Standard lead II of the same patient during an attack of supraventricular tachycardia. Note that the typical features of the WPW syndrome have disappeared.

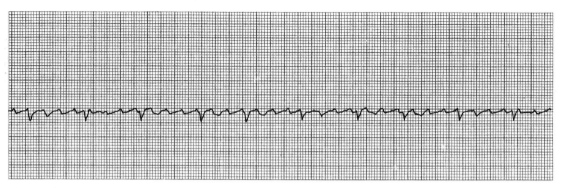

Fig. 1.2. Rhythm strip showing a ventricular rate of 87 beats/min in the presence of atrial flutter with a 3:1 block. (Courtesy of Dr D. Patterson.)

typically a fixed relationship between the atrial flutter waves and the ventricular response, which is never 1:1. This is spoken of as the degree of block, and may suddenly change either spontaneously or as a result of some manoeuvre like carotid sinus pressure or the use of drugs such as digoxin. A patient with a flutter rate of 150/min may have a ventricular rate of 75/min (2:1 block) and then change abruptly to 50/min (3:1 block). (See Fig. 1.2). In atrial fibrillation the atrial rate is more rapid and the ventricular response more irregular. An intermediate state of flutter-fibrillation may also occur. In any of these conditions there may be underlying rheumatic or ischaemic heart disease. These are also some of the arrhythmias which may follow myocardial infarction. Fever such as that due to pneumonia, pulmonary embolism, thyrotoxicosis or carcinoma of the bronchus with pericardial involvement are amongst the many other precipitating causes.

Difficulty in interpreting the ECG may occur in the differentiation of supraventricular tachycardia with bundle branch block from ventricular tachycardia. Hence the terms 'narrow complex' or 'broad complex' tachycardia are a more realistic and practical classification. (Table 1.1)

An important point here is to search hard for P waves which may be inverted and which sometimes occur within or after the QRS complex. These will indicate the supraventricular origin of the tachycardia. (Fig 1.3)

Ventricular tachycardia (VT) is a serious occurrence because of the danger that it leads to left ventricular failure and may progress to ventricular fibrillation and cardiac arrest. In broad complex tachycardia where it is unclear whether there is SVT with bundle branch block, or VT, it is better to treat for a presumed VT.

Although in the majority of patients ventricular extrasystoles, felt as a sudden thud or the heart missing a beat, are quite innocent, following myocardial infarction they assume greater significance. This is particularly so if they are multifocal, or if the ECG shows them to be occurring close to the T wave of the preceding complex, when there is a risk of the extrasystole inducing ventricular fibrillation. Again, prophylactic treatment will usually be indicated.

AMBULATORY MONITORING

There remains a number of patients in whom the nature of the palpitations will not have been eluci-

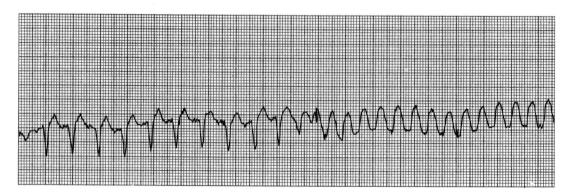

Fig. 1.3. Rhythm strip from a 24-hr ambulatory monitoring study showing transition from sinus tachycardia of 178 beats/min to ventricular tachycardia of > 250 beats/min. (Courtesy of Dr D. Patterson.)

dated on history, examination, and ECG. The use of ambulatory monitoring, in which a continuous 24-hour tape recording of the ECG is made while the patient continues normal activities, may be of great help in these cases. This may reveal dysrhythmias of which the patient is unaware, and also allows the patient to indicate on the tape when he is experienc- ing symptoms. This technique has also proved invaluable in the diagnosis of other types of 'attack' where a change in heart rhythm may be responsible (see Ch. 19, page 135). If arrhythmias occur so infre- quently that they are unlikely to be captured by 24-hour recording, an event recorder may allow a patient to record his ECG during an attack.

CLINICAL PROBLEM

T	P	BP	R
37	104	155/95	24

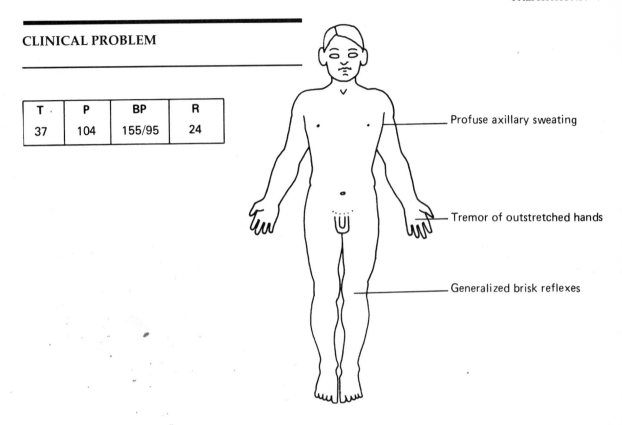

Profuse axillary sweating

Tremor of outstretched hands

Generalized brisk reflexes

A 33-year-old personnel manager was referred to hospital with the complaint of palpitations for the previous month. He had noticed that following exertion such as climbing stairs at home, he became aware of his heart beating rapidly but regularly. There was often an associated aching pain felt to the left of the sternum. Palpitations and pain would last for about 20 minutes and were accompanied by tremor and sweating of the hands. His wife had noticed that his shirts showed excess staining due to axillary sweating. The symptoms were by no means constant, and tended not to interfere with his work, but rather to occur in the evenings or at weekends when playing with his 8-year-old twin sons.

He was not taking any drugs. In the past he had taken vegetable laxatives for mild constipation, but for the last 2 months he had been having his bowels open twice each morning, passing soft formed stools, without the use of aperients.

Six months previously he had had an inferior myocardial infarction. He had been in hospital for 4 weeks and there had been no complications. On discharge from hospital he had been advised to reduce weight and had succeeded to the extent of his weight falling from 80 kg to 71 kg. He had also been advised to stop smoking and he was concerned that he had only been able to cut down from 35 to 20 cigarettes per day. He had returned to work 3 months prior to his present attendance.

On examination he was tense and nervous. His eyes were bright and staring and there was wrinkling of the forehead. There was a fine tremor of the fingers and profuse axillary sweating. The thyroid was not palpable and no bruit was heard over it. The pulse was 104/min and regular; all the peripheral pulses were palpable. Blood pressure was 155/95. The heart was not clinically enlarged and there were no added sounds or murmurs. All the limb reflexes were very brisk. The optic fundi were normal. No other abnormalities were found on clinical examination or urinalysis

Chest X-ray showed a normal cardiac silhouette and clear lung fields. ECG showed sinus rhythm. There were Q waves in leads II, III and AVF. The ST segments and T waves had returned to within normal limits compared with 6 months previously.

QUESTIONS

1. What are the likely causes of his present symptoms?
2. What investigations would you undertake?
3. What treatment would you recommend?

DISCUSSION

The patient is obviously worried that his present symptoms are a result of his previous myocardial infarction and represent a deterioration in his heart disease. The complications of ischaemic heart disease that have to be considered are angina and left ventricular failure. It is also possible that some form of paroxysmal tachycardia might be occurring.

The pain described does not have the typical features of angina. It comes on after, rather than during, exertion and it lasts too long. It is not situated in the characteristic site and does not show any radiation. Furthermore, it is not precipitated by a constant amount of physical exertion. Angina can present many atypical features and may be misinterpreted by the patient and even by the doctor as indigestion. However, in the majority of patients, close questioning will usually enable one to arrive at the correct diagnosis.

Pulmonary oedema or left ventricular failure is an unlikely diagnosis. There has been no cough or sputum, there is no gallop rhythm and on auscultation there are no abnormal signs in the lungs. There is nothing to suggest a ventricular aneurysm, the characteristic ECG sign of which would be persistence of elevation of the ST segments which, in this patient, have returned to normal.

This patient's palpitations are probably a result of sinus tachycardia. This is suggested by his observation that the pulse is regular. There is no abrupt onset to suggest paroxysmal attacks and, furthermore, the episodes are invariably associated with effort.

A sinus tachycardia is usually caused by an overactivity of the sympathetic nervous system. This may be mediated either directly by cardiosympathetic nerves or by circulating catecholamines. These catecholamines may be produced in excess, as in phaeochromocytoma or anxiety, or their action may be potentiated by thyroxine and triodothyronine as in thyrotoxicosis. In all three conditions the resulting stimulation of beta-adrenergic receptors will produce certain similarities in the clinical picture.

Thyrotoxicosis might be suspected in a patient with palpitations, sweating, tremor, brisk reflexes, nervousness, staring eyes, weight loss, and increased bowel activity. However, the sweating is here confined to the 'emotional' areas, and the weight loss probably represents the results of the dieting advised by his doctors. Furthermore the thyroid gland is not palpable and no bruit is present.

A phaeochromocytoma is also an unlikely diagnosis. There is no evidence of sustained hypertension in the heart size, fundi, or ECG. Intermittent paroxysmal discharge from such a tumour may also occur but the pattern of this patient's attacks is not typical.

In addition to these negative points, there are positive features to suggest that this patient's symptoms are due to 'effort syndrome'. The awareness of his response to exercise is giving rise to anxiety which is enhancing and prolonging this response. Such a situation is readily understandable in a young man with family responsibilities who has sustained a myocardial infarct. Additional anxiety has been created by his inability to stop smoking as recommended by his doctor. The setting of the attacks mainly in the family circle is another indication of the underlying anxiety.

Little further investigation is indicated. The ECG and chest X-ray were essential, if only for their reassuring effect on the patient. An effort-test ECG might be justified and would give the physician the opportunity to observe the patient's symptoms at first hand. Knowledge of the sleeping pulse rate would be valuable, for in anxiety it is normal, in contrast to the sustained tachycardia of thyrotoxicosis. A serum thyroxine (T4) or TSH estimation would also help to exclude this diagnosis. His blood pressure, raised at the time of examination, should be remeasured after a period of rest as there are no other findings to support a diagnosis of sustained hypertension. If doubt still persists, a non-invasive 24-hour ambulatory blood pressure profile could be obtained.

A simple screening test should be done to exclude phaeochromocytoma, such as the estimation of urinary vanillylmandelic acid (VMA).

Treatment of this patient requires sympathy with his predicament and the ability to provide effective reassurance. This cannot be simply supplied with pills but requires time to give an adequate explanation of the way in which the symptoms are produced. After this a short course of a tranquilizer, such as diazepam, may be given if necessary. Beta-adrenergic blocking drugs such as propranolol can give useful symptomatic relief and would frequently be given prophylactically following an uncomplicated myocardial infarction, having been shown to reduce mortality in the first year.

> Further investigations, including an effort test, did not reveal any abnormality. His wife measured his sleeping pulse on four successive nights and found it to be between 56 and 64 per minute. A diagnosis of 'effort syndrome' was made, and his symptoms settled after full discussion and the use of a mild sedative.

2. Heart failure

The diagnosis of heart failure is usually not difficult, but there may be much more difficulty in finding the underlying cause. A wide variety of primarily cardiac diseases cause heart failure and this may be their initial presentation as well as the terminal event. A number of non-cardiac diseases, in particular severe anaemia and thyrotoxicosis, may produce congestive heart failure as a major complication. Here, treatment of the failure may be singularly ineffective unless the systemic condition is recognized and treated. Because heart failure is the final pathway of many different pathological mechanisms, the relative importance of various independent but contributory factors may be difficult to arrive at. Many of these diseases are very common, for example coronary artery atherosclerosis, hypertension, and chronic bronchitis with emphysema. All three are common in the older age groups and often present independently in the same patient. The contribution of each can then be almost impossible to assess.

THE PATHOPHYSIOLOGY OF HEART FAILURE

The heart is a pump, and its function is to produce an output of blood of a volume and pressure adequate to perfuse the tissues and meet their immediate metabolic needs. The metabolic requirements of most tissues are relatively constant. The perfusion of the gut will vary with the needs of digestion, and that of the skin according to the necessity for heat loss and the maintenance of constant core temperature. The largest variable is the perfusion of the skeletal musculature, which alters greatly with physical activity. Even after there has been a compensatory reduction in blood flow elsewhere, for example to the gut, vigorous exercise will result in a rise in the cardiac output from a resting figure of 5–7 l/min to as high as 20 l/min. This capacity to increase output is the cardiac reserve, and in most people results mainly from an increase in heart rate. It will be progressively reduced in heart disease, so that commonly the patient in the earlier stages of his illness will only develop symptoms when he undertakes activities with which his cardiac reserve could previously cope.

When analysing the syndrome of heart failure it is useful to consider the heart as two quite separate pumps. The right heart operates against the normally low resistance of the pulmonary circuit, the average pressure in the pulmonary artery being only about 16/7 mmHg, in contrast to 120/80 for the systemic circuit. This difference in load is reflected in the anatomy of the right ventricle, which is well adapted to deal with an increase in volume work but less successful when confronted with pressure work. An example of this is atrial septal defect, where the right ventricle will usually cope for many years with an output much above that of the normal left ventricle. In contrast the thick-walled left ventricle is well adapted to produce high pressure and can thus cope adequately for a long time with such conditions as systemic hypertension or aortic stenosis. In aortic or mitral regurgitation, the left ventricle is called upon to deal with increased volumes of blood. It copes with this less well and once failure has developed, deterioration is usually rapid.

Many diseases involve either the right heart or left heart selectively. Indeed, individual chambers will often have to bear the initial consequences of some lesions. A simple example is left atrial failure resulting from mitral stenosis. This is generally true for valvular heart disease and also many examples of congenital heart disease. In conditions such as systemic hypertension or chronic lung disease, the initial stress will be laid upon the appropriate ventricle, but it is more useful to consider these simply as situations of left or right heart failure. Some diseases involve essentially the whole heart: for example, infective myocarditis, beriberi heart, and many cardiomyopathies. Heart failure is a frequent feature and both sides of the heart fail simultaneously.

Some confusion often occurs as to the exact meaning of the term congestive heart failure. Most commonly it is applied to the clinical situation of peripheral venous congestion, as shown by a raised jugular venous pressure associated with peripheral oedema, the assumption being that these signs are due to heart failure. This syndrome will occur with both right heart failure and biventricular failure, but not with pure left heart failure. In constrictive pericarditis similar signs occur even though the cause is not one of simple pump failure. Although the diagnosis of congestive heart failure is commonly made, it is by no means essential to use this term and it can be replaced by other less confusing descriptions.

In left heart failure the rising end diastolic pressure in the left atrium is transmitted back to the pulmonary veins and hence to the pulmonary capillaries. At this stage the increase in capillary hydrostatic pressure will predispose to pulmonary oedema. Further, the increased accumulation of blood in the lungs makes them less easily expanded, reducing the compliance. The pulmonary artery pressure will passively rise and so there will be an increased load upon the right heart which will ultimately lead to its failure. Active pulmonary arteriolar vasoconstriction may occur, which while reducing the pulmonary congestion, does so at the expense of increased strain upon the right heart. As cardiac failure develops and cardiac output falls there is an increase in sympathetic activity from the baroreceptors. Heart rate rises and there is peripheral vasoconstriction and constriction of the great veins, thus maintaining blood pressure and increasing venous return. Activation of the renin–angiotensin mechanism causes aldosterone release and salt and water retention, which contributes to oedema.

Left heart failure results either from an increase in left ventricular load (such as systemic hypertension, aortic stenosis or high output states) or from myocardial disease (ischaemia, myocarditis, cardiomyopathy, cardiac depressant drugs). Diastolic (as opposed to systolic) dysfunction of the left ventricle is increasingly recognized and may be due to hypertrophy and myocardial infiltration (amyloid). In left heart failure there is, in addition to pulmonary congestion, reduced exercise tolerance, fatigue and lethargy.

Heart failure may occur although the cardiac output at rest is normal or even high. This occurs when the needs of the body, even at rest, have been greatly increased, for example as a result of thyrotoxicosis, in anaemia, or if an arteriovenous shunt is short-circuiting a significant percentage of the output and so rendering it ineffective. This situation of increased output, resulting in what is often called a hyperkinetic circulation, is more likely to lead to cardiac failure when there is underlying coronary artery disease.

The sequence of events when heart failure has developed first on the right side is less obvious. The common causes of this situation are chronic lung disease and disease of the pulmonary vasculature, particularly pulmonary emboli. That heart failure is present is not in doubt, for the cardiac output is commonly reduced below the level necessary for adequate perfusion of the tissues even at rest. Furthermore, particularly in lung disease such as chronic bronchitis and emphysema, it is usual to find clinical features which suggest that the left heart is also failing. Thus there may be the complaint of orthopnoea and the signs of left ventricular enlargement with basal crepitations. Cardiac catheterization may also reveal the haemodynamic picture of left heart failure, but why has it occurred? If severe anoxia is present as a result of the lung disease this can depress left ventricular function and lead to failure. Furthermore in western society coronary artery disease is common and coronary perfusion may be reduced without the ischaemic heart disease having become clinically manifest. When it is combined with anoxia, a reduced cardiac output, and perhaps a tachycardia with resulting reduction in duration of diastole and reduced coronary filling, it may provide the necessary additional factor to produce left ventricular failure.

SYMPTOMS OF HEART FAILURE

In some ways the most important symptoms to the patient are those that result directly from the reduction in cardiac output. There is commonly a general reduction in vigour and drive, with tiredness and lethargy. Physical effort becomes curtailed and the patient's activities steadily more circumscribed. Although important, these are very non-specific complaints, which occur in a wide variety of other conditions. They are prominent in many psychiatric conditions, particularly depression, and as a result are of little value in making a diagnosis of heart failure. Impaired cerebral perfusion may, in the elderly, lead to a chronic brain syndrome with confusion, restlessness and disorientation. This commonly occurs as a result of cerebral atherosclerosis, but symptoms may first develop or become exacerbated only when there is the additional factor of a fall-off in cardiac output due to heart failure. Acute myocardial infarction may sometimes present in this way in old people, chest pain being completely absent. Impaired perfusion and anoxia of the brain may affect the normal rhythmic function of the respiratory centre, and Cheyne–Stokes respiration result. Symptoms tend to occur particularly at night. The hyperpnoeic phase may be very vigorous and wake the patient so that he complains of insomnia.

Perhaps the most useful of the common symptoms of heart failure is dyspnoea. It occurs chiefly as a result of pulmonary congestion, and is due in part to decreased compliance of the lungs. The respiratory centre will also be stimulated both directly and reflexly by arterial hypoxia and hypercapnia. Dyspnoea of cardiac origin is usually worse when the patient lies flat, so that at night he will usually sleep well propped up. This is called orthopnoea and is probably due to a redistribution of blood on lying flat such that a greater proportion is in the lungs, decreasing pulmonary compliance. Despite this, attacks of paroxysmal nocturnal dyspnoea may occur. Severe pulmonary oedema occurs as a result of sudden failure of either the left atrium or left ventricle. It often develops on a background of increasing left heart failure with progressive orthopnoea and recurrent attacks of paroxysmal nocturnal dyspnoea. It may develop without warning, either in association with a tight mitral stenosis, or as a result of myocardial infarction.

Pulmonary congestion predisposes to haemoptyses, which are usually small and may be recurrent. They are especially common in mitral stenosis.

Haemoptyses may also result from pulmonary infarction, which is a common occurrence in heart failure, usually as a result of phlebothrombosis in a deep vein in the legs, causing pulmonary emboli. In contrast haemoptyses are uncommon in states of pulmonary ischaemia such as Fallot's tetralogy. Congestion and swelling of the bronchi often gives rise to coughing, and cough may occur after exercise when the heart failure and pulmonary congestion have become more marked. Recurrent attacks of infective bronchitis will be a common feature in many cases of cor pulmonale but are also more likely in any situation where the lungs are congested. The wheezing dyspnoea that can result from either congestion and oedema ('cardiac asthma') or bronchitis may lead to the patient's symptoms being misinterpreted as being respiratory in origin (bronchial asthma). A careful analysis of the circumstances under which the dyspnoea occurs and the past pattern of the complaint will usually help to clarify the diagnosis.

As heart failure progresses systemic venous congestion will finally develop. In part this is due to the expansion of the blood volume that commonly occurs, particularly in association with cor pulmonale (see Ch. 3). It is also an important compensatory response maintaining cardiac output by increasing the diastolic filling pressure. The salt and water retention is mediated through the renin–angiotensin mechanism. This peripheral congestion is a major factor in producing oedema, which will be typically gravitational. It will be most marked in the legs, gradually ascending as the condition worsens. The swelling will be more obvious by the end of the day or after any prolonged period of standing, and will apparently disappear after rest. If very severe it may be associated with enlargement of the abdomen due to ascites. If ascites is marked but the peripheral oedema only modest, other causes of oedema, particularly liver disease, must be excluded and the possibility of constrictive pericarditis carefully considered (see Ch. 16). Congestion of the liver will increase its size and stretch the capsule, giving rise to pain and tenderness. If heart failure has developed rapidly this pain may be severe, sufficiently so on occasion to falsely suggest some primary intra-abdominal condition. Congestion of the rest of the bowel in association with some degree of hepatic dysfunction is probably responsible for the poor appetite commonly found in heart failure. This in turn frequently leads to tissue wasting and muscle weakness, although weight loss is commonly masked by the accumulating oedema fluid. Rarely, muscle wasting may result from an actual protein-losing enteropathy produced by the failure.

Two symptoms which commonly occur with heart disease are chest pain and palpitations. They are not however symptoms which occur as a direct consequence of heart failure even though they may be present in association with it as a result of the underlying disease. They are discussed elsewhere in Chs. 1 and 4.

PHYSICAL EXAMINATION

The physical signs reflect the changes already described. The reduction in cardiac output, although fundamental, is often not easy to detect. If failure is severe however there may be reduction in blood pressure and weakening of the pulse. The skin will be cold and pale in the usual low output state, but in the much less common situation of high output failure with a hyperkinetic circulation the skin will be warm and the pulse bounding. Reduction in perfusion with a slowing of circulation through the capillary bed leads to a greater extraction of oxygen and the clinical sign of cyanosis. This must always be looked for in the mucous membranes, for peripheral cyanosis alone is most commonly due to local factors such as cold and not to heart disease. Reduction in renal blood flow may lead to the formation of smaller quantities of more concentrated urine, while there may be some degree of reabsorption of oedema fluid at night, resulting in a loss of the normal diurnal rhythm of urine flow. Mental confusion and body wasting may be present.

Abnormalities of the pulse will usually be due to associated arrhythmias. Systemic hypertension commonly causes heart failure in western societies, probably as a result of associated coronary artery disease. A rise in blood pressure may occur however as a result of left ventricular failure, perhaps because of impaired perfusion of the brain stem. In a patient with heart failure a raised blood pressure may be the cause of the heart failure, secondary to it, or a coincidental finding. Hypertension in heart failure should not be regarded as the cause unless there is evidence of sustained, long-standing deviation of blood pressure, for example hypertensive retinopathy or left ventricular hypertrophy. An important sign of a failing left ventricle is pulsus alternans. Every other beat is weak due to impairment of ventricular contraction, the rate and rhythm being normal. The first heart sound will vary, being louder with the stronger ventricular contractions. The sign is best detected, however, by careful sphygmomanometry. As the occluding pressure falls the heart rate will be found to double suddenly once all the beats are transmitted. The heart is enlarged when in failure and this can usually be detected clinically. The apex beat will be displaced and the area of cardiac dullness increased. In cor pulmonale the enlargement may be less apparent, for the heart usually lies vertically and its dullness may be obscured by emphysematous lungs.

Pulmonary congestion will give rise to dyspnoea and orthopnoea, and may result in acute pulmonary oedema with the production of large quantities of frothy pink sputum. The increased barrier to diffusion and ventilation–perfusion mismatch will increase the hypoxaemia and cyanosis. The usual finding on examination of the lungs is bilateral basal rales, which may be more widespread if the failure is severe. The percussion note will usually be only a little impaired, and stony dullness should always suggest the presence of pleural effusion which may occur in heart failure. If pulmonary infarction has occurred a pleural friction rub may be heard.

Peripheral venous congestion due to a rise in right atrial diastolic pressure will be seen as an elevation of the jugular venous pressure. The patient must be examined lying at an angle of 45° to the horizontal, and on occasion the internal jugular may be more easily assessed than the external. Gross jugular distension with absence of venous pulsation may result from mediastinal obstruction, but this will usually be obvious from the associated facial oedema and the absence of cardiac signs. If the venous pressure is only a little elevated it can often be made more obvious by compression over the liver: hepatojugular reflux. If the right ventricle is grossly dilated there may be tricuspid regurgitation with a large V wave in the jugular venous pulse and a pulsatile liver. The liver will frequently be enlarged and is commonly tender, unless cardiac cirrhosis has resulted from long standing failure. Ascites should be looked for if the abdomen seems protuberant, the characteristic sign being dullness in the flanks which shifts on movement of the patient. It is especially common with constrictive pericarditis but is also more frequent when there is cardiac cirrhosis. Occasionally there may be a minor degree of splenomegaly, either due to passive congestion or secondary to the cirrhosis, but clinical detection may be difficult if ascites is also present. Peripheral oedema is a major sign of heart failure. It is usually obvious in the legs, but may be confined to the sacrum if the patient has been in bed.

While palpation and auscultation of the praecordium is of the greatest value in establishing the presence of heart disease and its nature, it is of less importance in the recognition of heart failure. Dilatation of one or more of the cardiac chambers is always present in failure and if either of the ventricles dilates considerably, functional incompetence may be produced at the mitral or tricuspid valve. It is impossible on clinical grounds alone to distinguish between functional and organic lesions of the atrioventricular valves, and

the loudness of the murmur correlates only poorly with its haemodynamic significance. The presence of such murmurs is therefore of limited diagnostic value, other than indicating that significant cardiac dysfunction is present.

Much attention has been paid to the variety of additional heart sounds that may occur in diastole, particularly when a ventricle is under strain or actual failure is present.

The third heart sound (S3) is produced in the ventricles by the tensing of the chordae tendinae and mitral valve cusps as the ventricle elongates during early rapid filling. It is probably present in most normal people under the age of 30 and can be heard in the majority with the stethoscope. Even if the heart is normal, if the ventricles contract more forcibly, for example as a result of anxiety or thyrotoxicosis, the third sound will be heard more easily.

If large quantities of blood flow into a dilated ventricle a pathological third sound is commonly produced. In timing and quality this is identical with the physiological third sound and can only be recognized as pathological from the circumstances under which it occurs. Increased ventricular filling is particularly a feature of disease, causing an increase in stroke volume, and an abnormal S3 is more likely with left-to-right shunts or incompetent valves such as severe mitral regurgitation.

The fourth heart sound (S4) occurs as a result of atrial contraction. It can be heard in some children and some very fit adults. In general it is not often detected for it is low pitched and soft and is commonly fused with the first heart sound.

If it is easily detected in an adult it is likely to be pathological. The circumstances which give rise to it will be a powerful atrial contraction associated with decreased ventricular compliance. The atria will also contract more vigorously if there is increased sympathetic tone. Ventricular compliance will be decreased

Table 2.1   Common causes of heart failure

Right heart failure	Left heart failure
Pulmonary hypertension secondary to left heart failure	1. *Left ventricular failure*
	Coronary artery disease
Cor pulmonale	Hypertension
Thromboembolic pulmonary hypertension	Aortic valve disease
	Mitral incompetence
Pulmonary hypertension due to congenital heart disease	Ventricular septal defect
	Patent ductus arteriosus
Atrial septal defect	Coarctation of the aorta
Pulmonary valve stenosis	2. *Left atrial failure*
Infundibular stenosis	Mitral stenosis
	Atrial myxoma

if there is myocardial fibrosis as a result of ischaemic heart disease, and also in rare conditions such as amyloid infiltration of the heart. Compliance is also reduced if there is systolic overload of the ventricle, as a result for example of systemic hypertension or aortic stenosis. Diastolic overload with an increased stroke volume will not produce this situation. If effective atrial contraction does not occur as a result of atrial fibrillation or gross atrial dilatation, or is not transmitted to the ventricle because of AV valve stenosis, then no S4 will be produced whatever the circumstances in the ventricle.

The term gallop rhythm refers to a characteristic cadence of at least three sounds in association with tachycardia. It may be due to a combination of S1, S2 and S3 called 'S3 gallop' (an older more confusing term was 'protodiastolic gallop'). Alternatively a gallop rhythm can be produced by the combination of S1, S2 and S4 called 'S4 gallop' (older less accurate terms were 'atrial gallop' and 'presystolic gallop'). With rapid heart rates S3 and S4 may occur simultaneously and this can produce a summation gallop, whether or not the individual sounds are abnormal. This is especially likely to occur in hypertensive heart failure.

INVESTIGATION OF CARDIAC FAILURE

Few investigations are of value in establishing the diagnosis of heart failure, for this is primarily a clinical diagnosis. Investigations will mainly be directed towards establishing the cause of the failure, and perhaps in quantifying the degree of abnormality present.

If there is pulsus alternans this may be associated with electrical alternans on the ECG, but again the clinical diagnosis will usually be obvious. The ECG may of course suggest the cause of the heart failure : ischaemia, infarction or hypertension, and will show any contributory arrhythmia.

The chest X-ray is the one investigation which can be helpful. It may show cardiomegaly unsuspected by clinical examination. Prominence of the upper lobe veins will indicate a rise in left atrial pressure, while there may be the typical features of pulmonary oedema, with perihilar shadowing and Kerley B lines and a pleural effusion. Cardiac ultrasound will indicate the degree of valvular dysfunction and of left ventricular dilatation. Nuclear angiocardiography can be used to determine the ejection fraction and stroke volume.

CLINICAL PROBLEM

T	P	BP	R
37.4	102 irreg.	120/90	28

Spider naevi

Obese

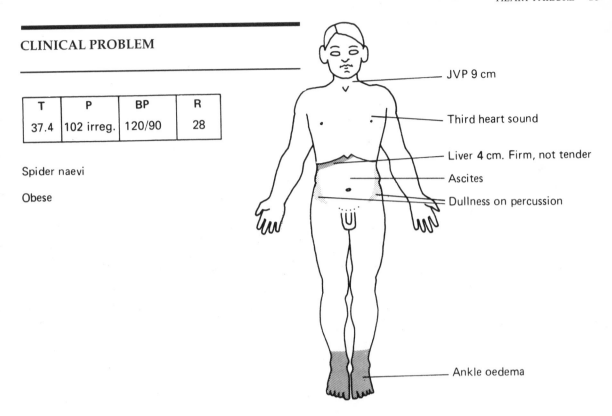

JVP 9 cm

Third heart sound

Liver **4** cm. Firm, not tender

Ascites

Dullness on percussion

Ankle oedema

A 52-year-old Greek Cypriot businessman presented to his general practitioner because of recent deterioration in his health. Over the previous 12 months he had felt increasingly tired and lacking in energy. His appetite had been worse and he had noticed occasional dyspepsia, particularly after heavy or fatty meals. His bowels had always been constipated and for the last 6 months he had noticed that he was losing bright red blood during and after defaecation. He had no other symptoms but on direct questioning he admitted that he occasionally had left-sided chest pain, which had occurred intermittently over the last 2 years, particularly in association with exercise.

Ten years previously he had suffered from epigastric pain which had occurred in association with meals for about 4 months. He had been told at the time he had a duodenal ulcer and his symptoms had improved with treatment. He smoked 30 cigarettes daily and drank several bottles of brandy weekly. In his family his mother suffered from mild diabetes mellitus, and one brother had had pulmonary tuberculosis as a young man.

Examination showed him to be very obese with a protuberant abdomen. He was a little pale. His pulse and blood pressure were normal. Proctoscopy revealed a moderate degree of piles. The general practitioner treated him with oral iron and referred him to a surgical Outpatients Department for injection of the piles. Here it was thought that the liver was palpable and also that some degree of ascites was present. He was accordingly admitted to a medical ward for further investigation.

On admission (see diagram) pulse 102 irregularly irregular. Blood pressure 120/90. Temperature 37.4. RR 28. He was in no obvious distress and was not orthopnoeic. The apex beat could not be felt, but the heart size was not increased on percussion. The heart sounds were quiet and a third sound could be heard. The JVP was raised 9 cm. There was dullness on percussion in the flanks and the liver was enlarged 4 cm, firm and not tender. There was a little ankle oedema. A few spider naevi were present over the upper chest but there were no other signs of liver failure.

Initial investigation: Hb 11g/dl. WBC $6.7 \times 10^9/l$. Differential normal. ESR 63 mm. Blood film showed hypochromia. MSU normal. Urea 3.1 mmol/l. Electrolytes normal. CXR: some degree of cardiomegaly with clear lung fields. ECG: atrial fibrillation with right bundle branch block.

QUESTIONS

1. What are the likely diagnoses?
2. What investigations would you undertake to establish the diagnosis?

DISCUSSION

The diagnosis is by no means obvious in this man. His history is very non-specific and his symptoms could be produced by many different disease processes. A striking feature of the history, however, in view of the signs found on examination, is the absence of any complaint of dyspnoea or orthopnoea. His story of long-standing constipation and the recent passage of bright red blood on the stool is very typical of piles and this is confirmed by the proctoscopy. A digital examination should be made and sigmoidoscopy should be performed as a routine. Blood loss from piles, although usually trivial, can on occasion be marked. It may certainly be sufficient to cause some degree of anaemia and this is especially likely in the elderly, where the diet may be poor and absorption of iron impaired.

It is difficult to evaluate the left chest pain. Despite its association with exercise its site makes it very unlikely to be angina.

A number of points must be considered in his personal history. He is a very heavy cigarette smoker which predisposes him to the development of both coronary artery disease and carcinoma of the bronchus. Furthermore, he admits to drinking several bottles of brandy weekly, which indicates that his alcohol intake is sufficient to cause significant tissue damage. Although the brunt of this insult will fall upon the liver, damage may also occur to the heart. Alcoholic cardiomyopathy is an uncommon but well recognized condition, and diagnosis can be difficult. It may occur as a result of deficiency of thiamine or as a result of the direct action of alcohol on the myocardium.

Tuberculosis is common in Cyprus and a family history of this disease is often given by Cypriot immigrants to this country. Pulmonary tuberculosis will not usually present any difficulty in diagnosis once a chest X-ray has been obtained. It should however be remembered that tuberculous pericarditis also occurs and may present with the signs of pericardial constriction many years after the initial infection.

His previous dyspeptic symptoms are difficult to evaluate. Duodenal ulceration has a tendency to recur and he has had recent indigestion. His anaemia may therefore be due to bleeding from the duodenum rather than the piles and it is impossible to exclude this possibility without further barium studies or gastroscopy.

The findings on examination reveal a significant rise in the systemic venous pressure and this could explain the hepatomegaly, ascites, and peripheral oedema. The firmness and lack of tenderness of the liver suggest that the venous congestion has been present for some time and that cirrhosis is present. This would in turn explain the raised ESR and the presence of a few spider naevi. If alcoholic liver damage were solely responsible for the hepatomegaly and ascites the raised JVP and other cardiac findings would require some further explanation. The cardiac abnormalities consist of atrial fibrillation, a third heart sound, with a raised JVP and the ascites and oedema already discussed. Many of the features of congestive heart failure are therefore present. He is obese and a heavy cigarette smoker and is therefore a candidate for ischaemic heart disease, a common cause of atrial fibrillation and heart failure. Against this interpretation is the absence of any symptoms or signs of left ventricular failure, with only minimal cardiac enlargement. There is, furthermore, no history or X-ray evidence of chronic pulmonary disease.

The combination of peripheral congestion and hepatomegaly and ascites, with the absence of dyspnoea or any evidence of pulmonary congestion, suggests a diagnosis of constrictive pericarditis. The absence of pericardial calcification on a straight chest X-ray does not exclude the diagnosis. The ECG findings are compatible with this diagnosis, although typically there should be low-voltage curves with widespread T-wave inversion. An ultrasound examination is essential in the assessment of pericardial disease and exclusion of valvular abnormalities.

Alcoholic cardiomyopathy usually produces a picture of biventricular heart failure and dyspnoea is an early and major symptom. Atrial fibrillation and ectopic beats are common and there is usually marked cardiomegaly.

In this patient further oblique views of the heart together with screening established the diagnosis of constrictive pericarditis, there being definite calcification with markedly reduced cardiac pulsation. The aetiology was assumed to be tuberculous and a successful result was obtained from partial pericardial resection.

3. Peripheral oedema

Oedema is due to the accumulation of excess fluid in the interstitial space. It can be caused in a variety of ways, and a simple classification is as follows:

1. *Generalized oedema* due to transudation of salt and water, e.g. hypoproteinaemic syndromes, congestive cardiac failure, acute glomerulonephritis.

2. *Local oedema* due to:
   a) increased permeability of small blood vessels, e.g. infection, trauma, burns, allergy.
   b) Oedema due to lymphatic obstruction, e.g. malignancy, filariasis, chronic infection.
   c) Oedema due to venous obstruction, e.g. thrombosis, infiltration with malignancy, external pressure.

GENERAL PRINCIPLES IN THE FORMATION OR INTERSTITIAL FLUID

In conditions where the small blood vessels are intact, the formation of interstitial fluid is governed by the familiar scheme proposed by Starling. The arterial hydrostatic pressure, in excess of tissue pressure, tends to cause transudation of salt and water out of capillaries, while the colloid osmotic pressure of the plasma proteins tends to draw fluid back in. There is thus an overall loss of fluid from the capillary at its arterial end, and reabsorption at the venous end. A small amount of protein is present in this transudate. A low colloid osmotic pressure or a raised hydrostatic pressure at the venous end of the capillary will tend to cause oedema. Increasing the tissue pressure (e.g. with an elastic stocking) or raising the colloid osmotic pressure when low (e.g. albumin infusion in cirrhosis) will inhibit oedema formation. Fluid accumulating in the interstitial space passes into thin-walled lymphatic vessels. From here it passes into the general circulation via the main lymphatic channels. Lymph vessels have valves and the passage of lymph is assisted by muscular activity and by negative intrathoracic pressure.

If small blood vessels are themselves damaged directly by thermal injury or infections or allergic reactions, there is loss of fluid from their lumen. The oedema thus formed has the qualities of an exudate, being rich in protein.

GENERALIZED OEDEMA DUE TO TRANSUDATION OF SALT AND WATER

Among the commonest causes of oedema are heart failure and the hypoproteinaemic states. Before discussing the clinical features it is worth considering in detail the mechanisms which are responsible for oedema formation in these conditions.

The control of the extracellular fluid volume, and the formation of oedema

The mechanisms involved in the control of extracellular fluid (ECF) volume are incompletely understood. Since the sodium cation is the most important osmotically active constituent of the ECF, the problem mainly concerns the factors leading to accumulation of sodium in the body and its excretion by the kidney.

About 85% of all the filtered sodium is reabsorbed in the proximal convoluted tubule. The remaining 15% is variably reabsorbed in the distal tubule, partly with chloride ions and partly in exchange for potassium and hydrogen ions. The regulation of sodium excretion is probably mainly concerned with this 15% and in this the role of adrenal steroids is very important. Aldosterone is the major adrenal mineralocorticoid hormone. The effect of aldosterone is on the distal renal tubule, causing sodium reabsorption and potassium excretion. This effect is blocked by spironolactone. Whether aldosterone has an effect on the proximal tubule is undecided. An important stimulus to aldosterone release comes from the renin–angiotensin system. Renin is produced in specialized cells in the juxtaglomerular apparatus. Any fall in ECF volume (e.g. due to haemorrhage or dehydration) results in release of renin into the blood. Here it acts on renin substrate (produced in the liver) to produce angiotensin I which is then converted to angiotensin II in peripheral tissues such as the lung by angiotensin-converting enzyme

(ACE). Angiotensin II is the stimulus for aldosterone release. Renal sodium reabsorption then occurs, the blood volume rises, and the release of renin diminishes. There is also a small effect produced by ACTH since aldosterone release is imperfect in hypopituitary patients.

The glomerular filtration rate (GFR) exerts a direct effect on sodium excretion. Any factors which tend to decrease GFR (such as a fall in blood pressure for any reason) increase the amount of sodium reabsorbed in the proximal convoluted tubule. The increased reabsorption of salt and water when GFR is reduced, is responsible for the appearance of greater concentration of the contrast in an intravenous pyelogram in patients with renal artery stenosis, when compared with the normal kidney. Marked fluctuations of GFR probably do not normally occur. However, methods are not sensitive enough to detect minor fluctuations which might still cause significant alterations in sodium excretion.

Distension of the great veins in the chest, or of the atria of the heart causes a water diuresis, probably mediated by inhibition of release of antidiuretic hormone (ADH). Vascular receptors in the right atrium also sense volume change in the circulation. Atrial natriuretic peptide (ANP) is produced by endocrine cells in the right atrium. Release of ANP counteracts volume expansion by causing natriuresis.

The way in which these factors operate in producing oedema can now be considered.

Hypoproteinaemic states. The major part of the colloid osmotic pressure of the plasma can be attributed to its albumin content. Hypoalbuminaemia may be due to failure of synthesis as in protein malnutrition (Kwashiorkor) and cirrhosis, or to increased loss as in nephrotic syndrome and protein-losing gastroenteropathy. There is a fall in colloid osmotic pressure and when the serum albumin falls below 25 g/l there is transudation of solutes (mainly salt and water) out of capillaries into the intercellular fluid space. When this compartment is expanded by about 10%, clinically evident oedema appears. There is loss of circulating fluid and a fall in plasma volume. Aldosterone is released and sodium and water reabsorption occurs in the kidney. In a normal person this would restore the plasma volume, but as long as hypoproteinaemia continues fluid thus reabsorbed is lost into the intercellular space and aldosterone secretion and further salt retention continues.

Cardiac failure. The mechanisms involved in causing oedema have been debated for a long time. The circulation can be regarded as a collapsible container filled with blood by the heart. It has a certain mean pressure within it on which the filling of the heart depends. (This pressure is about 7 mmHg when the heart stops beating.) When the heart fails this pressure falls, and a certain amount of fluid passes into the capillaries from the tissues. This expansion of the circulating volume improves the filling of the heart (and therefore cardiac output), but as the heart fails further, renal salt and water retention occurs as a result of stimulation of the renin–angiotensin system (see above and page 10) to keep the pressure within the circulation adequate to supply the failing heart. The blood volume is expanded – demonstrable as raised venous pressure – and the fluid retention is evident as oedema. In many patients with heart failure there is increased sympathetic activity, with a rise in peripheral vascular resistance. There is constriction of veins which reduces the capacity of the circulation and results in increased filling of the heart. Aldosterone plays a part in the accumulation of salt and water. The stimulus for aldosterone release in heart failure is reduced renal cortical blood flow which results in renin release. This reduction in blood flow is caused by selective renal cortical arterial constriction and reduced cardiac output. The raised venous pressure subsequently encourages oedema formation, especially in dependent regions. Whether oedema is pulmonary or systemic partly depends on where the rise in capillary pressure occurs. Left heart failure and pulmonary oedema will result from aortic and mitral valve disease, hypertension and ischaemic heart disease, whereas right heart failure will be caused by pulmonary disease. Right heart failure also commonly supervenes in long-standing left heart failure. In pulmonary disease, an elevated $p\text{CO}_2$ contributes to the formation of peripheral oedema by increasing capillary permeability.

Acute glomerulonephritis. It used to be thought that the oedema in this condition was due to hypersensitivity damage to small vessels. However, the oedema has the property of a transudate, not an exudate. Considerable sodium retention has been shown to occur in this condition as a result of the greatly decreased GFR. It is probable that this is the major mechanism accounting for the hypertension and peripheral oedema.

Idiopathic oedema. This condition affects women in early middle age. The oedema is dependent and fluctuates with position and also with the menstrual cycle. The cause is unknown, and the condition may be worsened by excessive diuretic therapy. The condition is not usually difficult to diagnose since no other signs of disease are present.

The clinical presentation

Peripheral oedema accumulates in dependent regions and areas where the skin is lax. Swelling of the ankles is usually the earliest sign. In hypoproteinaemic states and in glomerulonephritis there is often oedema of the face and hands, most marked after lying down. The patient with cardiac failure, on the other hand, is breathless and sleeps propped up; sacral oedema is therefore very common. Ascites may occur in all of these conditions, but it is especially likely to do so in cirrhosis of the liver where there is portal hypertension as well as hypoalbuminaemia. Ascites is also likely to occur in constrictive pericarditis. In this condition, as in tamponade due to pericardial effusion, there is great elevation of the venous pressure, which may rise rather than fall, on inspiration (Kussmaul's sign), and pulsus paradoxus.

Gross cardiac failure is usually easily diagnosed, but in the early stages diagnosis may be more difficult. The history is of fatigue and breathlessness, and on examination enlargement of the heart and signs of cardiac or pulmonary disease will be found (see Ch. 2).

Hypoproteinaemia will be diagnosed by estimation of the serum proteins. The patient with nephrotic syndrome will have heavy proteinuria. The features of cirrhosis may be present. Intestinal causes of hypoproteinaemia may require tests for malabsorption and small bowel radiology for precise diagnosis.

Acute glomerulonephritis will be suspected by its acute onset, the presence of hypertension and the finding of protein and red cells in the urine of a patient with oliguria.

Iatrogenic fluid overload occurs mainly in elderly patients, in those with impaired renal function, or in postoperative patients who have difficulty in handling a water load. If a patient on intravenous fluids becomes oedematous the reason is normally that too much fluid has been given too quickly to a patient who may have impaired cardiac or renal function.

Table 3.1 Investigation of peripheral oedema

A Generalized oedema

Chest X-ray – signs of heart failure, cardiomegaly
Plasma albumin – low in nephrotic syndrome, cirrhosis, malnutrition (in the western world this is likely to be due to chronic disease, especially cancer)
Blood urea and electrolytes – diminished GFR in renal disease or in severe cardiac failure

B Localized oedema

Chest X-ray – SVCO
Pelvic ultrasound or CT scan – pelvic tumours or lymphatic enlargement
Lymphangiography – abnormal lymphatic architecture, lymph nodes replaced by tumour
Venography – to confirm diagnosis of venous obstruction

OEDEMA DUE TO INCREASED PERMEABILITY OF SMALL VESSELS

Clinically, this form of oedema does not usually present a diagnostic problem, the cause of the subcutaneous swelling accompanying cellulitis or skin ulceration, for example, being obvious. Occasionally various kinds of allergic vasculitis such as erythema nodosum can be accompanied by a lot of oedema, and be mistaken for cellulitis.

A form of allergic oedema which may cause some confusion is angio-oedema. In this condition there is an exudation of fluid into the subcutaneous tissues especially involving the face, lips and eyelids, although any part of the body may be affected. The tongue may swell and palatal and laryngeal oedema occasionally occur. Urticaria is not usually present, and a history of allergy is often lacking. A hereditary form is described in which severe abdominal pain may accompany an attack and laryngeal oedema may be severe, with a high mortality. This form of the disorder is now known to be due to an inherited deficiency of the inhibitor of the activated first component of complement, and a low serum complement is usually found. Angio-oedema may be mistaken for acute glomerulonephritis or the nephrotic syndrome, in both of which there may be facial oedema. The abrupt onset and associated symptoms, and the lack of evidence of renal disease, serve to distinguish these conditions.

OEDEMA DUE TO LYMPHATIC OBSTRUCTION

Lymph vessels have a large collateral circulation, so that any block has to extend over a wide area for oedema to appear. Secondary deposits in lymph nodes may cause oedema in this way but usually the damage has been made more extensive by block dissection of nodes and radiotherapy, for example in the treatment of carcinoma of the breast. In some tropical countries filariasis is endemic. In affected patients chronic lymphatic obstruction may develop over the years. This is due to the widespread fibrosis in lymphatic channels caused by the adult worm, together with associated secondary infection. An additional feature may be involvement of the retroperitoneal lymphatic system causing leakage of milky lymph into the urine (chyluria).

The oedema of lymphatic obstruction has certain characteristic features. The affected region becomes brawny and thickened, and after oedema has been present for some time may not pit on pressure. The oedema has a very high protein content – up to 40 g/l. This is due to the slow accumulation of protein over a long period of time. Rarely an angiosarcoma may develop in a limb with long-standing lymphoedema.

OEDEMA DUE TO VENOUS OCCLUSION

Veins may be occluded from without by neoplasm and secondary deposits in lymph nodes. The major cause of venous obstruction however is deep venous thrombosis, which is a very common cause of oedema in the legs, and if the block is in the inferior vena cava, both legs may swell. Other signs of venous thrombosis and obstruction are often present: dilated superficial veins with delayed emptying; enlarged collateral veins – especially evident in superior vena cava obstruction; a bluish discoloration of the limb;

tenderness along the line of the veins. There may be evidence of a cause of local compression, such as a pelvic or abdominal mass, or a remote cause for venous thrombosis such as malignancy elsewhere causing thrombophlebitis migrans, or polycythaemia. The oedema due to venous occlusion may cause difficulty in diagnosis if the patient is seen after the acute episode has subsided and if the swelling is bilateral. Hypoproteinaemic states are usually easily differentiated, but congestive cardiac failure may be difficult to exclude, especially in the elderly with coexisting heart disease. Similarly residual dependent oedema may occur after the treatment of heart failure; this should not be treated by intensifying diuretic therapy, but with supportive stockings.

A particularly important cause of oedema due to venous obstruction is the syndrome of superior vena cava obstruction (SVCO). This condition is almost always caused by a tumour in the superior mediastinum. The commonest cause is lung cancer but lymphomas, thymomas and germ cell tumours are other causes (often curable). The patient's face becomes swollen, especially around the eyelids. A dusky discoloration of the skin develops. The neck veins may be hugely distended (and this can sometimes be mistaken for a fat neck). Dilated veins are usually visible over the shoulder and anterior chest. There are distended cutaneous venules typically seen round the lower rib cage under the breasts.

The chest X-ray commonly shows a mediastinal mass, but on occasions this may be difficult to see if there is a small but infiltrating carcinoma. The true position is then revealed by a CT scan of the upper mediastinum.

CLINICAL PROBLEM

T	P	BP	R
37	130	70/40	32

Central cyanosis

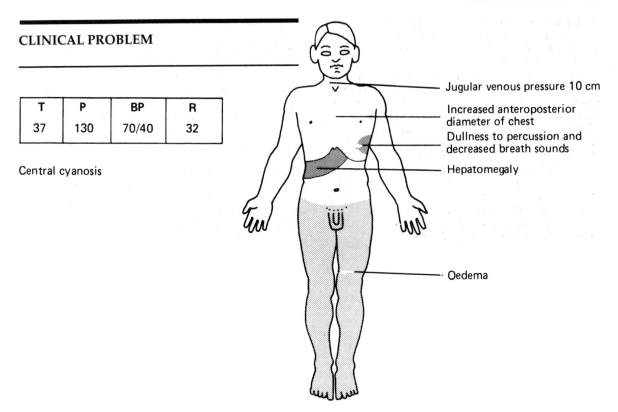

Jugular venous pressure 10 cm

Increased anteroposterior diameter of chest

Dullness to percussion and decreased breath sounds

Hepatomegaly

Oedema

A 65-year-old warehouse foreman was admitted to hospital complaining of severe breathlessness of 1 week's duration. This had come on rapidly over 24 hours. He had become severely breathless at night and had had to sleep propped up. Over the next few days both legs had become greatly swollen.

He had had a chronic productive cough for 15 years, worse in winter time when he had often been off work with acute bronchitis. In the preceding 12 months he had noticed swelling of both ankles towards the end of the day and increasing shortness of breath on exertion. Over the previous 3 months before admission he had had several episodes of haemoptysis, coughing up small quantities of fresh blood. He had never had chest pain. Before his recent deterioration he had noticed that he had lost about 3 kg in weight. He had smoked 30 cigarettes a day for 40 years and was a moderate beer drinker.

On examination he was dyspnoeic and cyanosed. Pulse 130 scarcely palpable, regular with a very small volume. Blood pressure 70/40. The jugular venous pressure was greatly elevated. The heart sounds were faint and the apex beat was not palpable. There was oedema of both legs up to the groins, and scrotal oedema. He was barrel-chested. The trachea was central and there was no finger clubbing. There was dullness to percussion with absent breath sounds at the left base extending into the axilla. In the abdomen, the liver was enlarged 8 cm below the costal margin and was tender, firm and with a smooth outline. There was no ascites.

QUESTIONS

1. What do you consider to be the possible causes of his sudden deterioration?
2. What investigations should be urgently undertaken?
3. What treatment would you undertake immediately?

DISCUSSION

The history is of chronic bronchitis in a cigarette smoker. The ankle swelling over the preceding 12 months suggests the onset of cor pulmonale. The 3-month history of weight loss and haemoptysis raises the possibility of the development of a bronchial carcinoma. There is a recent sudden deterioration with gross oedema, breathlessness, raised venous pressure and hypotension.

The signs in the chest are those of a pleural effusion. This would not entirely account for his recent deterioration. A myocardial infarction is a possible cause, but there is no history of chest pain, and this diagnosis does not fit in with the pattern of his previous illness. Pulmonary embolism must certainly be excluded. The swelling of the legs came after the onset of breathlessness which is not the typical sequence of events when deep venous thrombosis in the legs gives rise to pulmonary embolism. However it by no means excludes such a diagnosis and signs of venous thrombosis may follow the occurrence of the embolism. Similarly an embolus from thrombus in a pelvic vein or the inferior vena cava could explain his recent deterioration, hypotension and pleural effusion.

Superior vena cava obstruction, which is usually due to carcinoma of the bronchus, would give rise to raised jugular venous pressure but would not account for the oedema of the legs. Pericardial tamponade is a very likely diagnosis, and would account for the raised venous pressure, hypotension and rapid feeble pulse. One might expect to see paradoxical venous pulsation in the neck, and to be able to detect pulsus paradoxus by careful sphygmomanometry. In this patient, with a long history of smoking, haemoptysis, and weight loss, pericardial tamponade due to malignant infiltration from a bronchogenic carcinoma is highly probable. A carcinoma of the bronchus could also account for the pleural effusion.

Although any cause of hypoproteinaemia might cause oedema and a pleural effusion, this is very unlikely to be the cause in this case. Cirrhosis of the liver, nephrotic syndrome and malabsorption would not explain the hypotension, breathlessness and raised venous pressure, nor would these diagnoses account for his previous illness.

The most useful investigations in the immediate diagnosis would be a chest X-ray, ECG and cardiac ultrasound. A chest X-ray may show a carcinoma of the bronchus and an enlarged cardiac silhouette from heart failure or tamponade. It could also provide evidence of left heart failure, or diminished vascular markings in the case of a large pulmonary embolus. It will confirm the presence of a pleural effusion. An ECG may show evidence of myocardial infarction or the right ventricular strain pattern of pulmonary embolism. In this chronic bronchitic patient, right ventricular hypertrophy is likely to be present and of long standing. In pericardial effusion there may be low voltage tracing and the ultrasound will be diagnostic.

Other routine investigations such as a full blood count, plasma protein estimation and sputum cytology are not of immediate value. Aspiration and biopsy of the pleural effusion would be unhelpful in immediate management but could be of great value in diagnosis. A blood-stained pleural effusion is strongly suggestive of malignancy, but may occur in a minority of patients with pulmonary infarction (30% of cases). Examination of the fluid for carcinoma cells may give the diagnosis, as may the pleural biopsy.

If the presumptive diagnosis of pericardial tamponade is supported by the investigation, aspiration of the pericardial effusion under ultrasound control will be essential.

This man had a bronchial carcinoma infiltrating the pericardium, causing a haemorrhagic effusion. Aspiration brought temporary relief, but he died 12 hours later.

4. Central chest pain

All thoracic and many extrathoracic structures may give rise to central chest pain. These include muscles and joints of the chest wall, pleura, pericardium, lungs, heart, oesophagus, great vessels, stomach and gall bladder. In practice the first question to be answered is usually whether or not the pain is cardiac. If the pain is thought to be due to myocardial ischaemia, one must distinguish between angina, infarction or an intermediate state, and consider whether there is an underlying cause other than the common one of atherosclerosis. Even if the cause is atherosclerosis there may be precipitating factors that have led to the pain occurring at a particular time.

ISCHAEMIC HEART DISEASE

Angina and infarction pain have certain common characteristics. The pain is typically situated in the centre of the chest and may radiate to the neck and jaw (even, at times, mimicking toothache) and to the arms, usually the left. Patients often use the same adjectives to describe the two pains such as 'heavy', 'crushing', 'tight'. Those who have experienced both, invariably describe infarction pain as more severe. This is partly because of its longer duration. Pain which lasts more than 3–5 minutes at rest is unlikely to be angina, whilst conversely, infarction pain is rarely so brief.

Angina is commonly precipitated by exertion but this may not appear to be constant in degree because of variations in external temperature, speed of walking, or gradient. Other precipitants should not be ignored, such as the effect of emotion (watching boxing on TV for example), large meals and smoking. Sexual intercourse is another important precipitant and one which the patient may be reticent in discussing.

Infarction, by contrast, frequently comes on at rest or may awaken the patient. Rarely a patient gives a history of increasing angina over a short period of time, which is precipitated by less and less effort. This is known as crescendo angina or prodromal infarction, and will frequently culminate in frank myocardial infarction. This may subsequently relieve the previous disabling angina. It is important to recognize this condition as bed rest, nitrates, calcium antagonists, beta-blocking agents and aspirin may prevent infarction and allow the crisis to pass while a collateral circulation develops. The persistence of pain is an indication for urgent coronary arteriography with a view to immediate surgery or angioplasty. Rapid relief of chest pain by sublingual trinitrin supports a diagnosis of angina, as it will not influence infarction pain so dramatically.

The past history may be helpful if similar attacks have occurred. It may also suggest a particular aetiology which can then be confirmed on examination. The lower incidence of coronary artery disease in women before the menopause compared with men of the same age disappears after oophorectomy.

A family history is of interest but rarely of diagnostic value unless there is familial hyperlipidaemia. Recent heart disease in friends or relatives can, however, strengthen a cardiac neurosis in a susceptible subject. The occupation, social class, weight, smoking habits, and personality of the patient may contribute to atherosclerosis.

On examination there are no signs associated with angina, while if complications of infarction such as shock, pulmonary oedema or ventricular fibrillation occur the diagnosis will rarely be in doubt.

Although there are no physical signs of angina or uncomplicated infarction, there may be evidence of predisposing factors and underlying causes. These include obesity, hyperlipidaemia as shown by arcus senilis in young men, and xanthomata. Hypertension may not be present when the blood pressure is taken following infarction, but evidence of it may be found in the fundi, heart size and character of the apex beat. In aortic valve disease, particularly stenosis, angina is common, and once symptoms begin, downhill progress is usually rapid. Pure aortic incompetence raises the suspicion of tertiary syphilis. In syphilitic aortitis the coronary ostia may be stenosed and for this reason angina frequently occurs. Hyperthyroidism from a nodular goitre in the elderly may lack many of the features of thyrotoxicosis and can present as angina (masked thyrotoxicosis). A particularly dangerous situation is over-rapid replacement therapy with

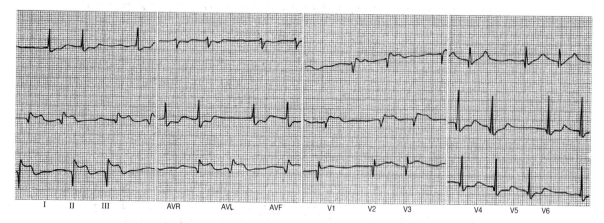

Fig. 4.1 Acute inferior infarction with Q waves and raised S-T segments in leads II, and III and AVF. There is complete heart block.

thyroxine in a newly-diagnosed case of myxoedema; myxoedema itself predisposes to ischaemic heart disease. Development of anaemia may unmask coexisting myocardial ischaemia. A sudden arrthymia such as supraventricular tachycardia, atrial flutter or fibrillation, or complete heart block may cause an abrupt reduction in cardiac output and cause ischaemic pain.

The most useful bedside test is obviously the electrocardiogram ECG (Figs. 4.1, 4.2). The changes associated with myocardial infarction (S-T elevation, Q waves and T-wave inversion) may take some hours to evolve and an early ECG may be normal. The emphasis in management nowadays is for the earliest pos-

sible administration of thrombolytic agents after myocardial infarction whenever feasible, and this treatment in turn may minimize or reverse the ECG changes.

Angina is frequently associated with a normal resting record. In this case, comparison with a tracing taken during a spontaneous attack is invaluable. However, such a record is rarely available. An effort test in which graded exercise is carried out on a treadmill following a predetermined protocol (e.g. Bruce protocol) will be helpful if the diagnosis remains in doubt. This may provoke the chest pain accompanied by S-T segment depression and tachy-

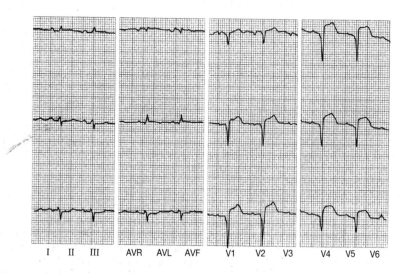

Fig. 4.2   Recent anterolateral infarction with QS waves and S-T elevation in leads V1–V6. (Courtesy of Dr D. Patterson.)

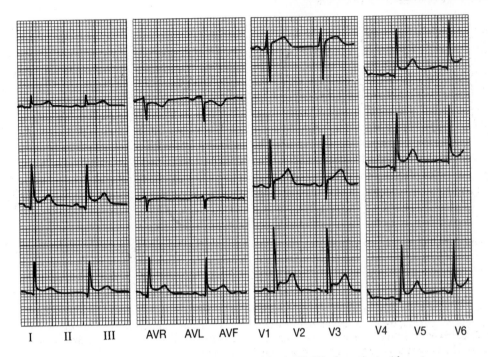

Fig. 4.3 Standard leads I, II, III, AVR, AVL, AVF and leads V1–V6 of a patient with acute pericarditis. The S-T segments are concave and raised

cardia in the ECG. Another use of the test in patients with angina or following infarction is to quantify the severity of the disease, which is of importance in selecting patients for angiography and possible surgery or angioplasty.

PERICARDITIS

Acute pericarditis from any cause may closely mimic myocardial infarction. One feature of the pain is that it may be worse on inspiration. This is probably due to associated pleural inflammation. Unlike myocardial infarction the pain may be modified by position, with relief on leaning forwards. The pathognomonic sign of pericarditis is a pericardial friction rub, which is qualitatively different from a murmur, being superficial and scratchy. One should be alert to the possibility of an associated pericardial effusion causing tamponade. The signs which would suggest this are pulsus paradoxus and a raised jugular venous pressure which may rise paradoxically on inspiration. A difficulty may be the transient pericardial friction rub which is occasionally heard in the first few days following myocardial infarction. In pericarditis the ECG will show S-T elevation in the presence of upright T waves and the absence of Q waves (Fig. 4.3). In contrast, following myocardial infarction T waves are initially upright, becoming inverted within 48 hours and, in addition, Q waves may be present.

ANEURYSM

A dissecting aneurysm may give rise to a tearing sensation radiating to the back. Usually there are accompanying signs such as hemiparesis, disappearance or inequality of pulses, and shock. Although atherosclerosis with hypertension is the commonest aetiology, it may occur in younger patients in the rare condition of Marfan's syndrome. A tall patient with arachnodactyly, lens dislocation, high arched palate and hyperextensible joints will suggest this possibility. The dissection may also extend in retrograde fashion to involve the ostia of the coronary arteries causing myocardial infarction. The characteristic appearance on chest X-ray is of widening of the mediastinum. Transoesophageal ultrasound is a major advance in the diagnosis of this condition.

Another way in which aneurysms may cause chest pain is when they involve the ascending aorta and give rise to pressure on other thoracic structures such as the sternum.

PULMONARY EMBOLISM AND INFARCTION

Pulmonary embolism may cause an acute occlusion of the pulmonary artery or a major branch. This typically causes sudden central chest pain, hypotension, dyspnoea, cyanosis, and right heart strain with failure. It has to be differentiated from myocardial infarction. A dramatic onset, the absence of signs in the chest, the

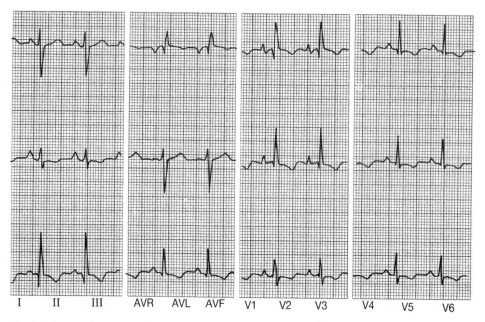

Fig. 4.4 Acute pulmonary embolism with $S_1 Q_3 T_3$ pattern in the standard leads and T–wave invasion in V1–V6 with partial right bundle branch block,(Courtesy of Dr D.Patterson.)

possible presence of deep venous thrombosis, and the electrocardiographic changes of right heart strain rather than those of myocardial infarction will point to the diagnosis (Fig. 4.4).

In pulmonary infarction smaller vessels are occluded. There are fewer haemodynamic changes and the clinical picture is of pleurisy and haemoptysis (see Ch. 8).

The same causes predispose to embolism and infarction as they both usually follow deep venous thrombosis. The embolus is composed of freshly formed thrombus which may break off before there are local signs of tenderness and swelling. For this reason one should be alert to early signs of thrombosis such as an unexplained slight rise in temperature in a patient bedridden as a result of injury, operation or myocardial infarction. Other factors predisposing to venous thrombosis are varicose veins and the contraceptive pill.

Should the condition recur without an obvious underlying cause the possibility of antiphospholipid antibodies predisposing to thrombosis should be excluded.

In pulmonary embolism there may be little abnormality on chest X-ray apart from the difficult sign of oligaemia of part of a lung field. In pulmonary infarction, by contrast, there may be a wedge-shaped infarct or linear atelectasis, with elevation of the hemidiaphragm and a pleural reaction. Isotope lung scanning is a valuable investigation. Most information is obtained if both ventilation and perfusion scans are done, which in pulmonary infarction will show impaired perfusion with normal ventilation. Pulmonary angiography may sometimes be necessary to confirm the diagnosis and as a guide to treatment.

SPONTANEOUS PNEUMOTHORAX

Sudden pain and dyspnoea, sometimes after a bout of coughing or straining, are the characteristic features of this condition, which can occur at any age. Dyspnoea may be disproportionate to the degree of lung collapse. Any underlying chronic chest disease will make the patient's distress greater. If there is associated cough the positive pressure of coughing may be transmitted to the pleural cavity and sometimes result in a tension pneumothorax, which may impair venous return and thereby cause cardiac embarrassment. Mediastinal shift to the opposite side shown by displacement of the apex beat or trachea may then occur, as well as hyperresonance on percussion and diminution of breath sounds. Chest X-ray is essential. A small pneumothorax can easily be missed and a film should be taken in expiration as well as the standard inspiratory film if the diagnosis is suspected. In a partial left pneumothorax a click or crunch may be heard with each heart beat, particularly when the patient lies on his left side.

OESOPHAGEAL PAIN

Gastro-oesophageal reflux disease (GORD) sometimes associated with a sliding hiatus hernia, may cause a wide variety of chest pains which at times may mimic cardiac ischaemic pain. Heartburn should easily be recognized. It occurs after meals or lying flat or bending, with relief on sitting or standing up, belching and taking alkalis. If there is associated oesophagitis, pain on swallowing hot or cold liquids, citrus juices or spirits may occur (odynophagia). Radiological examination can appear normal unless specific manoeuvres additional to the routine are performed. Demonstration of the reflux on barium swallow does not necessarily prove that it is the cause of symptoms. The acid perfusion test may reproduce oesophageal pain and can be of value in the difficult case. The seated patient, with a tube 8–10 cm above the oesophageal hiatus, is perfused with isotonic NaCl at 10 ml/min for 10 minutes and then 20 ml/min for 5 minutes at body temperature. Unbeknown to the patient, 0.1 M HCl is then substituted and perfused at both rates for 15 minutes each or until pain occurs, which can be relieved by 0.1 M NaHCO$_3$ (Bernstein test). Alternatively a pH electrode sited in the lower oesophagus can be used to see if symptoms correlate with episodes of reflux of stomach acid.

Oesophageal spasm may occur in relation to gastro-oesophageal reflux, and may also be responsible for the pain which is a feature of achalasia in its early stages. In this latter disease the denervated oesophageal muscle may be hypersensitive to cholinergic transmitters. This forms the basis of the edrophonium test where the drug is given during a barium swallow or whilst making oesophageal pressure recordings. Whereas normal subjects show no response, a positive reaction is a powerful sustained and often painful oesophageal contraction. Relief of chest pain by nitrates does not prove it to be cardiac, since oesophageal spasm may also respond.

SPINAL PAIN

Degenerative changes in the lower cervical or upper thoracic spine may give rise to pain which is referred to the anterior chest. A history of pain on exertion may suggest angina, especially as there may be root pain radiating to the arm; however, with care, it can be demonstrated that the pain can be clinically reproduced by certain movements. Above the age of 50 most cervical spine X-rays reveal degenerative changes irrespective of the presence or absence of symptoms, and the interpretation of abnormal findings, even in oblique views showing the outlet foramina can be difficult. Rarely, neoplastic deposits, vertebral collapse from osteoporosis or osteomalacia, or a paravertebral abscess may cause central chest pain. Herpes zoster can cause chest pain, usually in a root distribution, and there may be diagnostic difficulty before the rash appears.

CARDIAC NEUROSIS OR EFFORT SYNDROME
(see Ch. 1)

This condition should be diagnosed positively rather than by exclusion. Pain is only one of several symptoms, is usually situated at the apex of the heart, and is commonly associated with a superficial tenderness, often described as prickling. It is of long duration, not eased by rest and often comes on after rather than during exercise. There may be associated difficulty in breathing described as an inability to take a proper breath, palpitations, headaches, and fatigue.

CLINICAL PROBLEM

T	P	BP	R
36	120	150/90	36

Obese

Pallor of skin

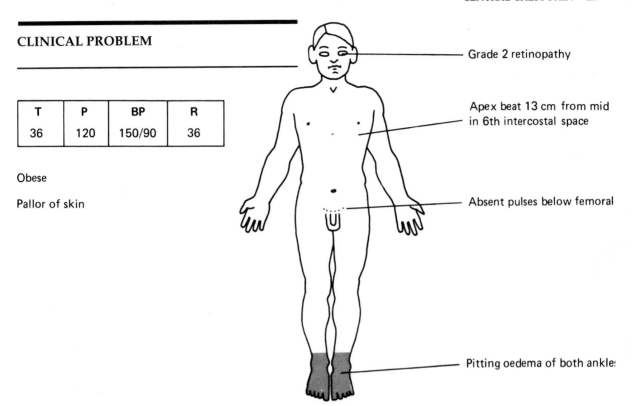

Grade 2 retinopathy

Apex beat 13 cm from mid in 6th intercostal space

Absent pulses below femoral

Pitting oedema of both ankles

A 52-year-old interior decorator was admitted to hospital complaining of severe central chest pain radiating to the back. This had come on suddenly as he had reached his bedroom on retiring after a late supper. At the onset of the pain he had a bout of coughing, but produced no sputum. He took a proprietary antacid that he kept by his bedside which made him belch, but did not relieve his pain. The pain persisted over the next hour until the emergency doctor arrived, and was associated with considerable breathlessness, together with cough productive of mucoid sputum containing flecks of blood.

He had been well until 6 years previously when he had developed bronchial asthma for which there was no obvious precipitating cause. Bronchodilators had been ineffective in controlling his wheezing and he had been treated since its onset with prednisolone, requiring a maintenance dose of 12.5 mg daily. He had gained 25 lb in weight and for the previous year had suffered indigestion particularly after fried food. Three months previously he had told his general practitioner that he had morning headaches and he had been found to be hypertensive (BP 180/125). Since then, he had been taking nifedipine with relief of his headaches.

On examination in hospital he was overweight with truncal obesity and striae in the flanks. He was distressed, pale and sweating. He was unable to lie flat, and had tachypnoea with poor movement of the chest wall. The trachea was central. There was loud generalized wheezing, more marked during expiration. The pulse was 120/min and regular, and BP was 150/90. No pulses were palpable below the femorals. The heart apex beat was displaced, being 13 cm from the midline in the 6th left intercostal space. Heart sounds were normal and no murmurs were heard. Ophthalmoscopy showed narrowing and tortuosity of the retinal arteries with arteriovenous nipping. The JVP was not raised. There was slight pitting oedema of both ankles. The remainder of the examination did not reveal any abnormality.

QUESTIONS

1. What are the possible causes of the chest pain?
2. What immediate investigations would you undertake?
3. What would be your immediate treatment?

DISCUSSION

This patient is a severe asthmatic, in that he requires a considerable dose of steroids to suppress his symptoms. Although he had a cough at the onset of his present illness, one cannot attribute his condition to asthma alone as this does not explain his chest pain. None the less the possibility that the chest pain is a complication of asthma or steroid therapy must be considered.

The most likely diagnosis is that of myocardial infarction. Hypertension and obesity resulting from steroid therapy would be predisposing factors. The site, onset and persistence of the pain are all in keeping with this diagnosis. Although infarction pain usually radiates to the shoulders, arms and neck, radiation to the back may sometimes occur. The development of breathlessness and orthopnoea, with wheezing and blood-flecked sputum suggests that left heart failure with pulmonary oedema has followed the infarction.

Spontaneous pneumothorax cannot be ruled out as the typical physical signs may not be obvious in an obese and distressed patient, and the occurrence of a pneumothorax following a bout of coughing is not uncommon. Pleural adhesions from past infections may prevent complete collapse of the lung and continued coughing could result in positive pressure developing in the pleural space. Both asthma and steroid therapy are considered to be factors predisposing to spontaneous pneumothorax.

A probable additional complication of steroid therapy in this patient is his dyspepsia. The pain of gastro-oesophageal reflux can closely mimic cardiac pain and radiate to the back. Antacids and belching usually give relief. One would not expect considerable breathlessness to be precipitated by oesophagitis.

The presence of pain in the back raises the possibility of a collapsed dorsal vertebra, resulting from osteoporosis induced by steroid therapy. Localized tenderness and aggravation of the pain by movement of the spine would then be expected, but are absent in this patient.

The pain associated with dissecting aneurysm of the aorta characteristically radiates to the back and often moves to the loin as the dissection progresses. Unequal, absent or delayed pulses of the major arteries may be found and neurological signs frequently result from occlusion of major branches of the aortic arch. Preservation of the femoral pulses with distal pulses being absent is not a feature of dissection. This can be explained in this patient by the presence of left ventricular failure, reduced cardiac output, peripheral vasoconstriction and the likelihood of peripheral vascular disease.

The possibility of polyarteritis nodosa must always be considered when a patient presents with late onset asthma. Asthma may be the only symptom present for some years before involvement of other systems such as the kidneys, and, rarely, the heart where it may cause myocardial infarction.

Pulmonary embolism must always be considered in the differential diagnosis of sudden severe central chest pain. The absence of signs of a deep vein thrombosis does not exclude the diagnosis. When haemoptysis occurs it is more likely to be due to a peripheral lung infarct causing pleuritic pain than to a massive embolism occluding the pulmonary artery or one of its major branches. In any event, signs of acute right, rather than left, heart failure would be expected, with elevation of the JVP. His mild ankle oedema, if long standing, is more likely to be due to nifedipine.

The essential immediate investigations in this patient are an electrocardiogram (ECG) and chest X-ray. The ECG would obviously be of great value in diagnosing myocardial infarction. However, since the patient has been admitted within a few hours of onset, changes may not yet have appeared on the ECG and the test should be repeated in that case. The value of the chest X-ray will be in excluding a pneumothorax for which films in both inspiration and expiration are necessary. Furthermore, signs of left heart failure and pulmonary oedema might be seen. These include engorgement of the upper lobe veins, basal septal (Kerley B) lines, and perihilar haze ('bats wing' shadow). The chest X-ray can be normal in dissecting aneurysm but may show widening of the mediastinum.

The most likely diagnosis in this patient is myocardial infarction and pulmonary oedema, for which conventional treatment would be intravenous aminophylline, a quick-acting diuretic such as frusemide, analgesia and oxygen. Although the history of bronchial asthma would rightly require caution in the use of these last two measures, none the less cardiac asthma is an indication for treatment with diamorphine and 100% oxygen. Thrombolytic agents (streptokinase or plasminogen activator with heparin and aspirin) should be considered in a recent proven myocardial infarction, to improve the prognosis. Any co-existing potential bleeding, such as a peptic ulcer would contraindicate their use. In addition the stress induced by the condition of the patient may fail to evoke an appropriate adrenocortical response due to adrenal suppression by steroid therapy. He should, therefore, be given intravenous hydrocortisone.

The ECG confirmed the presence of an acute anteroseptal myocardial infarction. The chest X-ray showed the features of pulmonary oedema and cardiomegaly.

5. Shock

The term 'shock' is used to describe a clinical state. Although the word is difficult to define precisely and is often used inaccurately, it remains useful because it characterizes a syndrome which is generally well recognized, and because there are mechanisms common to all causes underlying the disorder.

A shocked patient is pale and sweating with cold and often cyanosed peripheries. The blood pressure is low, the pulse rate is rapid, and the peripheral veins are collapsed. There is restlessness and mental confusion. A patient in this state would be generally regarded as being in shock. Difficulties arise if one or more of these features is lacking.

THE PATHOPHYSIOLOGY OF SHOCK

Haemorrhagic shock

The shock which results from haemorrhage has been widely studied, and is the easiest model for under-standing the circulatory abnormalities in a shocked patient (Fig. 5.1). In haemorrhagic shock, there is first a reduction in blood volume. Since the venous system contains the largest part of the circulating blood, the fall in blood volume causes a fall in venous pressure and a reduction in venous return to the heart. The cardiac output, which is dependent on venous return, falls, the stroke volume diminishes and the blood pressure falls. The fall in blood pressure threatens the cerebral circulation, and various circulatory reflexes are activated to counteract this. These originate in the carotid sinus and aortic arch, and the result is intense stimulation of the sympathetic nervous system, causing release of catecholamines with tachycardia and arteriolar vasoconstriction. The vasoconstriction is most marked in the skin and gut. The blood pressure is thus maintained but at the price of hypoxia in the vasoconstricted areas.

In animals undergoing experimental haemorrhagic shock, after a few hours of this intensive vasocon-

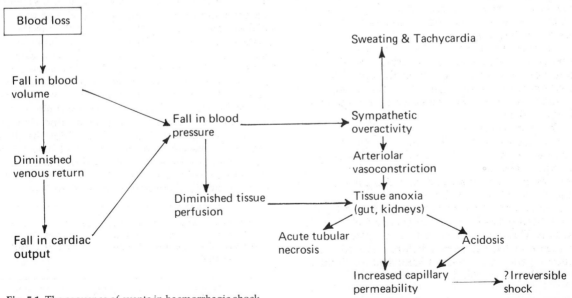

Fig. 5.1 The sequence of events in haemorrhagic shock

striction, restoration of the blood volume may no longer be effective treatment. At this stage, tissue damage in the splanchnic bed can be so great that fluid and blood are lost from the capillary network and further hypovolaemia results. The therapy of prolonged haemorrhagic shock has to take into account this disturbance in the microcirculation. In experimental haemorrhagic shock pressor agents will increase arteriolar vasoconstriction and worsen the situation, while drugs which block alpha-receptors given in addition to blood replacement cause splanchnic vasodilatation and can improve survival in experimental animals.

Irreversible shock due to haemorrhage alone is very uncommon in man. In cases of haemorrhage where shock is irreversible, other complicating factors such as tissue injury, burns and sepsis are usually present. Other mechanisms then contribute to the pathophysiology of shock.

a) *Pump failure.* Although primary pump failure is the major mechanism in cardiogenic shock, some degree of LV failure is also found in other shock states. Thus direct depression of myocardial function occurs in the toxaemia of septic shock, and impaired coronary perfusion in prolonged hypotension from any cause.

b) Increased peripheral vasoconstriction leads to tissue anoxia and contributes to mental confusion, bacteraemia (from gut-derived organisms) and oliguria. This process is exacerbated by arteriovenous shunting of blood past the capillary bed.

c) Anoxia leads to lactic acidosis and further depression of myocardial function.

Cardiogenic shock

Here the drop in blood pressure is primarily due to the failure of the heart as a pump. The arteriolar vasoconstriction which follows is mediated through the same mechanism as in haemorrhagic shock, and the same disturbance in small blood vessels in the splanchnic circulation can result. The fall in blood pressure is of especial importance to the damaged heart, because the heart is unique in that the coronary circulation fills in diastole and if the diastolic pressure is very low, there may not be enough pressure to open the coronary arteries to allow perfusion. Maintenance of diastolic pressure is therefore of especial importance in keeping an effective circulation through the coronary arteries to an already damaged myocardium.

Septic shock

Septic shock is also characterized by low blood pressure and cardiac output, sometimes accompanied by intense peripheral vasoconstriction, and reduced tissue perfusion. Two-thirds of cases are due to Gram-negative septicaemia. Lipid-A of endotoxin damages capillary walls and endothelial damage is accompanied by thrombocytopenia and disseminated intravascular coagulation (DIC – see Ch. 29). The endotoxin causes arteriolar vasoconstriction and pooling of blood in veins. The venous pressure falls and as a result there is a profound fall in cardiac output. Blood volume is not reduced at first, but later on there is reduction in blood volume due to loss of fluid from anoxic capillaries. The picture of shock in Gram-negative septicaemia is modified when it occurs in patients with hepatic cirrhosis. These patients are especially prone to this complication and often have a cardiac output greater than normal. The presence of bacteraemic shock may not result in reduction in cardiac output below the normal range. In shock caused by Gram-positive bacteraemia the picture may be identical with that produced by Gram-negative organisms. In some patients septic shock is accompanied by vasodilatation and increased capillary permeability leading to hypovolaemia. Endothelial damage in pulmonary capillaries leads to 'shock lung' with diffuse consolidation on chest X-ray and impaired gas exchange with progressive anoxia. All forms of septic shock are commoner in immunocompromised patients and in patients undergoing instrumentation, operation or with indwelling intravenous lines.

Anaphylactic shock

Anaphylactic shock is caused by the release of vasoactive compounds as a result of reaction of antigen with antibody in a previously sensitized person. Histamine, serotonin, bradykinin, and slow-reacting substance are all thought to play a part in the production of the shock, and histamine is probably the most important. The antibody is of the IgE class and exhibits the property of 'cytotropism', that is, it adheres to the surface of cells, especially mast cells in the skin, bronchial mucosa, and gut. The union of antigen and antibody takes place on the surface of the mast cells resulting in degranulation of the cell and release of vasoactive substances. Histamine causes bronchial constriction, and hypovolaemia due to capillary dilatation and loss of intravascular fluid. The release of vasoactive compounds also plays an important part in the severe shock which often occurs in acute pancreatitis, which is accompanied by considerable vasodilatation, with loss of intravascular fluid.

Consequences of shock

Whatever the cause of shock, a variety of secondary changes may accompany it. Tissue anoxia occurs, and with it local acidosis and the liberation of metabolites. There is subsequent systemic acidosis, the severity of which depends on the degree of stagnation of blood flow. Either hypoxia or acidosis or metabolites finally relax the precapillary sphincters so that more blood flows into the capillary bed. This results in further hypovolaemia and the formation of tissue oedema.

Renal blood flow is low as a result of hypotension, and glomerular filtration rate falls. Oliguria is therefore a common accompaniment of shock. If renal blood flow falls to very low levels, acute tubular necrosis may occur. Before this stage there is a rising blood urea and excretion of urine of low specific gravity.

Hypoglycaemia may occur in the late stages of shock, probably due to failure of hepatic production of glucose.

THE DIAGNOSIS OF THE CAUSE OF SHOCK

The cause of haemorrhagic shock is often self-evident, but gastrointestinal bleeding may be concealed, and must be excluded in any shocked patient where the cause is not apparent. A past history of peptic ulceration should be sought, and rectal examination may reveal melaena. A less obvious source of occult haemorrhage is retroperitoneal bleeding, either following abdominal surgery or spontaneously from an aortic aneurysm. Often the blood tracks along the large vessels and appears later as areas of bruising in the thighs and sacral region.

Bacteraemic shock is often overlooked. It is now recognized that this cause of shock is common, and must also be excluded in any patient where no other obvious source is present. A previous history suggestive of infection is often present, such as cholecystitis, pyelonephritis, cholangitis, or pneumonia. Ischaemia of the bowel due to vascular thrombosis, volvulus or strangulated hernia are other predisposing causes. Any form of peritonitis, especially faecal peritonitis, may be complicated by endotoxin shock. A careful examination of the abdomen is therefore essential, including rectal examination and listening for bowel sounds. Gram-negative septicaemia may also occur after major abdominal surgery, and here the differentiation between bleeding and endotoxin shock may be especially difficult. Gram-negative shock may occasionally occur following the relatively minor procedures of cystoscopy and termination of pregnancy.

Cardiogenic shock often occurs in the context of obvious myocardial infarction or pulmonary embolism, when the diagnosis is straightforward. However, elderly patients often present with the complications of myocardial infarction rather than with the characteristic chest pain. Shock may be the presenting feature of such a case, and an electrocardiogram must always be taken.

Anaphylactic shock is suggested by the clinical picture. There is usually a clear history of exposure to antigen – nowadays nearly always an injection of a drug or serum. The patient feels an itching, burning sensation within a few minutes. Bronchial constriction then develops with cyanosis, and there may be laryngeal oedema and stridor. The blood pressure falls and the patient may die quickly. Some patients live a few hours longer and may, during this time, develop urticaria. The cause of death is usually respiratory failure, but occasionally hypotension is the most prominent feature.

INVESTIGATIONS

A haematocrit is useful since if it is raised it suggests loss of plasma as in peritonitis, but if low suggests bleeding, unless haemodilution has not yet occurred (see Ch. 11). It is most useful as a baseline against which progress can be assessed. An ECG is essential. Chest X-ray may show pulmonary oedema in myocardial infarction, or an unsuspected pneumonia in an elderly patient. A straight X-ray of the abdomen may show gas under the diaphragm if there has been perforation of a viscus, or fluid levels in intestinal obstruction from volvulus or mesenteric thrombosis.

Blood cultures are essential if there is any possibility of bacteraemic shock. Cultures of sputum and urine should be taken if appropriate. The urine output must be carefully measured and sent for measurement of electrolytes and osmolality, as this will prove a useful baseline for further management. Plasma urea and electrolytes are essential, and a determination of pH and pO_2 will be helpful.

Lastly, hypoglycaemia can closely resemble shock, and blood sugar should be estimated if this is at all likely.

TREATMENT OF SHOCK

Volume replacement

Most causes of shock are associated with depletion of circulating blood volume. This is reflected in hypotension, collapsed veins, and a tachycardia. It is essential that blood volume is restored. This should be with blood or plasma in all cases except where loss of electrolytes is the main factor (as in acute dilatation of the stomach or intestinal obstruction). The filling pressure of the right heart is monitored by a central venous pressure (CVP) catheter. Left-sided filling pressure can be measured by the flow-directed Swan–Ganz catheter which lodges in the small pulmonary arterioles, but this is more hazardous. Pulmonary artery diastolic wedge pressure (PADP is normally 1–5 mmHg) usually reflects left-sided filling. A challenge with plasma or blood (200–300 ml) should not cause a rise of CVP or PADP of more than 3–4 mm Hg. If volume depletion has been a major contributory factor to the shock the blood pressure rises, and the pulse rate falls, the extremities become warm and the veins fill. Urine flow increases. If transfusion is too rapid or too great in amount, especially if the patient is elderly or has heart disease the CVP or PADP will rise rapidly.

Antibiotics

These lower mortality in experimental bacteraemic shock, and are mandatory in this condition. Gentamicin is an especially valuable antibiotic in Gram-negative shock. This and a broad-spectrum cephalosporin are a useful combination, as is the combination of cloxacillin, gentamicin and metronidazole against both Gram-positive and Gram-negative organisms. The key to successful antibiotic therapy lies in taking appropriate cultures before treatment is started.

Pressor and inotropic agents

The intense vasoconstriction accompanying shock is mediated through alpha-adrenergic nerves. Experimentally, the stagnation of the microcirculation resulting from this vasoconstriction can be improved by alpha-adrenergic blockade, and the mortality lowered. Pressor agents, on the other hand, by increasing vasoconstriction, do not improve the prognosis of experimental shock. This has led to the clinical use of alpha blockade in conditions of shock where effective peripheral circulation, as judged by warm extremities and good urine flow, has not followed adequate volume replacement. At low dose, dopamine enhances renal blood flow; at higher doses it is more positively inotropic and also causes increasing vasoconstriction.

Dobutamine is a positive inotrope, but causes peripheral vasoconstriction. Nor-adrenaline infusion is also often very effective at raising blood pressure in septic shock. Although it causes intense vasoconstriction, its use is often accompanied by restoration of urine output as the blood pressure rises.

Phosphodiesterase inhibitors (such as enoximone) may prove to have a useful role in enhancing myocardial contractility.

In anaphylactic shock, adrenaline should be given intramuscularly, and if necessary intravenously. An antihistamine, such as diphenhydramine, and hydrocortisone should be given, both intravenously.

Corticosteroids

Direct measurements of plasma cortisol have shown that hypoadrenalism is not a contributory factor in the hypotension of haemorrhagic and bacteraemic shock. In fact, plasma cortisol levels are usually greatly elevated. Nevertheless it is customary to give high doses of hydrocortisone (50–60 mg/kg) in bacteraemic shock, and in this dose, the drug is acting pharmacologically directly on blood vessels, reducing arteriolar vasoconstriction. It is not clear whether steroids improve prognosis or not.

Digoxin

In cardiogenic shock the use of digoxin depends on the presence or absence of other complications such as pulmonary oedema and arrhythmia. Some physicians regard shock as an additional indication for digitalization. Its value is uncertain.

Mechanical ventilation

Low cardiac output in shock results in tissue anoxia. If cardiac failure is present then there is, in addition, failure of oxygenation of blood in the lungs. In many cases of septicaemic shock the adult respiratory distress syndrome (ARDS – 'shock lung') develops. Hypoxaemia, deteriorating mental state, exhaustion, retention of secretions, may all lead to the necessity of assisting the patient's breathing by mechanical ventilation. This is a hazardous procedure and one which is best undertaken in a planned manner rather than as an emergency.

CLINICAL PROBLEM

T	P	BP	R
38	140	70/50	28

Slight central cyanosis

Peripheral cyanosis

Cold and sweating

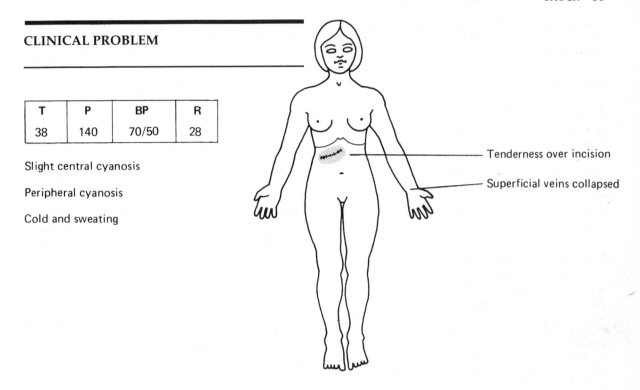

Tenderness over incision

Superficial veins collapsed

A housewife of 65 was admitted to hospital with a history of 5 days' fever, rigors and severe right upper abdominal pain. She had noticed dark urine over the same period and had lost her appetite. Previously she had always been well.

On examination on admission she was unwell, and had a temperature of 38.2°C. Blood pressure 140/90. Pulse 125 regular. The heart and lungs were normal. There was extreme tenderness in the right upper quadrant of the abdomen. At laparotomy a gangrenous gall bladder was removed which contained several stones. There was some free fluid in the abdomen, but no other abnormalities. Exploration of the common bile duct was negative.

Following the operation she made an uneventful recovery at first. However 2 days later she complained of nausea and of feeling unwell. These symptoms had come on over a period of a few hours. She had not had pain, cough or shortness of breath.

On examination (see diagram) she looked very ill. Temperature 38°C. Blood pressure 70/50. Pulse 140. Respiration 28/min. She was cold and sweating. There was marked peripheral cyanosis, and slight central cyanosis. The jugular venous pressure was not raised, and superficial veins were collapsed. The heart and lungs were normal. In the abdomen, there was residual tenderness over the region of the laparotomy. Bowel sounds were present. Rectal examination was normal. A urinary catheter was passed and 100 ml of residual urine obtained which contained a trace of albumin but no red cells or white cells.

QUESTIONS

1. What do you consider to be the probable diagnosis?
2. What investigations do you think are essential for immediate management?
3. What would your immediate management be?

DISCUSSION

This patient has become shocked in the early post-operative period, and the differential diagnosis must include intra-abdominal bleeding and Gram-negative septicaemia. The latter diagnosis is made more probable by the operation having been performed for an infective cause. Pulmonary embolism is less likely so soon after the operation, the patient has not complained of chest pain or dyspnoea, and the venous pressure is not elevated. Myocardial infarction should certainly be considered although the absence of chest pain makes this diagnosis less probable. Biliary peritonitis and pancreatitis are unlikely because she has not complained of pain, there is no abdominal tenderness and bowel sounds are present.

Investigations will include haemoglobin and white cell count. The presence of anaemia strengthens the probability of bleeding but its absence does not exclude it. A polymorphonuclear leucocytosis will point towards an infective cause. Tests for disseminated intravascular coagulation should be performed, including fibrin degradation products, platelet count, and prothrombin time examination of the blood film for fragmented red cells.

An ECG is essential since this may show changes suggestive of pulmonary embolism or myocardial infarction. A chest X-ray may show an area of diminished vascularity of the lung suggestive of pulmonary embolism, or changes of pulmonary infarction. The appearances of left ventricular failure due to myocardial infarction may be present.

Measurement of central venous pressure is essential both in diagnosis and in management. Since the correlation between right and left atrial pressures may not be good in severely ill patients, consideration should be given to inserting a Swan–Ganz catheter. A raised venous pressure is often found in pulmonary embolism, while haemorrhage and septicaemic shock are both accompanied by low venous pressure. During treatment, careful observation of the venous pressure will lessen the risks of fluid overload.

The urine should be cultured, and a centrifuged specimen examined under the microscope. Although there is nothing in the history and physical examination to suggest urinary infection, this must be excluded in any patient where the diagnosis of septicaemic shock is possible and where the cause is not immediately apparent. The blood urea and urinary sodium, urea, and osmolality should be measured. These measurements will probably not be of immediate value in management, but will be useful if the patient becomes oliguric, when it may be difficult to decide whether intrinsic renal damage is present. Blood cultures are essential. Cultures should also be taken from the drainage tube site.

Treatment must be started at once. The patient should be transfused with plasma or blood, depending on the haematocrit, until the venous pressure starts to rise. This will ensure that adequate blood volume replacement has been achieved. If the patient has uncomplicated haemorrhagic shock, the blood pressure will rise and the signs of peripheral circulatory failure will disappear. Irreversible haemorrhagic shock is very rare in man. Volume replacement is essential in septicaemic shock, and must be combined with antibiotic treatment without waiting for blood culture results. In the patient described here, where the shock might be due to haemorrhage alone it would be reasonable to transfuse the patient quickly and if there was not obvious clinical improvement after 1–2 hours, to start antibiotic treatment as well. Bactericidal antibiotics covering a wide range of bacteria must be given. Hydrocortisone will usually be given, although its value is unproven.

The patient had an *E. coli* septicaemia and was treated with blood transfusion, cloxacillin, gentamicin, and hydrocortisone before the results of blood culture were obtained. After 2 pints of blood her venous pressure rose, as did the blood pressure, without further deterioration. She was oliguric for a further 12 hours but with dobutamine urine output subsequently returned to normal.

6. Dyspnoea

Dyspnoea is a subjective feeling of difficulty in breathing. It can also be defined as an unpleasant sensation that increased respiratory effort is needed. Some include in the definition any condition in which increased respiratory effort is present, without it necessarily being unpleasant. In practice most physicians exclude the hyperpnoea which occurs in metabolic acidosis and the tachypnoea which occurs in acute anxiety. However, hyperpnoea may itself cause distress and the distinction is often arbitrary. The mechanism by which the sensation of dyspnoea is produced is not understood. It cannot be explained by disturbance in blood gas tensions alone, since many dyspnoeic patients do not have hypercapnia or hypoxia. It appears to originate from mechanical stimuli generated in the lungs, and is perhaps best explained by the patient recognizing that the work needed to inspire a given volume of air is inappropriately large. The relationship between the force exerted to expand the lung by a given amount and the amount of expansion achieved (length–tension relationship) is altered and the sensation of dyspnoea may arise because the force required has increased in relation to the volume achieved.

Various classifications of dyspnoea have been put forward, but from a practical point of view the most useful one is based on the pattern of onset and progression. This is shown in Table 6.1. The main pulmonary changes which give rise to a sensation of dyspnoea are airways obstruction, decreased lung volume and decreased elasticity of the lung. The most important cardiovascular abnormalities which cause dyspnoea are elevation of left atrial pressure and pulmonary embolism.

DYSPNOEA OF RAPID ONSET

The diagnosis of the patient who complains of the rapid onset of breathlessness can be difficult. In the history, the most important features are the rapidity of onset, the presence and nature of any pain, and the past medical history.

Severe dyspnoea occurring abruptly is very suggestive of pneumothorax or pulmonary embolism. In the former, there may be a history of sharp chest pain

Table 6.1 Classification of dyspnoea by its clinical presentation

A Dyspnoea of rapid onset
1. Pulmonary
Acute bronchitis
Pneumonia
Pneumothorax
Asthma
Inhaled foreign body

2. Cardiovascular
Left heart failure
Pulmonary embolism
Pericardial tamponade
High altitude

3. Psychogenic

4. Metabolic
Diabetic ketoacidosis
Uraemia
Poisons

B. Dyspnoea progressing over a few months
1. Pulmonary
Pleural effusion
Tumour (including lymphangitis carcinomatosa)
Pulmonary infiltrations and fibrosis
Tuberculosis

2. Cardiovascular
Congestive cardiac failure
Anaemia
Recurrent pulmonary embolism

3. Neuromuscular
Myasthenia gravis

C Dyspnoea which is slowly progressing
1. Pulmonary
Chronic bronchitis
Emphysema
Pneumoconiosis
Diffuse pulmonary fibrosis

2. Cardiovascular
Congestive cardiac failure
Recurrent pulmonary embolism

3. Mechanical
Gross obesity
Ankylosing spondylitis
Scleroderma

felt on the side of the pneumothorax. If the pneumothorax is large enough to cause severe dyspnoea, signs of shift of the mediastinum will usually be present. An exception is when a small pneumothorax complicates pre-existing pulmonary disease, such as chronic bronchitis or asthma. Pulmonary embolism usually occurs in patients who have a predisposing cause and there is little difficulty in distinguishing it from pneumothorax on history and physical signs. In massive embolism the chest pain is usually crushing. On examination there is commonly hypotension, cyanosis, and a gallop rhythm. There is usually no clinically detectable abnormality in the lungs in the early stages. The cause of the dyspnoea in massive pulmonary embolism is not known. Anxiety, hypoxia, and stimulation of stretch receptors in the pulmonary arteries are all possible factors.

Severe dyspnoea coming on over 1–2 hours is most likely to be due to bronchial asthma or left heart failure. The latter may be due to myocardial infarction or aortic or mitral valve disease. Bronchial asthma is usually easily distinguished from left heart failure by the history of previous attacks, by the absence of a history of chest pain and the absence of cardiac murmurs. The differential diagnosis may however be difficult at times, especially when the left heart failure gives rise to a wheezing dyspnoea. Pneumonia, particularly in a patient with chronic bronchitis, may cause severe dyspnoea. Usually the presence of pleuritic pain, cough with purulent sputum, and signs of consolidation make the diagnosis straightforward.

Pericardial tamponade may cause difficulty in diagnosis. There is often a clear history of an antecedent febrile illness, together with central chest pain typically relieved by sitting forward. However, tamponade can occasionally come on rapidly, particularly when due to involvement of the pericardium by malignant tumour, the commonest being carcinoma of the bronchus. In these patients there may be no history of previous febrile illness or chest pain. The patient with tamponade usually has a low blood pressure, pulsus paradoxus, and a raised jugular venous pressure. The jugular venous pressure may also rise paradoxically on inspiration (Kussmaul's sign). These features on history and examination usually serve to distinguish the condition from left ventricular failure and pulmonary embolism.

Hyperventilation due to metabolic acidosis may occasionally give rise to the complaint of breathlessness, but more often this is a relatively minor accompaniment of a self-evident illness such as diabetic ketoacidosis. Renal failure should be looked for and the urine examined.

Three poisons may make the patient hyperventilate: salicylate, due to a direct effect on the respiratory centre causing a respiratory alkalosis, followed by a metabolic acidosis; methyl alcohol and ethylene glycol, both of which are uncommon poisons, but which cause a profound metabolic acidosis.

In children, sudden breathlessness or stridor may be due to an inhaled foreign body. Signs of lobar collapse may be present, but physical examination may be of little help and a chest X-ray is essential.

Psychogenic dyspnoea may also be of a rapid onset. The dyspnoea usually has features which are unlike organic disease. The patient may complain of not being able to take a satisfactory breath in, or of a sensation of being suffocated. There may be obvious hyperventilation, more marked during examination, and symptoms of tetany may occur. The dyspnoea may occur after exertion rather than during it. The patient often does not seem to be in any distress at all. It is important to remember that psychogenic dyspnoea, due to anxiety, may be present in a patient who has organic disease of mild degree, for example ischaemic heart disease or pulmonary tuberculosis, and that this may be responsible for the initiation of the symptoms. Part of the treatment of psychogenic dyspnoea lies in being able confidently to exclude organic disease as a cause of the patient's symptoms and to convince the patient that this is so.

DYSPNOEA PROGRESSING OVER A FEW MONTHS

When dyspnoea is of gradual onset and becomes worse over a period of a few months a different differential diagnosis presents itself.

A pleural effusion may present in this way. Malignant effusions may be very large, and often present as breathlessness. Primary carcinoma of the lung is the commonest cause, but secondary tumours, lymphomas and pleural mesothelioma may be responsible. A pleural effusion large enough to cause dyspnoea will be accompanied by clear-cut physical signs (see Ch. 9). Pulmonary neoplasms may also give rise to dyspnoea by obstruction of a main bronchus, or by widespread lymphatic infiltration. Both pleural effusion and tumour are easily diagnosed by physical examination together with a chest X-ray.

Diffuse pulmonary fibrosis is a more difficult problem. The physical signs and radiological appearances can be very slight early on in the disease, although dyspnoea may already be a prominent feature. The diagnosis is easier if there is a disease present known to be associated with pulmonary fibrosis, such as sarcoidosis. Some help will usually be gained from pulmonary function tests (see below).

Although congestive cardiac failure is usually obvious as a cause of dyspnoea progressing over a few months, this is not always the case. Increasing breathlessness on exertion may be the earliest symptom of cardiac failure, and a careful examination may reveal cardiac enlargement or murmurs, which will suggest the diagnosis, even in the absence of raised venous pressure. A chest X-ray will usually show cardiac enlargement, and possibly signs of left heart failure such as distension of upper lobe pulmonary veins or septal 'B' lines (see Ch. 2).

Any cause of anaemia may give rise to breathlessness, and this is especially likely to occur if any other predisposing cause is present, for example ischaemic heart disease.

Recurrent pulmonary embolism may present a most difficult problem in diagnosis. There may be a history of deep venous thrombosis of calf or pelvic veins, of recent pregnancy, or of taking the contraceptive pill. The symptoms of pulmonary infarction, pleuritic chest pain and haemoptysis may be absent in a patient presenting with dyspnoea due to pulmonary hypertension from thromboembolism. The patient may complain of effort syncope and anginal pain. This is not always the case however, and this diagnosis must be kept in mind in any patient with breathlessness while the cause remains uncertain, for there is the possibility of arresting the progress of the disease by anticoagulation.

Physical examination may reveal an enlarged heart with a left parasternal heave. The second sound in the pulmonary area may be accentuated and an ejection click after the first sound is sometimes present. No abnormality is found in the lungs in most cases.

A chest X-ray may show enlargement of the cardiac shadow. The clinical and radiological signs of pulmonary hypertension do not occur until two-thirds of the vascular tree has been obliterated. The changes of right ventricular hypertrophy and strain may be seen on the ECG. A lung scan will usually be helpful even in the absence of physical signs, and in the presence of the frequently normal chest X-ray. Areas of diminished perfusion of the lung may be shown, and if present greatly strengthen the diagnosis. This appearance is not by any means diagnostic of infarction: infection, collapse, cysts may all cause similar changes. It is important therefore to obtain ventilation images, ideally with radio krypton, to confirm the presence of perfusion–ventilation mismatch. The diagnosis of thromboembolic pulmonary hypertension is supported by finding raised right ventricular and pulmonary artery pressures and by showing obliteration of pulmonary arteries on angiography.

The main difficulty in diagnosis in patients with dyspnoea which is progressing over several months is when physical examination and chest X-ray are both normal. It is then that lung scanning and the more complex lung function tests can be of considerable value, as the differential diagnosis includes one of the various causes of diffuse pulmonary fibrosis and pulmonary thromboembolism. In this group of patients, it may be tempting to attribute dyspnoea to psychological causes, but this diagnosis should not be made by exclusion alone. Other features suggestive of a psychiatric disorder should be present.

DYSPNOEA WHICH IS SLOWLY PROGRESSING

Chronic lung disease of any kind normally presents in this way. Chronic bronchitis and emphysema, widespread bronchiectasis, diffuse pulmonary fibrosis, pulmonary thromboembolism, pneumoconiosis, tuberculosis will all be suggested by typical features of history and by radiological appearances. In the majority of patients there is no difficulty in discovering the cause of the dyspnoea. However, the physical signs and radiological appearances of emphysema may not be marked, and some patients with emphysema have little cough or wheeze but have a main complaint of breathlessness. Appropriate lung function tests, particularly the measurement of diffusing capacity, are indicated.

Diffuse pulmonary fibrosis can cause dyspnoea over a long period of time without abnormal physical signs being present. Points to note on examination are the presence of cyanosis, and the amplitude of the chest movements which are typically restricted. Clubbing of the fingers and rales at the lung bases are often present. A right ventricular impulse and loud second sound in the pulmonary area indicate right ventricular enlargement and pulmonary hypertension. This may follow thromboembolic disease or destructive disease of the lung from any cause.

INVESTIGATION OF A PATIENT WITH DYSPNOEA

Chest X-ray

Most cases of dyspnoea will have an obvious cause, and the pattern of investigation is self-evident. A chest X-ray is the most helpful investigation. It may show enlargement of the heart, pulmonary infiltration, pleural effusion, tumours, collapse or consolidation. In fibrosing alveolitis the X-ray may be normal at the outset, but soon shows shadowing in acute cases. In the chronic disease there is a mottled appearance more marked in the lower zones, with areas of translucency. There is an overall loss of lung volume with elevation of the diaphragm. In emphysema, the classical changes are low flat diaphragms with a narrow heart shadow. The ribs are horizontal and there are diminished peripheral lung markings. Bullae may be present. Small pneumothoraces can easily be missed and if this diagnosis is suspected, films should be obtained in full expiration as well as full inspiration.

Lung function tests

Spirometry is a valuable investigation. A reduced forced vital capacity (FVC) is found in any condition which restricts the expansion or contraction of the lung. Reduction of lung volume has this effect and occurs in recurrent pulmonary infarction, large pleural effusions and after pneumonectomy. Restriction of expansion of the lung also occurs in pul-

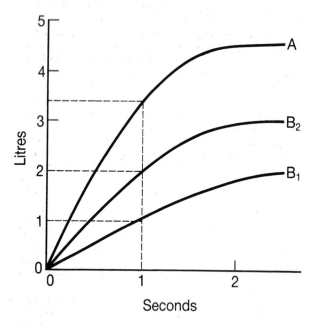

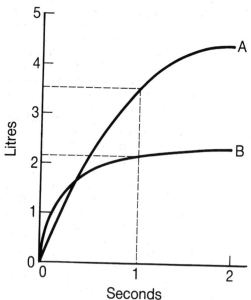

Fig. 6.1 A. Normal spirogram

$$\frac{\mathrm{FEV}_1}{\mathrm{FVC}} = 3.4/4.6 = 74\%$$

B. Obstructive ventilatory defect , before (B_1) and after (B_2) bronchodilator inhalation. The airways obstruction is partially reversed.

$$B_1\,\frac{\mathrm{FEV}_1}{\mathrm{FVC}} = 1.1/2.0 = 55\%$$

$$B_2\,\frac{\mathrm{FEV}_1}{\mathrm{FVC}} = 2.0/3.0 = 66\%$$

Fig. 6.2 A. Normal spirogram

$$\frac{\mathrm{FEV}_1}{\mathrm{FVC}} = 3.5/4.4 = 80\%$$

B. Restrictive ventilatory defect

$$\frac{\mathrm{FEV}_1}{\mathrm{FVC}} = 2.1/2.3 = 90\%$$

monary fibrosis from any cause, when the muscles of respiration are weak as in myasthenia gravis, and when there is an external restriction to full respiratory movements such as is caused by the rigid thoracic cage in ankylosing spondylitis. Airways obstruction from any cause will also reduce FVC. The ratio of forced expiratory volume in one second (FEV_1) to FVC is, however a better measure of air-

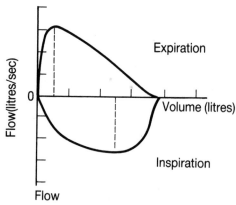

Fig. 6.3 A. Normal flow/volume loop

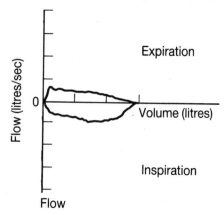

Fig. 6.3 B. Flow/volume loop showing upper airways obstruction in a patient with carcinoma of the larynx (preoperative).

ways obstruction. In asthma, for example, the FVC may be only slightly reduced, but the FEV_1 greatly so. This is called an obstructive ventilatory defect (Fig. 6.1 B). Therefore spirometry should always be repeated after inhalation of a potent bronchodilator to assess the degree of reversibility. Obstruction to airways is not a cause of dyspnoea which creates great diagnostic difficulty, and spirometry is more useful as a guide to treatment rather than as an aid to diagnosis. The conditions reducing FVC but without causing airways obstruction will inevitably give rise to a reduction in FEV_1 but the ratio of FEV_1/FVC will be normal (Fig. 6.2 B). Another simple, but less accurate, measure of airways obstruction is the peak flow rate (PFR). In diffuse pulmonary fibrosis a restrictive ventilatory defect may be detected when clinical examination has been unhelpful. On the other hand normal spirometry, even when corrected for age, sex and height, does not exclude organic disease unless the patient's previous level of performance is known. Flow/Volume loops, plotting the rate of flow against the total volume of air moved, in both expiration and inspiration are of value in analysing more fully obstructive and restrictive defects and in addition may allow the separation of obstruction due to lower airways disease from the less common obstruction due to upper airways pathology. Indeed the characteristic shape of the Flow/Volume curve may be the first indication of the true site of the lesion.

Blood gases

Blood gas tensions are of great help in certain circumstances. In recurrent pulmonary embolism there is shunting of deoxygenated pulmonary arterial blood. This may give rise to a low pO_2 if the process is widespread. The pCO_2 is normal or low since the patient hyperventilates slightly in response to the low pO_2. On exercise the patient hyperventilates greatly but becomes even more anoxic, and this is a valuable diagnostic test in distinguishing these patients from those with hysterical overbreathing who have a normal pO_2 on exertion. Hypercapnia does not occur because of the greater solubility of CO_2 allowing free diffusion of CO_2 across the alveolar–capillary membrane. In diffuse pulmonary fibrosis there is also a low pO_2 but this tends to occur later in the disease. Early on there is a fall in pO_2 on exercise, with an accompanying hyperventilation and fall in pCO_2. Later the pO_2 is very low and the patient is clinically cyanosed. The low pO_2 is probably partly due to shunting of blood and partly to a diffusion defect.

Estimating the transfer factor (diffusing capacity) may be of value. It is usually the earliest functional abnormality in diffuse pulmonary fibrosis. Any disease where there is a great loss of alveolar surface area (such as in emphysema) or where there is a restriction of the free diffusion of oxygen (such as in pulmonary oedema) will cause a low transfer factor. The test is unreliable in the presence of airways obstruction. Tests of pulmonary compliance (or of elasticity) are occasionally helpful in the diagnosis of diseases such as diffuse pulmonary fibrosis, where the compliance is decreased because of the increased rigidity of the lungs.

If a patient with dyspnoea has no abnormality on physical examination, chest X-ray and lung scan, and has normal ventilatory capacity, normal blood gases before and after exercise, normal transfer factor and compliance, then the physician can be fairly confident that no organic disease is likely to be present. Whether these patients should have their symptom labelled 'psychogenic' is another matter. Some will go on to develop obvious organic disease with the passage of time.

CLINICAL PROBLEM

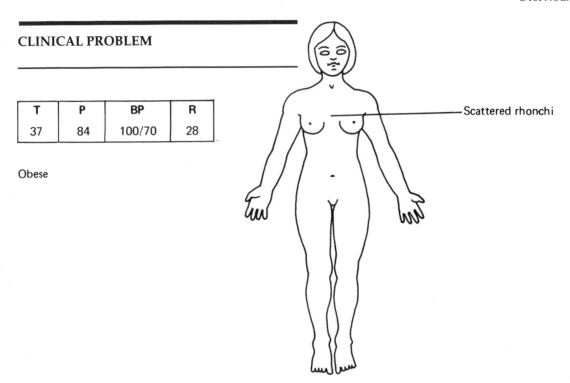

T	P	BP	R
37	84	100/70	28

Obese

Scattered rhonchi

A housewife of 35 complained of increasing breathlessness on exertion over a period of 9 months. She had reached the point where she could climb only 10 stairs before having to stop, but had not had orthopnoea or paroxysmal nocturnal dyspnoea. A slight morning cough which was productive of mucoid sputum had developed, but there had been no haemoptysis. Her third pregnancy 1 year previously had resulted in a normal delivery, followed by resumption of normal menstruation. Previously she had enjoyed good physical health.

After the birth of her child she had suffered from a depressive illness associated with poor sleep and considerable anxiety over her children. She had felt unable to cope with her domestic responsibilities, and was particularly anxious in case she became pregnant again. However her religious beliefs prevented her from accepting contraceptive advice. During this illness her appetite had been poor and she had lost a little weight. Her sleep was disturbed and she had lost all sexual interest. This illness had responded completely to supportive treatment from her family

doctor and a 4-month course of tricyclic antidepressants. After her recovery her appetite had increased and she had gained 10 kg in weight. She had been overweight since the birth of her first child 9 years previously. She smoked 20 cigarettes a day.

On examination she was rather anxious but not dyspnoeic at rest. She was considerably overweight at 86 kg, her height being 5 feet 7 inches. There was no evidence of cardiac failure; blood pressure was 100/70. Pulse 84/min regular. The heart was not enlarged clinically, the heart sounds were faint, and no murmurs could be heard. In the lungs there were occasional rhonchi, and rales which cleared on coughing. The rest of the examination was normal.

QUESTIONS

1. What are the most likely causes of her breathlessness?
2. Which investigations would prove of most value?

DISCUSSION

The history is suggestive of an organic cause for her breathlessness. Her depression resolved completely, yet her symptoms progressed. There are none of the emotional accompaniments of breathlessness which are common in patients with psychogenic dyspnoea. Thromboembolic pulmonary hypertension is a likely cause of this patient's dyspnoea, despite the absence of confirmatory physical signs, as these may be masked by her obesity. When progressive dyspnoea develops in relation to recent pregnancy or abortion the possibility of chorioncarcinoma metastasizing to the lungs must also always be considered. Progressive dyspnoea over 9 months in a young woman who has previously been well, is most unlikely to be due to chronic bronchitis and emphysema, even though she is a cigarette smoker and occasional rhonchi can be heard in her chest. Her weight gain is an inadequate explanation of dyspnoea of this severity. She has not had nocturnal dyspnoea or any other feature of heart failure on history or examination, and there is nothing to suggest a cause for left ventricular failure. Diffuse pulmonary fibrosis can present in this way and is a possible diagnosis.

A full blood count must be part of the initial investigation to exclude anaemia as a cause of dyspnoea. A chest X-ray is the most helpful investigation. In this patient the cardiac shadow may be enlarged due to right ventricular enlargement as a result of pulmonary hypertension. Enlargement of the pulmonary arteries is another sign of pulmonary hypertension which may be present in patients with recurrent pulmonary emboli or diffuse pulmonary fibrosis. Diminished peripheral vascular markings, so called 'pruning' of pulmonary vessels, is also found in pulmonary hypertension. A diffuse reticular shadowing is a common feature of diffuse pulmonary fibrosis, and is often most obvious in the lower zones, especially early in the disease. Somewhat similar X-ray appearances can be seen in lymphangitis carcinomatosa, commonly from a primary in breast or bronchus. The low flat diaphragms characteristic of emphysema, and the septal 'B' lines of left ventricular failure are not likely to be present in this patient.

Examination of the sputum is unlikely to be helpful in this case although malignant cells should be looked for as she is a heavy smoker. ECG may show right ventricular hypertrophy and strain in pulmonary thromboembolism and diffuse pulmonary fibrosis. Spirometry will show a restrictive ventilatory pattern in both these disorders. Blood gas studies at rest, after exertion, and after breathing 100% oxygen will help to differentiate between psychogenic dyspnoea on the one hand and thromboembolism or pulmonary fibrosis on the other. Isotope lung scan will usually show areas of diminished perfusion in pulmonary embolism even if the chest X-ray is normal. A ventilation scan should confirm that there is ventilation–perfusion imbalance. Although there was nothing to suggest a valvular lesion clinically and she had recently successfully undergone a full-term pregnancy, cardiac ultrasound combined with Doppler assessment can be valuable in any case of unexplained dyspnoea, and may show cardiac pathology, particularly valvular such as mitral stenosis, unsuspected on clinical examination. Breathlessness developing in patients who are HIV positive may be the first symptoms of AIDS presenting with pneumocystis pneumonia. Initially the chest X-ray may appear normal and more complex tests are often necessary to establish the diagnosis.

In this patient the chest X-ray was normal but blood gases and lung scan were suggestive of either pulmonary thromboembolism or diffuse pulmonary fibrosis. Right heart catheterization confirmed the presence of pulmonary hypertension and angiography showed this to be due to pulmonary thromboembolism.

7. Cyanosis and hypoxia

Cyanosis is caused by the presence of an excess of deoxygenated haemoglobin which is visible in the small vessels of the skin and mucous membranes. Hypoxia means that there is insufficient oxygen available for the normal metabolic requirements of the tissues. The term hypoxaemia is used when the partial pressure of oxygen in the blood is reduced. If this reduction is of sufficient severity, cyanosis results. It is useful to describe cyanosis as central or peripheral, as different mechanisms may be responsible for these two appearances.

Central cyanosis is a bluish discoloration of the lips, tongue and conjunctivae. It is due to desaturation of arterial haemoglobin.

Peripheral cyanosis is a bluish discoloration of the skin of the hands or feet and of the nail beds. It is always present when there is central cyanosis, but may occur without there being central cyanosis if there is diminished or slowed blood flow through the region in question. Abnormal peripheral cyanosis must be looked for when the skin is warm, since it may occur normally in the cold. Whereas peripheral cyanosis may be a purely local phenomenon, central cyanosis means that there has been a failure of oxygenation of blood in the lungs, and that hypoxaemia is present. (An exception is methaemoglobinaemia discussed below.)

THE TRANSPORT OF OXYGEN BY THE RED CELL

An understanding of the causes of hypoxia depends on knowledge of the way in which oxygen is carried by red cells. A common mistake is to confuse the partial pressure of oxygen in the blood on the one hand with the saturation of haemoglobin with oxygen on the other. The partial pressure of oxygen (pO_2) in the blood of a normal individual depends on the partial pressure of oxygen in the inspired air. The normal pO_2 of inspired air is 21.3 kPa (160 mmHg) and the partial pressure of oxygen in the arterial blood (paO_2) is about 13.3 kPa (100 mmHg). If the subject breathes 100% oxygen from a face mask the inspired pO_2 may rise to 53 kPa (400 mmHg) and the paO_2 will show a similar rise.

The saturation of haemoglobin with oxygen refers to the amount of oxygen the haemoglobin is carrying as a percentage of its total carrying capacity. The haemoglobin is normally fully saturated at a paO_2 of 12 kPa (90 mmHg) and breathing 100% oxygen does not cause any increase in oxygen-carrying capacity even though the paO_2 rises. Breathing high concentrations of oxygen results in displacement of nitrogen dissolved in the plasma. The paO_2 is high because of the dissolved oxygen. This is carried in physical

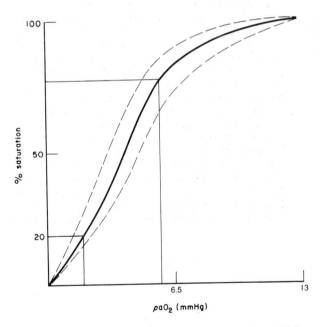

Fig. 7.1 Oxygen dissociation curve. The haemoglobin is 100% saturated when the paO_2 is above 12.0 kPa. When the paO_2 falls below 6.0 kPa cyanosis is usually visible if there is a normal haemoglobin concentration. Below 6.0 kPa a slight reduction in paO_2 leads to marked desaturation of the haemoglobin. A paO_2 below 2.0 kPa is incompatible with life. When the curve is shifted to the right more oxygen is liberated for a fall in paO_2 from 13 kPa to 5 kPa. The converse is true when the curve is shifted to the left.

solution in the plasma but does not contribute materially to the oxygen-carrying capacity of the blood. As the pa_{O_2} falls below 12 kPa (90 mmHg) a most important change occurs in the saturation of haemoglobin. At first there is a gradual but slight decrease in saturation, but below a pa_{O_2} of about 6 kPa (45 mmHg) the saturation of haemoglobin falls sharply for a relatively small fall in pa_{O_2}. In health this means that oxygenated haemoglobin relinquishes its oxygen as it passes through the tissues where the p_{O_2} is low. This relationship between p_{O_2} and saturation is known as the oxygen dissociation curve and is shown in Fig. 7.1.

Cyanosis is usually detectable when the saturation of haemoglobin with oxygen is 65% or less in an individual who is not anaemic. This degree of desaturation occurs when the pa_{O_2} of the individual is 6.5 kPa (50 mmHg) or below. Therefore the presence of central cyanosis means that at best the pa_{O_2} is 6.5 kPa (50 mmHg). Furthermore, central cyanosis also means that a further small reduction in pa_{O_2} will lead to a large increase in the amount of deoxygenated haemoglobin present as predicted by the oxygen dissociation curve. It is difficult to detect cyanosis in a severely anaemic person and conversely cyanosis is more obvious for a given pa_{O_2} when it occurs in a polycythaemic individual.

There are several factors which alter the oxygen dissociation curve. These alterations result in greater or lesser amounts of oxygen being liberated in the tissues, and change the pa_{O_2} at which cyanosis appears.

When the dissociation curve is shifted to the right the same fall in p_{O_2} in the tissues results in a greater release of oxygen from haemoglobin. On the other hand in the lungs less uptake of oxygen will occur for a given p_{O_2}. The curve is shifted to the right by acidosis, whether it is respiratory or metabolic in origin (see Fig. 7.1).

A shift of the curve to the left has the reverse effects, with diminished release of oxygen in the tissues as the p_{O_2} falls and increased uptake at a lower p_{O_2} in the lungs.

A product of red cell glycolysis, 2,3-diphosphoglycerate (DPG) is present in large amounts in the red cell. This metabolite exerts a strong influence on haemoglobin and the oxygen dissociation curve. A decrease in DPG increases the affinity of haemoglobin for oxygen, shifting the curve to the left. Such a decrease in DPG is caused by systemic acidosis, so that this effect opposes the direct effect of acidosis, and the oxygen dissociation curve is unaffected overall. A practical point is that when a systemic acidosis is reversed abruptly, the direct effect of acidosis is reversed at once, while the DPG effect takes several hours to return to normal. During this time the curve will be shifted to the left and haemoglobin will 'hold on' to its oxygen, aggravating tissue hypoxia. Both

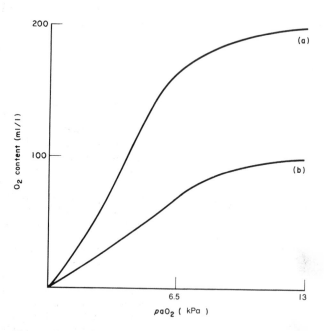

Fig. 7.2 Oxygen-carrying capacity of haemoglobin in normal (a) and anaemic (b) individuals. In the example shown the haemoglobin is 8 g/dl. The shift of the curve to the right enables more oxygen to be released to the tissues.

anaemia and hypoxia on the other hand cause a rise in red cell DPG, and the curve shifts to the right allowing a greater release of oxygen in the tissues, which partly compensates for the diminished oxygen supply (see Fig. 7.2).

Although the degree of saturation of haemoglobin with oxygen is what determines the presence of cyanosis, desaturation is not the only cause of hypoxia. In Table 7.1 the causes of hypoxia are classified. Anaemia causes tissue hypoxia because there is diminished oxygen content of the blood, even though the haemoglobin is fully saturated (Fig. 7.2). The causes and diagnosis of anaemia are dealt with in Ch. 28 and will not be discussed further.

Table 7.1   The causes of tissue hypoxia

A. Failure of oxygenation of blood in the lungs

1. Pulmonary causes
Ventilation/perfusion inequality
  chronic bronchitis and emphysema
  multiple emboli
  pneumonia
  asthma
  pulmonary fibrosis
Loss of surface area for diffusion
  emphysema
  pulmonary infarction
  pulmonary fibrosis
Severe hypoventilation
  chronic bronchitis
  severe asthma
  primary alveolar hypoventilation
Alveolar–capillary diffusion defect
  left heart failure (pulmonary oedema)
  diffuse pulmonary fibrosis
  lymphangitis carcinomatosa

2. Cardiac causes
Right-to-left shunt
Cardiac failure

3. Low inspired pO_2
High altitude

B. Diminished oxygen-carrying capacity of blood
Anaemia
Methaemoglobinaemia
Sulphaemoglobinaemia

C. Inadequate release of oxygen in tissues
1. Poor perfusion of tissues
Shock
Peripheral vascular disease
Cold

2. Decreased red cell 2,3-DPG (systemic acidosis – see text)

D. Failure of uptake by tissues
Tissue poisons, for example cyanide

THE PRODUCTION OF CYANOSIS IN PULMONARY DISEASE

There are several reasons why patients with lung disease become cyanosed. The most important is an abnormality of the relationship between ventilation and perfusion of alveoli (V/Q abnormality). In a normal alveolus, CO_2 diffuses out of the pulmonary arterial blood and is exhaled. Oxygen crosses the alveolar wall by diffusion and is sufficient in quantity to oxygenate all the blood perfusing that alveolus. If there is alveolar hypoventilation with normal perfusion, or normal alveolar ventilation with shunting, there will be a failure of oxygenation and desaturated blood will reach the systemic circulation. Normal oxygenation in other parts of the lung cannot compensate for this. (The events are shown in fig. 7.3.) On the other hand, localized areas of alveolar hypoventilation will not cause a rise in pCO_2 in the pulmonary venous blood since the remaining alveoli are normally ventilated and any tendency towards CO_2 retention is rectified. Abnormalities of the ventilation/perfusion relationship occur patchily throughout the lungs in chronic bronchitis, emphysema, pulmonary fibrosis and in severe asthmatic attacks. In acute massive pulmonary embolism, blood is diverted from the obstructed pulmonary artery through other vessels and over-perfusion of the remaining lung results, causing cyanosis.

In lobar pneumonia the affected alveoli are full of exudate, and the perfusing blood is not oxygenated, again causing cyanosis. The severity of the infection and the degree of mental confusion correlates closely with the degree of desaturation.

Oxygen diffuses less readily than CO_2 and if there is a loss of surface area for gas transfer, hypoxia will be a more prominent feature than hypercapnia. A loss in surface area occurs after pneumonectomy, in emphysema, diffuse pulmonary fibrosis and multiple pulmonary infarction.

Diffusion of oxygen is also impaired in pulmonary oedema, and this accounts in part for the cyanosis often seen in this condition. In left heart failure, however, the blood flow through the lungs is not normal, and overperfusion of relatively underventilated areas, such as the upper lobes, occurs and contributes to the cyanosis. Although the hypoxia in diffuse pulmonary fibrosis is often ascribed to a diffusion defect ('alveolar–capillary block'), this is probably not an important factor. There is considerable disturbance of the ventilation/perfusion balance in affected areas of the lung, and conventional tests such as carbon monoxide transfer for 'diffusion' defects do not distinguish between these two mechanisms.

Generalized hypoventilation of all alveoli also causes hypoxaemia. This is a less important cause of hypoxaemia than the other mechanisms. A reduction in ventilation from 5 l/min to 3 l/min will lower

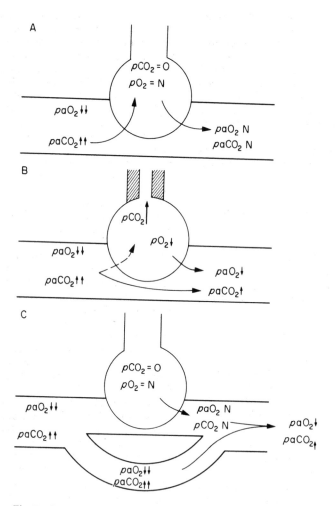

Fig. 7.3 In patients with V/Q abnormalities the final blood gas concentrations will be determined by the relative proportions of these three situations

A. Deoxygenated blood with a high pa_{CO_2} perfuses the alveolus which contains air with no CO_2 and high po_2. Normal diffusion occurs and the efferent blood is fully oxygenated with a lower pa_{CO_2} (N = normal)

B. Deoxygenated blood with a high pa_{CO_2} perfuses the underventilated alveolus which contains air with a subnormal po_2 and a raised pco_2 due to obstruction of air flow. The CO_2 cannot be adequately eliminated. If there are enough normally ventilated alveoli to allow CO_2 to be eliminated on subsequent circulations, the pa_{CO_2} will not rise overall. On the other hand, the hypoxaemia cannot be corrected by an increased uptake in other alveoli and the patient may be cyanosed.

C. There is normal ventilation but diminished perfusion with intrapulmonary shunting. The shunt allows deoxygenated blood with increased CO_2 to bypass the alveolus. As in B, cyanosis may occur but CO_2 can be eliminated in other normal alveoli on subsequent circulation

pa_{O_2} from 12 to 8 kPa (90–60 mmHg) at which point the haemoglobin will still be 85% saturated. However, alveolar hypoventilation is the most important cause of hypercapnia, and in the example quoted the pa_{CO_2} will have risen from 5.3 to 9.3 kPa (40–70 mmHg). Dangerous hypercapnia is thus present without the patient being cyanosed. Ventilation–perfusion abnormalities and loss of surface area for diffusion do not affect elimination of CO_2 as mentioned above.

Occasionally major vascular shunts occur in the lungs and cause cyanosis. These include vascular tumours and fistulae.

THE PRODUCTION OF CYANOSIS IN HEART DISEASE

If a major right-to-left intracardiac shunt exists, cyanosis is of course inevitable, and the condition is easily distinguished from pulmonary disease. Diagnosis of the cause of the shunt depends on clinical examination and investigation. The shunt may be at any level:

a) In the great vessels: patent ductus arteriosus or aorticopulmonary window with reversed shunts, transposition of the great vessels.
b) In the ventricles: ventricular septal defect with reversed shunt, Fallot's tetralogy, single ventricle.
c) In the atria: atrial septal defect or patent foramen ovale with reversed shunt. Anomalous pulmonary venous drainage.

In cardiac failure the cyanosis is due to a combination of redistribution of blood flow and impaired diffusion as already described. Many patients with raised venous pressure and peripheral oedema are suffering from cardiac failure secondary to chronic respiratory disease, especially chronic bronchitis and emphysema (cor pulmonale). In these patients left heart failure may not be present, and cyanosis can be attributed to the lung disease.

THE DIAGNOSIS OF THE CAUSE OF CENTRAL CYANOSIS

In the vast majority of cyanosed patients the cause is clear from the history and clinical examination. Tissue hypoxia may itself give rise to symptoms and signs irrespective of the underlying cause. The elderly in particular tolerate hypoxaemia poorly, especially if there is an impaired circulation due to atherosclerosis. Hypoxia of the tissues causes lassitude and fatigue, often followed by excitability, and if severe, coma and death. In hypoxaemia, underlying arterial disease may result in specific symptoms developing: angina, cardiac failure, intermittent claudication, dementia. These symptoms may occur regardless of the cause of hypoxaemia and do not help to make the diagnosis.

The great majority of cyanosed patients are suffering from respiratory or cardiac disease. An exception is those patients who have developed methaemoglobinaemia as a result of drugs, of which phenacetin is the commonest cause. Methaemoglobin does not combine with oxygen and hypoxia can result if the concentration of methaemoglobin is high. The patient's colour is slatey-grey rather than blue. There is an absence of cardiac or respiratory disease and the abnormal haemoglobin can be demonstrated spectroscopically.

The history in patients with pulmonary disease will usually be of dyspnoea on exertion, cough and sputum. An exception is in thromboembolic pulmonary hypertension in which the onset of dyspnoea and cyanosis may be insidious, without cough or sputum. Cardiac failure will present with the usual symptoms. Cor pulmonale is a common cause of cyanosis, and the hypoxaemia caused by the chronic respiratory disease is one of the factors which exacerbates heart failure, by the direct effect of myocardial hypoxia, and by causing pulmonary arteriolar vasoconstriction.

Examination may show signs of chronic obstructive airways disease: widespread rhonchi, use of accessory respiratory muscles, increased anteroposterior diameter of the chest with reduced expansion, and decreased liver and cardiac dullness. Clubbing of the fingers and basal rales may occur in diffuse pulmonary fibrosis. Left heart failure may be present as shown by rales at the lung bases, cardiac enlargement, and gallop rhythm, together with the signs of a cause of left heart failure such as myocardial infarction, mitral or aortic valve disease or hypertension. When there is a right-to-left intracardiac shunt present there may be clubbing of the fingers and physical signs of right ventricular enlargement and pulmonary hypertension. A murmur associated with atrial or ventricular septal defect or patent ductus may be present.

There is little difficulty, in most patients, in deciding whether the cause of cyanosis is cardiac or pulmonary. The main exception is in the elderly bronchitic who has evidence of ischaemic heart disease and signs which might indicate left heart failure. In these patients the discovery of the cause of cyanosis is usually academic, since both cardiac and pulmonary disease will be treated. In general, cardiac failure should not be attributed to chronic bronchitis and emphysema, unless the pa_{CO_2} is elevated. A practical point is that in the correction of cyanosis in these patients 100% oxygen should not be used, because of the danger of CO_2 narcosis. Oxygen should be administered at first in low concentration, monitoring the pa_{CO_2} to assess the response to treatment.

In patients with long-standing respiratory or cardiac disease, a secondary polycythaemia is often present. Cyanosis in these patients may therefore be detected when the pao_2 is above 6.6 kPa (50 mmHg).

INVESTIGATION OF CYANOSIS

Investigation of cyanosed patients is directed towards finding the cause and assessing the severity of the hypoxaemia. A chest X-ray will clearly be necessary and may show evidence of pulmonary or cardiac disease. An ECG will provide evidence in right atrial and ventricular hypertrophy in cor pulmonale and in right-to-left intracardiac shunts. Right bundle branch block is usually present when there is an atrial septal defect. Cardiac ultrasound with Doppler measurements and colour-flow mapping are now the preferred method of diagnosis and quantitative assessment of intracardiac shunts. Polycythaemia may be present and this implies long-standing hypoxaemia of any cause.

Measurements of blood gas tensions are of great help if the cause of cyanosis is in doubt. The pao_2 will be low provided the cyanosis is not caused by methaemoglobinaemia or sulphaemoglobinaemia. If the $paco_2$ is low this suggests that the patient is hyperventilating in response to hypoxia due to a cardiac cause, diffuse pulmonary fibrosis or pulmonary thromboembolism. If the $paco_2$ is raised, then alveolar hypoventilation is occurring and this is usually due to chronic bronchitis and emphysema. When there is mixed cardiac and pulmonary disease there is no definite way of deciding the contribution of each to the cyanosis but this is not normally a distinction of clinical importance.

Further investigation of pulmonary or cardiac disease may be necessary (see Ch. 6 on investigation of dyspnoea). Continuous non-invasive monitoring of tissue oxygen saturation by oximetry is of great value in determining whether the condition of a hypoxic patient is deteriorating and thus the need for assisted ventilation. Such monitoring during sleep may reveal episodes of hypoxia due to sleep apnoea.

CLINICAL PROBLEM

T	P	BP	R
37	100 irreg.	100/80	28

Central cyanosis

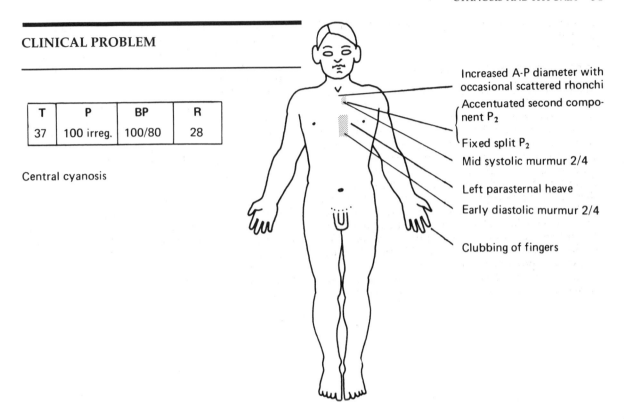

Increased A-P diameter with occasional scattered rhonchi

Accentuated second component P_2

Fixed split P_2

Mid systolic murmur 2/4

Left parasternal heave

Early diastolic murmur 2/4

Clubbing of fingers

A 50-year-old bank manager presented with a history of increasing shortness of breath of 2 years' duration. He had noticed a decline in his exercise tolerance over the preceding 5 years, but this had not become severe until 2 years previously, since when even moderate exertion had proved difficult. He was able to walk as far as he wished on the flat, but had to stop on any slight incline and after 12 stairs. He had smoked 20 cigarettes a day for 30 years, and had had a morning cough productive of mucoid sputum for many years. There was no history of swelling of the ankles.

In the past he had always been well. However, he had been turned down for service in the army at the age of 18, when a cardiac murmur had been noticed. This was not investigated in detail at that time, except for a chest X-ray which was reported as normal.

On examination he was cyanosed both centrally and peripherally. The pulse was 100/min and irreg-ularly irregular. Blood pressure 100/80. There was no evidence of cardiac failure. The apex beat was not displaced, but there was a prominent left parasternal heave. The second sound in the pulmonary area showed a marked fixed split, with accentuation of the pulmonary component. There was a moderately loud ejection murmur heard over the pulmonary area, while a diastolic murmur could be heard down the left sternal border. The trachea was central and there was slight clubbing of the fingers. The antero-posterior diameter of the thorax was increased, and respiratory movements were restricted. There were occasional rhonchi in both lungs. The rest of the physical examination was normal.

QUESTIONS

1. What are the likely causes of cyanosis in this case?
2. How would you distinguish between them?

DISCUSSION

This patient has been a heavy cigarette smoker for many years, and has signs suggestive of chronic bronchitis and emphysema. In addition he has a cardiac lesion with an arrhythmia which is probably atrial fibrillation. The signs point to a diagnosis of pulmonary hypertension. Pulmonary hypertension of this severity is unlikely to have developed as a result of chronic bronchitis without there being a past history of cardiac failure, and without signs of carbon dioxide retention being present, such as tremor, warm hands and a full-volume pulse. The physical signs, fixed split of the second sound, and systolic and diastolic murmurs in the pulmonary area, strongly suggest a diagnosis of atrial septal defect (ASD). It is not uncommon for atrial septal defects to present in middle age at a time when pulmonary hypertension develops and the shunt reverses. Clubbing will then usually develop. Cyanosis and clubbing in this patient are probably due to reversed flow through such a defect. The fact that a cardiac murmur had been noticed 32 years previously supports this diagnosis. The physical signs are not likely to be due to mitral stenosis, although tight mitral stenosis can be present without a mitral diastolic murmur being audible. There is however no opening snap, there is fixed splitting of the second sound, and the murmurs of increased pulmonary blood flow and pulmonary regurgitation due to the long-standing pulmonary hypertension.

This patient has both cardiac and pulmonary causes of breathlessness and cyanosis, and investigation is necessary to decide the role which each plays in his condition. A chest X-ray would be helpful. It will usually show low flat diaphragms in emphysema, and may show any other pulmonary disease which might contribute to breathlessness such as bronchiectasis or pulmonary fibrosis. The heart will be enlarged and the pulmonary arteries prominent. If there is a right-to-left intracardiac shunt there will be oligaemic peripheral lung fields. If there is an ASD without reversal of flow, there will be pulmonary plethora. However cardiac and pulmonary artery enlargement with 'pruning' of peripheral pulmonary vessels could be attributed to severe chronic bronchitis and emphysema. If this were the case, carbon dioxide retention should be present, and spirometry would show a severe ventilatory defect.

Estimation of $pa\text{CO}_2$ and $pa\text{O}_2$ and spirometry are therefore essential investigations. The $pa\text{O}_2$ will be low for the patient is cyanosed, but no conclusions about the cause of cyanosis can be drawn from the degree of desaturation. It will indicate the severity of either the pulmonary or cardiac lesion. If the $pa\text{CO}_2$ were normal or low then the diagnosis of ASD with reversed shunt is strongly supported. If there were great elevation of $pa\text{CO}_2$ there is clearly severe pulmonary disease although this would not rule out an ASD being present as well. Spirometry will show reduction of FVC and a proportionately greater reduction of FEV_1 in severe chronic bronchitis and emphysema (see Ch. 6). Modest reductions of FEV_1 and FVC are not associated with hypoxaemia or hypercapnia.

An electrocardiogram would be of some help. It will show atrial fibrillation, and in the case of ASD there will be right bundle branch block. These will obscure the effects on the heart which may result from chronic lung disease, that is P pulmonale, and right ventricular hypertrophy and strain. A cardiac ultrasound is essential. This will show the defect and Doppler analysis will indicate the size of the shunt.

This man had mild chronic bronchitis and emphysema and an ASD with a reversed shunt. Investigations showed $pa\text{CO}_2$ 5.32 kPa (40 mmHg), $pa\text{O}_2$ 6.4 kPa (48 mmHg), FEV_1/FVC = 2.2/3.6 litres. After 100% oxygen the $pa\text{O}_2$ was 7.0 kPa (54 mmHg). ECG showed right bundle branch block and atrial fibrillation and ultrasound confirmed the presence of an ASD with a reversed shunt.

8. Haemoptysis

This common symptom usually brings the patient quickly to a doctor. It is generally recognized by the patient that it may be the initial presentation of serious disease and needs adequate investigation and explanation. This need for investigation usually results in the referral of the patient to hospital, although in the majority of cases admission will not be necessary.

A very large number of conditions can cause haemoptysis, and the symptom may arise from both disease confined to the lungs and some systemic disorders. It can be a very early symptom of disease, so that if initial investigation is negative follow-up of the patient is needed for at least a further 6 months, with repeated chest X-rays. Even with full initial investigation and careful follow-up, in most patients with haemoptysis where initial investigation has not revealed the cause, no further abnormality will develop and the haemoptysis will settle spontaneously. Some of these patients have chronic bronchitis.

One must first establish that the patient's complaint is truly the coughing up of blood from the lungs. This is not usually difficult, particularly as haemoptysis is commonly associated with other symptoms such as cough or sputum which will point to disease of the lungs. A common description of true haemoptysis is of blood suddenly 'coming into the back of the throat'. It is of particular importance to differentiate this from vomiting of blood. There is the occasional patient who is unable to describe his symptom clearly and considerable confusion results, and in such cases one may unavoidably be forced to investigate both alternative sources of bleeding!

Another problem is to recognize bleeding from the upper respiratory tract, or from the mouth. It is obligatory to examine these areas and obvious lesions such as ulcers, naevi or carcinoma may be seen. Sometimes the patient confuses bleeding from unhealthy gums with haemoptysis, although usually the relation of such bleeding to teeth cleaning and the appearance of the gums resolves the problem. The deliberate production of a little blood, for example by biting the cheek, is not difficult and very occasionally this symptom may be a feature of malingering. The diagnosis is always difficult to prove and even if suspected should not prevent the simpler investigations being carried out.

THE CLINICAL HISTORY

The symptom of haemoptysis must first be established. One should enquire whether the blood is bright red in colour, how much has been produced and whether it is associated with sputum. A history of recent trauma should be sought. Indirect damage as from blast injury, as well as the more obvious direct damage, as may occur in a game of rugby football, may present shortly afterwards as haemoptysis. The duration of the symptom is important as the causes of small infrequent haemoptyses over many years tend to be different from those of a single large recent bleed.

The other main respiratory symptoms should be carefully asked for: cough, sputum, chest pain, shortness of breath, and wheeze. These may point to the underlying cause. Thus cough and purulent sputum suggest infection, while pleuritic chest pain in association with haemoptysis always raises the possibility of pulmonary infarction. Tuberculosis commonly presents with haemoptysis, which can be of any degree. Other more general symptoms suggestive of systemic disease may be present, and one must ask if there has been fever, night sweats, weight loss, and bleeding into other sites, such as skin, urine or bowel.

The past medical history may be important. Chest disease in childhood, followed by recurrent cough and sputum suggests bronchiectasis, which may subsequently give rise to bleeding at any age. In some cases small haemoptyses are the major feature and there is little in the way of purulent sputum, so called bronchiectasis sicca. There are a number of cardiac causes of haemoptysis. Rheumatic fever in childhood may cause mitral stenosis in which recurrent haemoptyses are common. Any cause of left ventricular or left atrial failure can give rise to haemoptyses.

Pulmonary embolism from deep-vein thrombosis has a tendency to be recurrent and a past history of venous thrombosis or pulmonary embolism is very important. The deep venous thrombosis in a leg or pelvic veins which is the source of embolus is often clinically silent. A history of any factor known to predispose to venous thrombosis, such as childbirth, the contraceptive pill, a recent operation or injury, or any other form of immobilization, is of obvious importance.

In the family history there may be some bleeding tendency such as haemorrhagic telangiectasia or a defect of coagulation. A history of pulmonary tuberculosis or of respiratory symptoms suggesting such a diagnosis may be obtained in a member of the family or a close associate.

In children an important condition is inhalation of a foreign body. This will lead to bronchial obstruction and collapse, and can cause haemoptysis. In adults a detailed smoking history is essential. It is surprising how often the heavy smoker who stopped his habit only days previously will say he is a non-smoker and not mention his previous smoking.

PHYSICAL EXAMINATION

The general appearance may suggest some serious disease such as disseminated malignancy, but the majority of patients complaining of haemoptysis appear in good health. One may observe the typical mitral facies, while sometimes a carcinoma of the bronchus has already produced mediastinal obstruction with oedema and swelling of the face and neck, and engorgement of the veins draining into the superior vena cava. There may be purpura as a result of a generalized bleeding disorder, and in an elderly patient one should always consider the possibility of scurvy. Clubbing is an important sign in both carcinoma and chronic suppurative lung disease, and may also be seen in advanced pulmonary tuberculosis. Hypertrophic pulmonary osteoarthropathy may occur, usually as a result of an underlying carcinoma. On clinical grounds it might be misdiagnosed as early rheumatoid arthritis.

The pulse may be small and irregular due to atrial fibrillation in mitral stenosis. In severe hypertension nose bleeds may occur and can masquerade as haemoptysis. The fundi should be examined for hypertensive changes and may show haemorrhages due to a bleeding disorder. The mouth, gums and throat will be examined. The most important signs are likely to be in the chest. Bronchitis, bronchiectasis or pneumonia may give their typical signs, while evidence of apical disease suggests tuberculosis. Collapse of a lobe or lung in a child suggests an inhaled foreign body, while in an adult it is more likely to be due to carcinoma or adenoma. A localized wheeze may be present over the underlying obstruction.

A pleural rub may be due to infection but is also a common feature of infarction. There may be other features suggestive of pulmonary thromboembolism, such as the signs of pulmonary hypertension.

Localized tenderness of the chest wall will suggest a fractured rib, especially if the pain is made worse on 'springing' the chest. Very rarely the signs of an aortic aneurysm may be present. The signs in the heart of possible relevance will be those of mitral stenosis or other causes of left heart failure. In tight mitral stenosis the murmur may be absent. The legs must be examined for evidence of deep venous thrombosis. In addition to tenderness and oedema one should also look carefully for increased filling of the superficial veins, with increased warmth.

INVESTIGATION

By far the most important aid in diagnosis is the chest X-ray, both PA and lateral. In the majority of cases where any firm diagnosis is reached it can be made on the clinical findings and chest X-ray alone. Tuberculosis, carcinoma, pneumonia, lung abscess and aneurysm will usually be obvious, while bronchiectasis and pulmonary infarction can often be suspected. Fractured ribs may also be seen, although these can often be surprisingly difficult to demonstrate on X-ray, and on occasion an isotope bone scan can be of the greatest value in clearly demonstrating them. The cardiac outline may suggest mitral stenosis or there may be cardiac enlargement due to left ventricular failure from any cause. If there is any suspicion of valvular disease, then cardiac ultrasound is essential.

Reliable sputum cytology is obviously of the greatest value in the diagnosis of carcinoma, and may allow a firm diagnosis to be made even though the chest radiograph is normal. Examination of the sputum for acid-fast bacilli is unlikely to be positive in the presence of a completely normal chest X-ray. A more common problem is the patient with haemoptyses who has apical fibrosis, probably due to old healed tuberculosis. The occurrence of haemoptyses does not necessarily imply that the disease is active, and serial chest X-rays will usually be needed to answer this question. The area of damaged lung may be the site of bronchiectasis or there may be a cavity containing a mycetoma. On chest X-ray the mycetoma may give a characteristic appearance of a solid ball within a cavity surrounded by a crescent-shaped air shadow. The sputum may show aspergilli. The sputum must be examined and cultured for tubercle as a routine in all cases of haemoptysis. Routine microscopy and culture of the sputum for other pathogens will rarely be of value, except in the diagnosis of *Klebsiella* pneumonia which is commonly associated with haemoptyses.

An ECG may show right heart strain, suggesting pulmonary embolism. (see Fig 4.4 (page 26)) Atrial fibrillation may be present, with clot formation in the right atrium leading to pulmonary embolism and thus haemoptysis. If a pleural effusion is present it should be aspirated and the pleura biopsied. The

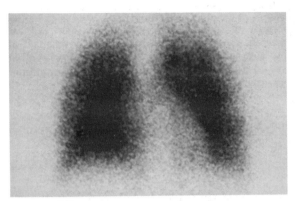

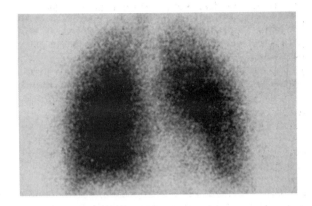

Fig. 8.1 Lung scans
A. Normal perfusion scan showing homogeneous distribution of technetium

B. Normal ventilation scan in the same patient showing homogeneous distribution of inhaled krypton

effusion caused by a pulmonary infarct often contains an excess of eosinophils, while biopsy will often show both tuberculosis and carcinoma when these involve the pleura (see Ch. 9).

Bronchoscopy is of the greatest value if either foreign body or neoplasm is suspected. It will enable a more precise diagnosis to be made and most foreign bodies can be removed. Tumours can be biopsied and the rarely occurring adenoma may be diagnosed. Often it will be obvious that the carcinoma is inoperable, so that thoracotomy can be avoided. Even if no tumour is seen, bronchial secretions can be aspirated for cytology and culture. Bronchography may be needed occasionally to establish the diagnosis of bronchiectasis and delineate its

extent. This is now far less important than in the days when surgery was the treatment.

In any patient where pulmonary embolus is suspected, a radioisotope lung scan should be done. Gross defects of perfusion may be seen due to single or multiple emboli, even in the presence of a completely normal chest X-ray. Ideally a ventilation lung scan should also be done at the same time, but this is not always available. In pulmonary embolism, when ventilation and perfusion scans are performed at the same time, areas of underperfused but normally ventilated lung may be revealed. When the chest X-ray is abnormal and only a perfusion scan is available, it is difficult to distinguish between pulmonary embolism and other lung diseases (see Figs. 8.1, 8.2).

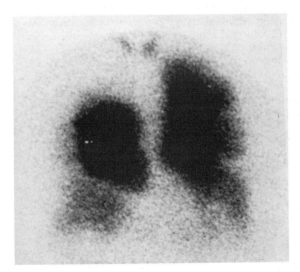

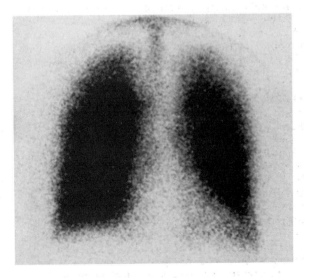

Fig. 8.2 Lung scans
A. Abnormal perfusion scan showing multiple areas of diminished perfusion in a patient with multiple pulmonary emboli

B. Ventilation scan in the same patient showing normal distribution of inhaled krypton. This disparity between ventilation and perfusion is typical of pulmonary embolism

Pulmonary angiography is an excellent means of diagnosing pulmonary emboli, but because it is an invasive procedure it is rarely performed. It will also reveal the rare condition of pulmonary angioma.

In a considerable number of patients all investigations prove negative, the cause is never found, and the bleeding settles spontaneously. In some cases, occasional haemoptyses continue, often because of some degree of bronchiectasis, but fortunately these haemoptyses are usually small. If all the simple tests are negative, pulmonary emboli should be carefully considered as in this condition effective treatment is possible.

CLINICAL PROBLEM

T	P	BP	R
38·8	90	160/100	26

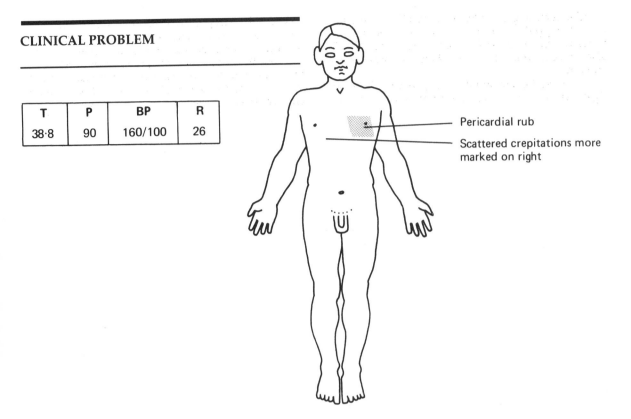

Pericardial rub

Scattered crepitations more marked on right

A 47-year-old schoolteacher presented to his general practitioner with the complaint that for the previous few weeks he had been coughing up small quantities of blood. Over the same period of time he had noticed some cough with a moderate quantity of yellow sputum, and had felt increasingly unwell. On direct questioning he admitted to progressive shortness of breath over the preceding month, so that he was unable to climb the three flights of stairs to his flat without stopping. After exertion he had noticed a tendency to wheeze, and this symptom only gradually settled with rest. Throughout this time his appetite had been poor and he had lost about 5 kg in weight. He smoked 10 cigarettes daily and drank only moderate quantities of alcohol. In his family, his father had suffered from chronic bronchitis for a number of years.

On examination, he looked ill but was not cyanosed or dyspnoeic at rest. Temperature 38.8°C. Pulse 95/regular. Blood pressure 150/90. In the chest, there were scattered crepitations present in most areas, together with some prolongation of expiration. The initial chest X-ray was reported as showing bilateral basal consolidation, more marked on the right.

He was treated with amoxycillin, salbutamol and choline theophyllinate, but showed little improvement. A week later he was still feverish and continuing to have small haemoptyses. He was admitted to hospital.

In addition to his presenting symptoms he was now complaining of central chest pain which was worse on deep breathing. He had also noticed aching in the knees and elbows, with some stiffness but no swelling.

On examination, T 38.8°C, BP 160/100, P 90 (see diagram). On auscultation the crepitations were more marked, particularly over the right lower lobe. In the cardiovascular system there was now an obvious pericardial rub, but no signs of tamponade. The fundi were normal. There was no evidence of arthritis. On routine testing the urine revealed a trace of protein and a weakly positive test for blood.

QUESTIONS

1. What do you consider to be the more likely diagnoses?
2. What further investigations are indicated?

DISCUSSION

Recurrent haemoptyses always deserve full investigation. It is unlikely that they will occur due to simple bacterial infection alone and the chest X-ray of this patient is open to many other interpretations. Haemoptysis may occur in an acute attack of bronchitis, but is unusual, and would not be expected to continue for a number of weeks. Thus despite the presence of cough, sputum and fever, this is unlikely to be the diagnosis. The wheeze and shortness of breath might suggest asthma and yellow sputum containing large numbers of eosinophils may be produced in this condition. A little blood staining in association with the rusty sputum of pneumococcal lobar pneumonia can occur, but the pattern of the illness in this patient, its slowly progressive time course and the mild fever, do not support this diagnosis. Blood-stained sputum is a common feature of *Klebsiella* pneumonia but again such an illness is more acute, the patients are mostly older and debilitated and the changes are usually in the upper lobes.

The symptoms of fever, haemoptysis and weight loss also suggest a tuberculous infection, but the chest X-ray appearance would be highly unusual, and the acute pericarditis is not typical of this diagnosis.

At this age, carcinoma of the bronchus is common, and may infiltrate the pericardium and cause acute pericarditis, which commonly progresses to tamponade.

Rarer conditions that can give rise to an illness of this type are polyarteritis nodosa or one of the related syndromes such as Wegener's granulomatosis.

Wheezing and haemoptysis are common features of pulmonary polyarteritis, whereas in bronchial asthma itself, haemoptysis is rare. The likelihood of systemic disease is increased by the presence of the pericarditis although a pleuropericardial friction rub is not uncommon in pyogenic infections of the left lung. There is nothing in the history or examination to suggest pulmonary emboli.

Investigation must obviously include a full blood count and ESR. The chest X-ray should be repeated and the pericarditis confirmed electrocardiographically. The sputum should be examined for acid-fast bacilli and malignant cells, and for eosinophils.

Renal disease is a common feature of polyarteritis and is suggested by the slight rise in blood pressure and the trace of protein and blood in the urine. It should be excluded by full examination of the urine and measurement of the blood urea and creatinine. However, in pulmonary polyarteritis renal involvement may not occur for some months or years.

Investigation of this man showed a mild degree of anaemia, with a neutrophil leucocytosis and a very high ESR. There was also eosinophilia. The sputum contained eosinophils rather than pus cells. No acid-fast bacilli or malignant cells were present in the sputum. There was moderate proteinuria together with microscopic haematuria. The blood urea was normal. The gamma globulin was markedly raised on serum electrophoresis, but the ANF test was negative. The ECG showed widespread S-T elevation consistent with pericarditis. The anti-neutrophil cytoplasmic antibody test (ANCA) was positive. Renal biopsy finally established the diagnosis of polyarteritis nodosa.

9. Pleural effusion

Pleural effusion is a sign of underlying disease and is not a diagnosis in itself. It may, however, be the earliest sign of disease or a prominent feature of a disorder where other signs and symptoms are not helpful in diagnosis. The differential diagnosis of the cause of a pleural effusion is a common problem in general medical practice.

PHYSICAL SIGNS

The effusion, which is an accumulation of fluid in the pleural space, must have a volume of about 500 ml before it can be reliably detected on physical examination. The most characteristic finding is stony dullness on percussion, with absent or diminished breath sounds, and decreased voice sounds and vocal fremitus. The dullness extends horizontally into the axilla and this is a point of differentiation of effusion from lower lobe consolidation or collapse. Above the effusion, a small area of bronchial breathing is often present. If the effusion is large there may be shift of the mediastinum away from the effusion with displacement of the apex beat and trachea. These are signs of fluid in the pleural cavity, but fluid may also accumulate in the interlobar fissure or above the diaphragm (infrapulmonary effusion) and here cause no detectable physical signs.

RADIOLOGICAL APPEARANCES

The smallest effusions are shown on a chest X-ray as filling-in of the normal costophrenic angle, often described by radiologists as a pleural reaction. Larger effusions have a concave upper surface and the shadow extends further upwards in the axilla. This appearance, often described as fluid 'rising' in the axilla, is due to the fluid being seen edge on. A common misconception, which arises from this appearance, is that the impairment of percussion note also should rise in the axilla. Infrapulmonary effusions have a similar radiological appearance to a raised hemidiaphragm, but when the patient lies on one side, the fluid moves in position unless it is encysted. Interlobar effusions appear as an opacity in the lung fields which may simulate a pulmonary tumour. When a large pleural effusion is present, the hemithorax may be completely obscured. An important practical point is that the upper limit of a pleural effusion is often underestimated on a chest X-ray compared with the physical signs. When deciding on the level at which to aspirate an effusion, the extent of dullness to percussion is often the better guide.

THE CAUSES OF PLEURAL EFFUSION

A collection of pleural fluid may be due to exudation or transudation. The distinction is made on the basis of the underlying disease, and on the protein and cell content of the fluid. Exudation is due to inflammation of the pleura and is characterized by a protein content of more than 30 g/l and the presence of cells. Transudates are due to the loss of fluid from the pleural capillary bed and are caused by the same conditions that cause oedema elsewhere in the body (see Ch. 3).

Pleural exudates

The majority of pleural effusions are exudates, and usually they occur as a complication of pulmonary disease which has already been diagnosed. The following are the main causes to be considered:

Pulmonary infarction. This condition often presents considerable difficulty in diagnosis. One of its common accompaniments is a pleural effusion, which is usually small, and which may be the only physical sign that infarction has occurred. It is often said that the effusion is haemorrhagic, and although this is sometimes the case, especially soon after the infarction, it is more commonly straw-coloured. The effusion contains neutrophils and lymphocytes and occasionally, large numbers of eosinophils. Aspiration and examination of the fluid can never confirm the diagnosis of a pulmonary infarction. This will usually be based on evidence of a source of embolism elsewhere, such as deep venous thrombosis in the legs or pelvis. Examination of the fluid is helpful in cases where the effusion is the only sign of disease and the differentiation between infarction and malignant or tuberculosis effusion must be made.

Pneumonia. Pleural effusion may complicate bacterial pneumonia, although it is very rare in virus pneumonia. Post-pneumonic effusions may become the seat of pyogenic infection resulting in an empyema. Usually, the effusion develops after a patient with bacterial pneumonia has already been started on treatment with antibiotics. If an empyema develops, the patient's condition will deteriorate, with increasing fever. In such a case the fluid must be aspirated completely and is usually straw-coloured with numerous neutrophils. The fluid must always be cultured, although it is often sterile. Complete aspiration of the effusion, together with appropriate antibiotic therapy usually results in cure. A bacterial pneumonia, particularly if complicated by pleural effusion, may be the first sign of an underlying bronchial neoplasm. In such cases the fluid must be examined for malignant cells and a pleural biopsy performed. The suspicion of an underlying carcinoma is strengthened when an apparently straightforward post-pneumonic effusion recurs repeatedly after aspiration.

Malignancy. The commonest cause of a malignant pleural effusion is a primary carcinoma of the bronchus involving the pleura. This may be the first evidence of the tumour. The effusion is often large, causing a shift of the mediastinum, and may accumulate very rapidly, causing dyspnoea. If there is underlying collapse of the lung due to the tumour, the mediastinum may paradoxically be shifted to the side of the effusion. The bronchial carcinoma has usually been previously diagnosed, and other signs due to the primary tumour or its metastatic spread will commonly be present. Aspiration reveals fluid which is usually blood-stained, but may be straw-coloured. It often reaccumulates rapidly after aspiration. This is a feature of pleural effusion which always suggests malignancy. There may be malignant cells in the effusion but their absence does not exclude the diagnosis, as success in finding and identifying the cells reflects the care and skill with which the fluid is examined. Furthermore, effusions may occur in carcinoma of the bronchus without there being involvement of the pleura by malignancy. They may result from an associated pneumonia or lymphatic obstruction. A pleural biopsy is valuable if the diagnosis has not been established previously.

Other pulmonary tumours may cause pleural effusions. Metastatic tumours may involve the pleura at a time when the primary site is unknown. Similarly an effusion may be the first indication of recurrent tumour after the primary has been excised. The effusion may be bilateral, and metastases may be visible in the lung fields. Malignant lymphomas may involve the pleura and the chest X-ray may show other features suggestive of this diagnosis such as enlarged hilar and mediastinal nodes. Cytology may suggest the nature of the underlying neoplasm. Primary malignant tumours of the pleura are uncommon, but pleural mesothelioma is being seen more often as a result of

people being exposed to asbestos dust. Other radiological signs of asbestosis, such as fibrosis in the lower zones and calcified pleural plaques, may be present.

Tuberculosis. Tuberculous pleural effusions are caused by a combination of direct tuberculous infection of the pleural space, and a state of hypersensitivity to the tubercle bacillus. Effusions may accompany primary infections in young children, but are uncommon. In these patients, the effusion is often accompanied by radiological signs suggestive of the diagnosis, such as a primary focus or enlarged hilar nodes. The pleural aspirate often contains tubercle bacilli. In adolescents pleural effusion may be the sole sign of the disease, although they may go on to develop further signs of the infection if left untreated. In adults infection of the pleural space with tubercle bacilli is uncommon, but can occur as a complication of established pulmonary disease such as tuberculous bronchopneumonia, or following rupture of a cavity into the pleural space.

The effusion can be very large, and acid-fast bacilli may be seen in the centrifuged deposit after aspiration. Culture of the fluid for the bacillus must be carried out, and repeated culture increases the chance of success. It is in the diagnosis of tuberculous pleural effusion, that pleural biopsy, repeated if necessary, is of the greatest value. The Mantoux test is always positive in these patients since the effusions are in part due to hypersensitivity.

Connective tissue disease. Rheumatoid arthritis may occasionally be accompanied by pulmonary complications and these are commoner in men. The commonest complication is pleural effusion, and although this usually develops in a patient with established disease, it may be the presenting feature. On aspiration the fluid is clear, with a high protein content. A low glucose concentration may be found. Biopsy is needed if tuberculosis or malignancy are possible causes of the effusion. In rheumatoid arthritis biopsy usually shows chronic inflammation without distinguishing features, although sometimes appearances similar to rheumatoid granulomata are found. Pleurisy with a small effusion also occurs in systemic lupus erythematosus.

Other causes. A pleural effusion may arise as a result of disease below the diaphragm, such as a subphrenic or hepatic abscess. Although the diagnostic signs of the primary disorder will usually be present, difficulty may arise in the diagnosis of subphrenic abscess. The patient may complain of shoulder-tip pain with no signs other than fever and a pleural effusion.

Acute pancreatitis may be accompanied by a pleural effusion. The mechanism of its formation is obscure, but it is usually blood-stained and has a high concentration of amylase.

Actinomycosis is exceedingly rare as a cause of pleural effusion, but it may present in this way.

Pleural transudates

The general principles underlying the formation of pleural fluid are the same as those in the formation of interstitial fluid elsewhere in the body. The main causes of pleural transudates are:

a) Congestive cardiac failure. This is the commonest cause, and other signs of congestive cardiac failure will usually be present. The effusions are usually small and bilateral. When unilateral the effusion is usually right-sided and can be very large. The chest X-ray will show other features of cardiac failure such as enlargement of the heart shadow, and upper lobe venous distension. Pleural effusion may occur in constrictive pericarditis and this diagnosis will be strongly suggested by calcification in the pericardium.

b) Hypoproteinaemic states. Cirrhosis of the liver, nephrotic syndrome, and malabsorption syndrome are the commonest causes of hypoproteinaemia. There is usually considerable salt and water retention as well. All of these conditions may be accompanied by pleural effusion, but the underlying disease is usually obvious, and the plasma albumin concentration is low.

Chylous pleural effusions

Perforation of the thoracic duct leads to the accumulation of lymph in the pleural space and a chylous pleural effusion. Most cases are the result of trauma or of surgery, but chylothorax can also be caused by malignant infiltration of the thoracic duct by primary or secondary tumours and lymphomas. The signs are those of a large pleural effusion, which reaccumulates rapidly after aspiration. The fluid has a milky appearance and the protein content is high. Repeated aspiration leads to lymphopenia and profound protein loss.

INVESTIGATION OF A PLEURAL EFFUSION

Many pleural effusions have causes which are clinically self-evident, and little further investigation is required. A great deal of information will be obtained by routine investigations such as full blood count, chest X-ray and sputum culture and cytology.

There remains the not uncommon clinical problem where a patient has a pleural effusion without clinical evidence of any underlying disease, and examination of the sputum and chest X-ray have not contributed to the diagnosis. In these patients, aspiration of the pleural fluid is essential.

Biopsy of the pleura and aspiration are usually performed at the same time. The fluid should not be aspirated too quickly, and about 500 ml of fluid can be withdrawn without risk to the patient.

Blood-stained effusions suggest malignancy, although pulmonary infarction is occasionally a cause. Clear watery fluid is found in transudates, and purulent fluid in an established empyema. The protein content of the effusion helps to distinguish transudates from exudates, although this is seldom a point at issue.

Bacteriological culture for pyogenic organisms is always essential, but a positive culture does not rule out malignancy as a cause of the underlying disease. Culture for tubercle bacilli is mandatory whenever an effusion is aspirated for diagnostic purposes.

The cells in the effusion should be examined. Numerous neutrophils suggest pyogenic infection, while large numbers of lymphocytes are usually found in a tuberculous effusion. Of interest is the finding of large numbers of eosinophils in some pleural aspirates. If there is no associated blood eosinophilia, then the commonest cause of eosinophilic effusion is pulmonary infarction. Other causes are pneumonia, malignancy and trauma. It is suggested that breakdown products of red blood cells are the cause of the eosinophil infiltration, but the finding is none the less unusual in cases of haemorrhagic effusion.

The chest X-ray should always be repeated after aspiration to see if any underlying abnormality has thereby been revealed.

These investigations will normally have been successful in discovering the cause. Occasionally further investigation may be necessary, especially if it is felt that there is an underlying carcinoma. In these cases bronchoscopy may be helpful, especially if specimens are taken for cytology at the time of examination.

CLINICAL PROBLEM

T	P	BP	R
39	96	120/80	30

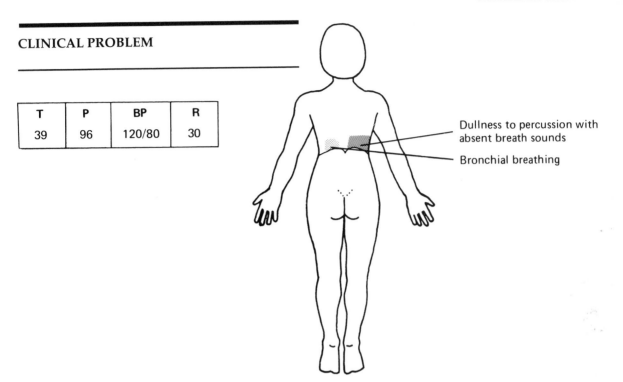

Dullness to percussion with absent breath sounds

Bronchial breathing

A woman of 55 had suffered from bronchial asthma for 10 years and had been treated with corticosteroids for 7 years. During this time she had had recurrent upper abdominal pain, which was alleviated by alkalis and occasional courses of cimetidine. For 2 months before admission she had been feeling unwell, tiring easily, with a cough which troubled her during the day but which was unproductive of sputum. She was a non-smoker. One week before admission her asthma worsened, and she increased her prednisolone to 40 mg/day. This produced improvement and she had reduced the dose to 20 mg/day by the time of admission. Two hours before admission she had developed sudden severe upper abdominal pain, and collapsed in the railway station on the way home.

On examination she was very ill; BP 90/60, T 37°C, P 160/min. In the chest there was generalized expiratory wheeze, and dullness to percussion at the right base posteriorly, extending into the axilla. There was general abdominal rigidity with diffuse tenderness. Bowel sounds were absent. Before laparotomy, she was given hydrocortisone, which was continued postoperatively. At operation there was free fluid in the abdomen, and a small perforation of a posterior duodenal ulcer. The perforation was sutured.

She made a good initial postoperative recovery, but on the third postoperative day she developed a pyrexia of 39°C which persisted. She was found to have dullness at the right base with absent breath sounds and an area of bronchial breathing at the left base. She was treated with amoxycillin and erythromycin, initially intravenously for 7 days, with improvement of the signs at the left base but without any effect on those at the right. A chest X-ray at this time showed a right pleural effusion, patchy shadowing at the left base, air under the diaphragm, and a calcified hilar lymph node.

QUESTIONS

1. What are the most probable reasons for her right pleural effusion?
2. What are the investigations which would be most helpful in diagnosis?
3. What would be your immediate management of this case?

DISCUSSION

This asthmatic patient has taken a high dose of steroids for many years, and has suffered from a perforated ulcer which is a hazard of this form of treatment. It is probably significant that it followed an increase in the dose. She had been feeling unwell for several weeks prior to the acute emergency, and at the time of admission already had signs of a right-sided pleural effusion. The likely cause of this patient's effusion is pulmonary tuberculosis or malignant disease, either primary of the lung or due to secondary deposits. Malignant pleural effusion may be the initial presentation of an occult primary carcinoma, and carcinoma of the breast is a possibility even though the breasts may appear clinically normal.

Although subphrenic abscess may follow perforation of a duodenal ulcer, and pulmonary embolism may follow any operation, these do not account for her previous ill-health and the signs of pleural effusion before surgery. A previous pyogenic infection may have caused a pleural effusion but this is an unlikely cause of chronic mild ill-health. On the other hand, tuberculosis is an important complication of long-term steroid therapy which may light up a previously quiescent focus. Such a focus is suggested by the hilar calcification. For this reason many physicians would give such a patient isoniazid while on steroids. There is nothing to suggest cardiac failure as a cause of the effusion.

The most important investigation is aspiration of the pleural effusion with pleural biopsy. The fluid must be cultured for acid-fast bacilli as well as pyogenic organisms. It should also be examined for malignant cells. If these investigations are negative, and if the effusion persists, the aspiration and biopsy should be repeated. Radioisotope lung scan may be of considerable value in the diagnosis of pulmonary embolism. This is not a likely diagnosis in this case, and it could be misleading in this patient who has abnormalities in both lungs clinically and radiologically. The sputum must be examined for tubercle bacilli, and malignant cells. A full blood count will be done, but is unlikely to be of diagnostic help. The Mantoux test ought to be positive in view of the hilar calcification, could be strongly positive if there is active disease, but might be suppressed in a patient on steroids. It is therefore of no value in diagnosis.

The best immediate management of this case would be to continue her steroids because she is recovering from a stressful operation and has been on this treatment for 7 years. Physiotherapy and continuation of antibiotics will be needed for her left basal pneumonia which is already improving. Her pleural effusion will not need treatment until its cause has been found.

> Aspiration of the effusion revealed a turbid fluid with numerous lymphocytes. A biopsy revealed tuberculosis. Culture of the fluid grew tubercle bacilli sensitive to all first-line drugs. One year after treatment she was quite well and chest X-ray showed residual right-sided pleural thickening.

10. Dysphagia

The symptom of difficulty in swallowing often results in an immediate request for a barium swallow and endoscopy. Although both these investigations may prove necessary, a surprising degree of precision in diagnosis can often be achieved by careful history-taking. The ability to ask the right questions requires some knowledge of the underlying physiology of swallowing and the ways in which different disease processes interfere with it. Not only will a diagnosis based on history enable the appropriate confirmatory test to be undertaken, but it may also lead to earlier diagnosis and treatment. Generally speaking, physical examination will be of secondary importance to the history, but may show evidence of disease in other parts of the body such as the central nervous system.

PHYSIOLOGY OF SWALLOWING

Solids are first masticated, which requires sound teeth, efficient bite, adequate lubrication with saliva and an absence of painful lesions of the tongue and mouth. Swallowing begins with the soft palate meeting the base of the tongue to enclose the bolus. By a piston-like action of the tongue the bolus is then propelled backwards into the pharynx while the soft palate moves backwards and upwards to close off the nasopharynx. Failure of the latter mechanism leads to regurgitation through the nose. As the bolus moves backwards so the epiglottis is tilted over the glottis, the larynx rising to meet it, resulting in closure of the airway and inhibition of respiration. Failure of this mechanism will lead to inhalation of food or liquid at the time of swallowing. This is in contrast to inhalation occurring later, due to regurgitation of food some time after a meal or at night. A slight delay occurs as the upper oesophageal sphincter (cricopharyngeus muscle) then relaxes. Normally this sphincter is closed with a high resting pressure of about 30 mmHg (see Fig. 10.1). Incoordination of relaxation is said to be an aetiological factor in the formation of a pharyngeal pouch as the high pressures generated in the pharynx during swallowing cannot be transmitted onwards into the oesophagus. Instead, there is bulging at the site of dehiscence in the posterior pharyngeal wall. This failure of relax-ation may be visualized by pooling of barium in the valleculae and pyriform fossae.

Following relaxation the cricopharyngeus imme-diately contracts, producing a pressure twice that of its resting value. This ensures that the primary oesophageal peristalic wave which generates a pres-sure of 30 mmHg cannot cause reflux. With the momentum gained from pharyngeal contraction and peristalsis the bolus takes approximately 9 seconds to reach the lower oesophagus and is greatly assisted by gravity. Hence, to detect the earliest defects in peristalsis, as in systemic sclerosis, an anti-gravity barium swallow is essential.

Whereas primary peristalsis is initiated by the vol-untary act of swallowing, secondary oesophageal peristalsis occurs as an unconscious reflex in response to distension of the oesophagus by any remaining food particles. Although there is probably no true anatomical lower oesophageal sphincter, there is an area of relatively high pressure (about 15 mmHg) in the lower 7 cm of the oesophagus. This physiological sphincter lies partly above the diaphragm and partly in the 4 cm below it. The subdiaphragmatic portion, to which is transmitted the positive intra-abdominal pressure, is crucial in preventing gastro-oesophageal reflux, since any rise in intra-abdominal pressure affects intragastric and intra-oesophageal pressures equally. One or two seconds after primary peristalsis starts, the gastro-oesophageal sphincter begins to relax to allow the bolus to enter the stomach. However, the pressure does not fall to the intra-gastric level (5 mmHg), otherwise reflux could occur since there is a negative pressure at rest in the intrathoracic oesophagus. Failure of relaxation at this site is the cause of the symptoms of achalasia. The hydrostatic pressure of food and liquid accumulating in the lower oesophagus can finally overcome the tone of the sphincter in achalasia.

CAUSES OF DYSPHAGIA

It is logical to consider causes of dysphagia from above downwards. Emphasis will be on the points in the history, examination and investigations which allow the various causes to be differentiated (Fig. 10.2).

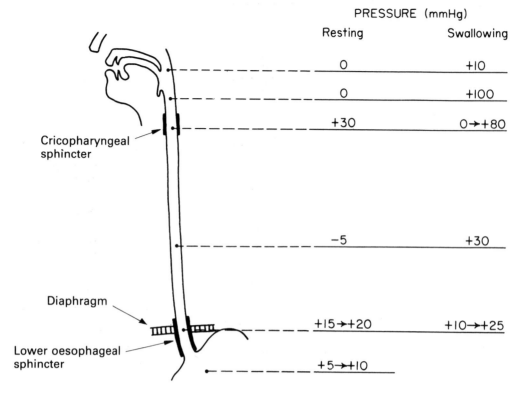

PRESSURE (mmHg)

	Resting	Swallowing
	0	+10
	0	+100
Cricopharyngeal sphincter	+30	0→+80
	−5	+30
Diaphragm / Lower oesophageal sphincter	+15→+20	+10→+25
	+5→+10	

Fig. 10.1 Representative pressures at rest and swallowing

Psychogenic

The patient is usually a woman suffering from anxiety, often with a hysterical personality. The complaint is of an inability to swallow rather than any discomfort during swallowing. Dryness of the mouth, associated with emotion, may exacerbate the condition. Sometimes attention may have been drawn for the first time to a small goitre, the patient then becoming aware of a 'lump in the neck'. This, in turn, engenders fear, which expresses itself as inability to swallow. It should be remembered that dysphagia due to goitre is exceptional, though it can occur with sudden haemorrhage into a cyst in a multinodular goitre.

Sjögren's syndrome

The features originally described were dryness of the eyes (keratoconjunctivitis sicca) and mouth (xerostomia), salivary gland enlargement, and arthritis of the rheumatoid type. There may also be lymphadenopathy, hepatosplenomegaly, purpura, Raynaud's phenomenon and peripheral neuropathy. However, ocular and oral involvement (the 'sicca' syndrome) may be the sole manifestation. Dryness of the mouth, sufficiently severe to interfere with chewing and swallowing, will be present with a red tender tongue, cracked lips and swollen salivary glands. The dryness and grittiness of the eyes due to lack of tear formation by the involved lacrimal glands can be demonstrated by the Schirmer test. In this test one end of a strip of blotting paper is placed under the lower eyelid and fails to become moistened.

Inflammatory and neoplastic conditions in the mouth

Most painful conditions of the mouth and tongue are usually self-evident from the history and examination. The premalignant condition of leucoplakia and its sequel, carcinoma of the tongue, will interfere with swallowing. Glossitis may be associated with various nutritional deficiencies, lack of iron being the most important. Infections, such as tonsillitis, peritonsillar abscess, pharyngitis, and severe caries can all cause pain. Although the recently edentulous patient may not actually complain of dysphagia, considerable weight loss, obviously due to decreased food intake, can occur.

Mechanical causes

A foreign body (fishbones are notorious) may lodge in the tonsillar bed or pyriform fossa. Although the pain

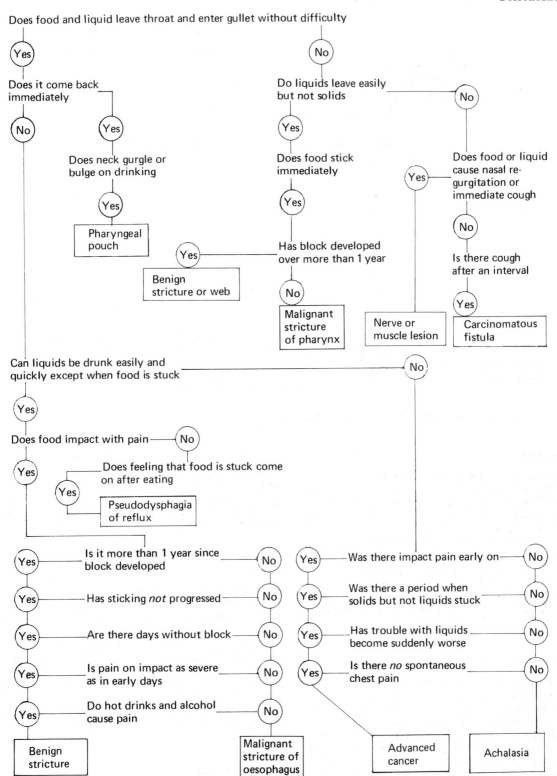

Does food and liquid leave throat and enter gullet without difficulty

Yes — Does it come back immediately

No ┐

Yes — Does neck gurgle or bulge on drinking

Yes → Pharyngeal pouch

No — Do liquids leave easily but not solids

Yes — Does food stick immediately

Yes ┐

Yes → Benign stricture or web

Has block developed over more than 1 year

No → Malignant stricture of pharynx

No — Does food or liquid cause nasal re-gurgitation or immediate cough

Yes → Nerve or muscle lesion

No — Is there cough after an interval

Yes → Carcinomatous fistula

Can liquids be drunk easily and quickly except when food is stuck ———————— **No**

Yes

Does food impact with pain — **No**

Yes

Does feeling that food is stuck come on after eating

Yes → Pseudodysphagia of reflux

Yes — Is it more than 1 year since block developed — **No**

Yes — Has sticking *not* progressed — **No**

Yes — Are there days without block — **No**

Yes — Is pain on impact as severe as in early days — **No**

Yes — Do hot drinks and alcohol cause pain — **No**

Yes — Was there impact pain early on — **No**

Yes — Was there a period when solids but not liquids stuck — **No**

Yes — Has trouble with liquids become suddenly worse — **No**

Yes — Is there *no* spontaneous chest pain — **No**

Benign stricture

Malignant stricture of oesophagus

Advanced cancer

Achalasia

Fig. 10.2 A guide to the diagnosis of dysphagia

impairs swallowing, the original event may have been unnoticed. A much more dubious cause of dysphagia is the protrusion of lower cervical intervertebral discs onto the posterior oesophagus. As with the attribution of other symptoms to cervical spondylosis, the diagnosis should not be lightly made, as radiological changes in the neck are common from middle age onwards and are generally asymptomatic.

Neuromuscular causes

In most instances dysphagia will be only one part of a more widespread neurological disturbance which, considered as a whole, will indicate the underlying disease. The neurological control of swallowing is complex. There is no clearly defined anatomical centre controlling swallowing, but the medulla oblongata is of great importance in this respect and is also concerned with interrelated actions such as chewing, licking, gagging, coughing, sneezing, vomiting, belching and breathing. These activities are influenced by afferent impulses from the cerebral cortex, glosso-pharyngeal nerves and various branches of the vagus. The motor outflow is via the cranial nerve nuclei (V, VII, IX ambiguus, X, XI and XII) and the upper three cervical segments. In cerebellar disorders, coordination of swallowing, and of speech, with breathing is no longer automatic, and failure of the glottis to close at the right moment may cause choking.

The various bulbar causes of dysphagia include infections such as diphtheria and poliomyelitis. Other causes are the malformation of syringobulbia, which may be associated with platybasia and the Arnold–Chiari malformation, the bulbar palsy of motor neurone disease, the pseudobulbar palsy of bilateral strokes, and the variable weakness of myasthenia gravis. In this type of dysphagia, difficulty arises when liquids, and to a lesser extent solids, leave the throat to enter the gullet. There is no problem usually in initiating swallowing, but fluid will immediately either regurgitate through the nose, or cause coughing by entering the larynx. This contrasts with the few seconds delay between swallowing and coughing when the patient has an oesophagotracheal fistula.

Pharyngeal pouch

Although food and liquid are swallowed easily, they may be regurgitated immediately or on bending over or turning the head. A bulging in the neck may be noticed which may gurgle on drinking. The patients are often elderly and the chief hazard is of recurrent aspiration pneumonia. Confirmation of the diagnosis is by barium swallow.

Sideropenic dysphagia

In this condition of many synonyms (Plummer–Vinson, Paterson–Brown–Kelly), epithelial changes due to iron deficiency sometimes cause glossitis but, more importantly, affect the upper oesophagus. Here there may be a web of fine membrane affecting only the anterior wall or encircling the oesophagus. The complaint is of solids, but not liquids, sticking in the throat immediately on swallowing (i.e. without aware-ness of an interval). A delay between swallowing and the sensation of sticking indicates an obstruction lower in the oesophagus since passage of the bolus down the oesophagus may take up to 10 seconds, whereas emptying of the pharynx is virtually instantaneous. A general point is that localization of obstruction is more accurately made by timing impact rather than by taking the level indicated by the patient. The latter is notoriously unreliable as the sensation may often be felt some distance above the true site. The patient with a web will usually give a surprisingly long history of months or years because symptoms may only occur with a particularly large bolus and therefore may be intermittent.

Associated with the web, the patient, generally a middle-aged woman, may have spoon-shaped nails (koilonychia), glossitis, cheilitis, splenomegaly and a hypochromic anaemia. The association between web and carcinoma at the same site is no longer thought to be strong. Generally malignant strictures, which are rare in the upper oesophagus, have a short and progressive history. Confirmation of the diagnosis of a web is by the characteristic findings on barium swallow and oesophagoscopy, and by the associated haematological abnormalities.

External pressure

These are rare causes of dysphagia, occurring at mid-oesophageal level and rarely amounting to total obstruction. Vascular causes are aneurysm of the arch of the aorta or an aberrant right subclavian artery arising from the left side of the aorta passing posterior to the oesophagus and causing an indentation on barium swallow (dysphagia lusoria). Medias-tinal nodes involved with secondary malignancy, usually from the bronchus, generally produce other symptoms and signs before such a mobile structure as the oesophagus is compressed. Inflamed nodes, usually due to tuberculosis, may become adherent and produce a traction diverticulum, although this seldom causes dysphagia.

Systemic sclerosis

Although lower oesophageal involvement can often be demonstrated, symptoms are relatively rare and mild. However, heartburn and acid regurgitation are common and may be severe. Impairment of peri-stalsis, with failure of the gastro-oesophageal physi-ological sphincter to close, occurs early in the disease. It contributes to gastro-oesophageal reflux disease (GORD) rather than dysphagia because of the role of gravity in swallowing. The defect can best be shown by an anti-gravity barium swallow. Later in the disease, narrowing of the lower oesophagus with slight dilatation above it is seen, usually due to a peptic stricture resulting from the long-standing associated reflux oesophagitis. Evidence of the disease elsewhere such as scleroderma of the hands and face, Raynaud's phenomenon, arthritis, pulmonary and renal involvement may be present, in addition to disordered small bowel peristalsis causing diarrhoea and the stagnant loop syndrome. Often it is these other clinical features that suggest the diagnosis and lead to a barium swallow.

Achalasia

This disease is often diagnosed only after much delay, and cardiomyotomy (Heller's operation) is frequently considered too late in its natural history. This is regrettable because little can be done to help a patient who has reached the stage of megaoesophagus to lead a normal life again. The disease is due to an idiopathic degeneration of the ganglion cells of Auerbach's plexus, although an identical lesion is seen in Brazil in Chagas' disease caused by the neurotoxin of *Trypanosoma cruzi*.

In the early stages of denervation the muscle is hypersensitive to endogenous and exogenous cholinergic substances which result in spasm, causing dysphagia and pain. Although swallowing, particularly of iced drinks, sometimes provokes pain, it also may occur spontaneously but transiently at any time of day or night. Radiation of the pain to the neck, together with its intensity, may erroneously suggest a cardiac cause. Although food and liquid leave the pharynx normally the failure of peristalsis and relaxation of the sphincter will slow their progress. Therefore neither food nor liquid can be taken rapidly in the early stages. When the patient reaches the mega-oesophagus stage, the large capacity of the gullet may make it possible to drink fast while it fills. Indeed, the hydrostatic pressure generated as the mega-oesophagus fills may overcome the sphincter. The patient often learns the value of forcible drinking to facilitate passage of food into the stomach. Unlike a carcinoma, dysphagia for both solids and liquids is often present from the outset and for a long time. The rapid progression from solid to liquid dysphagia is more suggestive of a stenosing lesion. Pain on eating solids is also much more a feature of carcinoma. Diagnosis in the early stages may be helped by the cholinergic hypersensitivity (see Mecholyl test, Ch. 4). In the later stages, plain chest X-ray may show a widened mediastinum with a fluid level, loss of gastric air bubble, and evidence of repeated episodes of aspiration pneumonia from spillover. A barium swallow is still the most important investigation and will show disordered peristalsis and oesophageal

dilatation with a funnel-shaped obstruction. Carcinoma occurs in 10% of patients with long-standing achalasia.

Benign oesophageal stricture

Apart from the rare and usually obvious cases due to drinking corrosives, benign strictures invariably are due to reflux oesophagitis. This, in turn, is usually associated with a sliding hiatus hernia, where the intra-abdominal portion of the oesophagus is pushed into the chest, removing one of the important anti-reflux defences. A history of flatulent dyspepsia, heartburn and regurgitation made worse by bending or lying flat, together with persistent iron deficiency anaemia may precede dysphagia. Although most peptic strictures occur in the lower oesophagus one might be surprised to find them as high as mid-oesophagus. Liquids can usually be drunk rapidly but food will stick; however, this is a slowly progres-

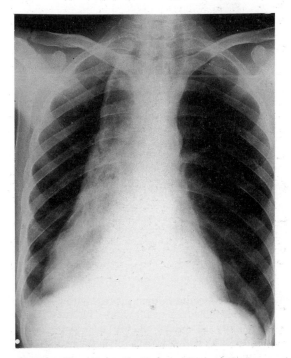

Fig. 10.3 Chest X-ray of a 64-year-old man with a long history of difficulty in swallowing and repeated episodes of right basal pneumonia. Gross widening of the mediastinum, containing gas shadows to the right and left of the trachea and irregular opacification within it adjacent to the right heart border; the right costophrenic angle is blunted. The appearances are those of mega-oesophagus due to long-standing achalasia of the cardia, giving rise to 'spillover' aspiration pneumonia. The patient died of carcinoma of the oesophagus.

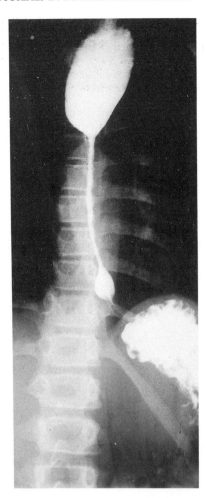

Fig. 10.4 Barium swallow in a young child who, 8 weeks earlier, had drunk bleach, a corrosive agent. A lengthy stricture involving the lower half of the oesophagus with dilatation above it is seen. The surface of the lining of the stricture is slightly irregular because of the accompanying oesophagitis. (Courtesy of Dr Hakhamaneshi).

Carcinoma of oesophagus

Carcinoma of the fundus encroaching on the gastro-oesophageal junction may be silent until it produces its own variant of dysphagia. Difficulty in swallowing solids occurs at the beginning of each meal, but after a few pain-producing mouthfuls the rest of the meal passes with relative ease. This can be differentiated from achalasia by the time course, the pain, and the dysphagia for solids alone in the early stages (Figs. 10.3, 10.4).

The more common lower oesophageal malignant strictures differ from benign strictures by spreading

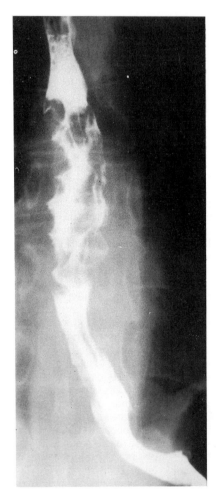

Fig. 10.5 Barium swallow in a middle-aged man with a short history of dysphagia for solids and weight loss. An area of irregularity due to multiple filling defects associated with loss of peristalsis and delay in transit of barium is seen. The cause was a fungating squamous-cell carcinoma of the oesophagus. (Courtesy of Dr Hakhamaneshi).

sive and initially, intermittent process with periods of days with trouble-free swallowing. This may be due to variability in reflux of the acid–pepsin juice provoking oesophageal spasm. Such spasm, described radiologically as tertiary contractions or corkscrew oesophagus, may in turn give rise to a pseudo-dysphagia with a sensation of food sticking, coming some minutes or more after meals. Pain from associated oesophagitis (odynophagia) may be provoked by hot drinks or alcoholic spirits. The diagnosis is confirmed by barium swallow and oesophagoscopy.

along the oesophagus at the same time as spreading circumferentially (Fig. 10.5).

Although the history is very much shorter and progresses more rapidly, impaction pain may be most marked at the outset, dimishing with time (unlike a benign stricture). This may be partly spurious, as the patient stops attempting to swallow solids, but also occurs because of replacement of sensitive mucous membrane and peristaltic muscle by tumour above the stricture. Unlike a peptic stricture, dysphagia occurs with each meal from the time of the first symptom. The stage of inability to swallow liquids may be soon reached, and the patient regurgitates.

CLINICAL PROBLEM

T	P	BP	R
37	104	190/100	22

Tongue smooth and shiny

Skin pale, dry and lax

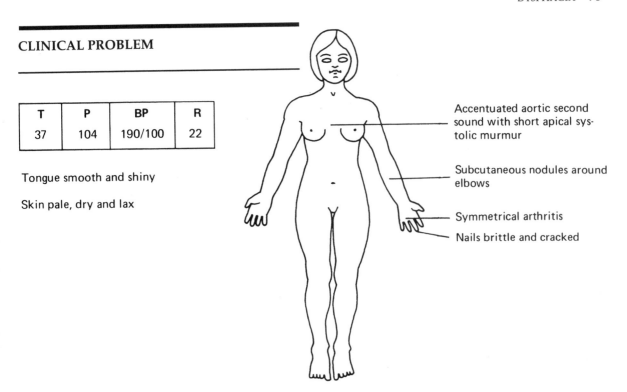

Accentuated aortic second sound with short apical systolic murmur

Subcutaneous nodules around elbows

Symmetrical arthritis

Nails brittle and cracked

A 52-year-old widow was referred from a chest clinic with the complaint of intermittent difficulty in swallowing for 3 years. She had noticed that toast and meat especially seemed to stick at the level of the manubrium some seconds after swallowing. At first the symptom occurred only about twice a week, usually at the beginning of a meal. She said that occasionally about 5 minutes after a large meal there was a heavy sensation 'as if something was stuck' at the lower end of the sternum. She had always been able to swallow liquids rapidly, without pain. In the preceding 4 months the difficulty in swallowing had occurred more frequently. Her weight had fallen from 95 kg to 89 kg. There had been no vomiting or heartburn. For some years she had found that it was uncomfortable to lie on her left side at night.

For the previous 6 months she had noticed increasing breathlessness on exertion, together with tiredness. There was no cough or sputum, but at the end of the day her ankles were sometimes swollen.

She had been attending a rheumatology department for 9 years for rheumatoid arthritis, which had led to marked deformity of her hands. This had initially been treated with salicylates alone, but for the previous 5 years she had also been taking a low dose of prednisone.

On examination she was obese. She was not orthopnoeic. The skin was pale, dry and lax and the nails were brittle and cracked. The tongue was smooth, moist and shiny with loss of papillation. In the cardiovascular system, the pulse was 104/ minute, regular and of good volume. Blood pressure was 190/100. The apex beat could not be localized, there was a short systolic murmur in the apical region, and the aortic second sound was accentuated. There was a symmetrical polyarthritis involving the metacarpophalangeal joints of both hands with ulnar deviation, the proximal interphalangeal joints, and the elbows and shoulders. Both ankles and knees were slightly affected. There were subcutaneous nodules around the elbow joints.

The following investigations had been performed in the chest clinic:

Haemoglobin 7.9 g/dl; MCV 72 fl; MCH 24 pg. film shows anisocytosis, microcytosis and hypochromia
WBC $8.7 \times 10^9/1$ with normal differential
ESR 32 mm in 1 hour
Chest X-ray: Cardiothoracic ratio 17:30 cm
Lung fields clear
Spirometry: $\dfrac{FEV_1}{FVC} = \dfrac{1.6}{2.0}$ litres

Stools positive for occult blood

QUESTIONS

1. What are the likely diagnoses?
2. Which other investigations would be helpful in diagnosis?

DISCUSSION

This patient was referred to the chest clinic because of breathlessness. This is due to her anaemia which has the characteristics of iron deficiency. Obesity is a contributory factor and could also account for the mild restrictive ventilatory defect seen on spirometry. Her cardiomegaly is due to the anaemia and mild hypertension.

The cause of the anaemia is probably the occult blood loss. The dysphagia is long-standing while the symptoms of anaemia are recent. This suggests that the anaemia is the result of whatever is producing dysphagia. It is unlikely that she has longstanding iron deficiency causing the dysphagia (so called sideropenic dysphagia).

The most likely cause of the dysphagia is an oesophageal stricture. Despite the patient localizing the site of obstruction to the manubrial region it is quite possible that the stricture is at the lower end of the oesophagus. The sensation of food sticking within seconds of swallowing, particularly of rough solids, suggests an organic stricture, although there may be some additional element of spasm. The feeling of 'something stuck' at the lower end of the sternum is very likely to be pseudodysphagia due to oeso-phageal spasm due to gastro-oesophageal reflux. This symptom is most likely to occur after meals, when it is thought that the falling level of gastrin causes the gastro-oesophageal sphincter to relax and allow reflux. Reflux may also occur at night because the horizontal position removes the protective effect of gravity, and patients often complain that their symp-toms are worse when they lie on their left side. The stricture is most probably benign and due to fibrosis secondary to the peptic oesophagitis. A malignant stricture is unlikely in view of the length of the history. The recent deterioration and weight loss is probably due to a worsening of the stricture but could be due to the development of a carcinoma, which is more likely to occur in a patient with chronic oesophagitis, when it may be an adenocarcinoma arising from a Barrett's lining (gastric columnar epithelium replacing the squamous epithelium).

She has no skin changes of scleroderma and the deforming polyarthritis with typical rheumatoid modules is against this diagnosis. There is nothing to suggest the diagnosis of Sjögren's syndrome and the dysphagia is not due to a dry mouth. Achalasia is unlikely as she has always been able to swallow liquids rapidly. In addition there has been no spon-taneous pain, no evidence of spillover disease in the lungs and nothing to suggest mega-oesophagus, on the chest X-ray.

Barium swallow and meal examination is therefore the essential investigation. It is usual for it to precede the equally important oesophagoscopy, as the latter may be dangerous if performed as a blind procedure. Oesophagoscopy allows direct inspection of the in-flamed oesophagus, visualization of reflux, biopsy of the mucosa and stricture and, if benign, its dilatation.

This patient had a sliding hiatus hernia with gastrooesophageal reflux and a benign stricture. Her anaemia was due to the oesophagitis and aggravated by the treatment of her rheumatoid arthritis.

The authors would like to thank Dr D A W Edwards for the basis of the algorithm on Dysphagia.

11. Haematemesis and melaena

Acute gastrointestinal haemorrhage remains one of the commonest medical emergencies. It is rather disappointing to note that annual mortality figures over the past 15 years have shown little improvement in the figure of 5%–10%. Closer analysis reveals that this, in part, may be due to a changing disease pattern in that more patients are falling into the categories that carry a high risk. Many of these deaths could be deemed unavoidable and such improvement as is now beginning to be seen is not so much attributable to high technology medicine in diagnosis and treatment as careful attention to detail by a team approach involving skilled and experienced physicians and surgeons. The published data suggest this can best be done in a designated combined medical–surgical gastrointestinal unit.

Old age is the predominant mortality risk factor since it is associated with an increased incidence of other disorders, such as chronic bronchitis and ischaemic heart disease, which give bleeding from peptic ulcer in the over-50s a poorer prognosis (Table 11.1). Although varices and gastric carcinoma are each responsible for only 3% of bleeds (Fig. 11.1) they carry mortalities in the region of 45% and 35% respectively (Fig. 11.2). Their combined mortality is greater than that from duodenal ulcer, which is the commonest cause of bleeding.

As gastrointestinal haemorrhage occurs with varying severity from a variety of causes, one problem in management is how extensive the diagnostic procedures should be in the early stages. Accurate diagnosis leads to the identification of the patient who is at great risk. As one cannot separate treatment from diagnosis in this situation, both will be discussed below.

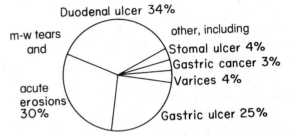

Fig.11.1 Causes of gastrointestinal bleeding (excluding 10% undiagnosed)

Urgent treatment may sometimes have to precede and establishment of a firm diagnosis. In over 10% of patients, a precise diagnosis may never be made. This somewhat unsatisfactory state of affairs can be tolerated in younger patients since this group carries a good prognosis. Now that early gastroscopy is performed, it is found that many of the previous undiagnosed group have acute ulcers, erosions or so-called Mallory–Weiss (M-W) tears at the gastro-oesophageal junction caused by the trauma of repeated vomiting. These lesions will usually only be seen in the first 48 hours.

ESTABLISHING THAT GASTROINTESTINAL BLEEDING HAS OCCURRED

This is rarely in doubt, although patients can sometimes be remarkably uncertain as to whether blood has been coughed or vomited. Occasionally blood

Table 11.1 The prevalence and mortality of gastric and duodenal ulcer haemorrhage related to age

| | Under 60 years | | Over 60 years | |
	No. of cases	deaths	No. of cases	deaths
Gastric ulcer	57	1 (1.8%)	98	25 (26%)
Duodenal ulcer	122	1 (0.8%)	88	9 (10.2%)

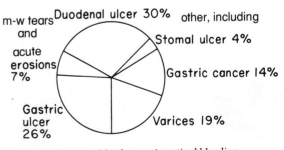

Fig 11.2 Causes of fatal gastrointestinal bleeding

from the upper respiratory tract, for example from a nose bleed, may trickle into the pharynx. If the material produced is acid on testing, it strongly suggests a gastric origin, although in carcinoma of the stomach or acute erosion, there may be associated achlorhydria. Haematemeses are almost always associated with some degree of blood in the stools, from a frank tarry melaena to dark stools which give a positive reaction on testing for occult blood. A source of confusion here is the black stool associated with oral iron therapy or with bismuth-containing antacid tablets. As in all other fields of medicine there are malingerers who say they have vomited blood, or may go to some lengths to simulate it. Passage of fresh blood per rectum without haematemesis usually suggests a source in the colon or rectum.

CONSEQUENCES OF HAEMORRHAGE

The important factors are the amount of blood lost and the rate at which it is lost. The effectiveness of the patient's compensatory mechanisms will depend on his age, and the extent of any associated cardio-respiratory and cerebrovascular disease . Acute blood loss may be superimposed on chronic.

Initially the problem is more one of reduction in circulating volume, i.e. shock, rather than impaired oxygen-carrying ability, i.e. anaemia. The more rapid the bleeding the more likely the patient is to present as haematemesis and, conversely, slower haemorrhage presents as melaena. In one series, patients presenting with haematemesis had twice the fatality rate of those presenting with melaena alone (12.0% versus 5.4%). By the time the adaptive mechanisms break down, with rapid pulse and fall in blood pressure, a young patient can have lost up to 50% of his circulating volume. After such a severe bleed, haemodilution occurs over the next 24 hours. This means that the initial haemoglobin concentration may be normal and will only be a true estimate of blood loss 24 hours after the event. By then, in the more severe cases, replacement by transfusion will have been initiated. In the absence of routine rapid and accurate blood volume estimation, the decision regarding transfusion is based on the age and condition of the patient, his pulse rate and blood pressure. In addition an initial haemoglobin concentration below 10 g/dl is usually regarded as an indication for transfusion. There is a risk of overtransfusion and the precipitation of left heart failure and pulmonary oedema. This is particularly so in the elderly, especially if previous anaemia has resulted in a high output state. In these patients it may be valuable not only to examine regularly the lung bases and jugular venous pressure, but to monitor the central venous pressure during transfusion, adjusting the drip rate accordingly. Where rapid transfusion is required and the patient is bordering on heart failure, a short-acting diuretic such as frusemide should be given intramuscularly. Digoxin may also be needed, especially if atrial fibril-

lation is present. Transfusion will combat shock and prevent ischaemic damage to other organs. Cerebral infarction and myocardial infarction may, however, occur, and the characteristic pain of the latter may be obscured. A moderate rise in blood urea is a common finding attributed to the 'protein meal' effect of blood in the gut. However, in addition, renal blood flow is reduced and, rarely, acute renal failure may occur. In a cirrhotic patient, bleeding from varices, there will be a reduction in hepatic blood flow. This, together with the 'protein meal' may precipitate liver failure and portosystemic encephalopathy. Retinal ischaemia can cause acute changes resembling malignant hypertension, and may result in optic atrophy. A further important reason for replacing blood loss, is that 15% to 20% of patients either continue to bleed or rebleed after admission, producing a dangerous deterioration in patients who have previously managed to compensate for the initial blood loss.

The hazards of blood transfusion are well known. When large volumes of blood are transfused there is the additional risk of inducing a bleeding tendency. There are many related causes for this, such as reduction in clotting factors in stored blood and the binding of calcium by the citrate used as an anticoagulant. To prevent this, fresh frozen plasma may be necessary after large and rapid transfusions, especially in patients with cirrhosis.

DIFFERENTIAL DIAGNOSIS

After establishing that gastrointestinal haemorrhage has occurred, blood should be taken for grouping, cross-matching, haemoglobin estimation and examination of the blood film. An intravenous infusion is set up at this stage. Before proceeding further a full history should be taken from patient and relatives and a complete examination must be performed to try and establish the cause of bleeding as well as its effects. Although acute and chronic peptic ulcers (including the 25% presumed to be acute erosions) are responsible for 90% of admissions the less common causes comprising about 10% must always be considered, since specific treatment may be indicated.

Many patients will give a history of preceding gastrointestinal symptoms, and some will have had a previous bleed, which will probably have been investigated resulting in a diagnosis of the underlying cause. However, a worrying trend in recent years with the increasing use of non-steroidal anti-inflammatory drugs (NSAIDs) in elderly arthritic patients is that the first manifestation of the presence of a peptic ulcer may be when it bleeds or perforates.

Duodenal ulcer

Most patients will give a history of epigastric pain occurring before meals, waking them at night, and relieved by food, milk, alkalis and belching. Ulcer pain often disappears when haemorrhage occurs; in fact if the patient continues to have severe or worsening pain after bleeding it should alert one to the relatively rare combination of events – haemorrhage and perforation. Other pointers to the diagnosis of duodenal ulcer are a positive past history, and a family history of the disorder. The patient's personality is often conscientious and ambitious, and there is frequently a history of recent stress.

Gastric ulcer

This is a much less common form of peptic ulcer than duodenal ulcer. However, gastric ulcers seem to have a greater likelihood of bleeding, and constitute 25% of all cases of gastrointestinal bleeding, compared with duodenal ulcer which contributes 35% of all cases. Gastric ulcer occurs with greater frequency in the aged and this is a high risk group who will benefit from early surgery. Pain occurs usually after food, often making the patient afraid to eat and resulting in a loss of weight. Vomiting may relieve pain. When a gastric of duodenal ulcer is seen at early gastroscopy it may also reveal stigmata of recent haemorrhage (SRH), such as thrombus adherent to the ulcer, or a visible vessel or red spot within it. These indicate an increased risk of continuing or recurrent bleeding.

Acute ulcers and erosions

A positive diagnosis can only be made by direct visualization by gastroscopy in the acute stage of the illness. The findings vary from a generalized haemorrhagic gastritis (diffuse gastrostaxis) to multiple or single acute superficial ulcers involving the gastric, duodenal or oesophageal mucosa. Only exceptionally is there a bleeding artery of significant size in the base of the ulcer, and there is unlikely to be further bleeding. Drugs and alcohol seem to play an increasingly important part in causing acute erosions. Many patients will have taken one of the 40 prescribable aspirin preparations or, more likely, one of the many 'over the counter' remedies. While it may be argued that they would not have taken aspirin if they were not already feeling unwell, none the less the drug may be sufficient to convert simple indigestion into a haematemesis. Although it is now well known that long-term aspirin ingestion, as in rheumatoid arthritis, is associated with chronic blood loss of about 5 ml per day, it is not yet completely clear how either chronic or acute bleeding is caused by the aspirin. Other NSAIDs such as indomethacin or corticosteroids may also give rise to haemorrhage. Although a history of dyspepsia is a contraindication to anticoagulant therapy, this may be a cause of bleeding, either due to the prothrombin time getting out of control, or because of an associated gastric disturbance. In these patients vitamin K should be given in spite of a slight risk of rebound thrombosis from rapid reversal of anticoagulation.

In acute erosion there will usually be a history of a short period of preceding dyspepsia. The patient may have with him tablets or a steroid or anticoagulant clinic card. Examination will be noncontributory.

Oesophagitis

Reflux oesophagitis often associated with a sliding hiatus hernia, is a relatively common cause of iron deficiency anaemia due to chronic blood loss in obese elderly women. They frequently give little or no history of flatulent dyspepsia or acid regurgitation ('heartburn'). The problem of whether reflux oesophagitis causes acute bleeding can only be resolved by early gastroscopy, but it is probably unusual. Occasionally an ulcer may occur in the oesophagus of a patient with a sliding hiatus hernia, at the junction of secretory columnar epithelium and the normal squamous epithelium ('Barrett ulcer'). A rolling hiatus hernia with a fixed loculus above the diaphragm occurs less commonly but is more likely to bleed.

Mallory–Weiss syndrome

A tear occurs at the lower end of the oesophageal mucosa as a result of prolonged or severe vomiting. The point in the history which should arouse suspicion is that the patient has had a bout of vomiting often after a drinking binge, or in the first trimester of pregnancy, but only at the end of the bout did the vomit contain fresh blood. A definite diagnosis can only be made by oesophagoscopy.

Stomal ulcer

Following both partial gastrectomy or vagotomy and pyloroplasty for bleeding from a peptic ulcer there is a risk of later bleeding in up to 5% of cases. This will usually be due to a stomal ulcer or recurrence of the original ulcer if left behind. A history of ulcer dyspepsia will generally be obtained, though surgery may have modified the location of the pain.

Carcinoma of the stomach

This was formerly thought to be a cause of chronic rather than acute blood loss. However it is presenting more frequently as a cause of acute haemorrhage, particularly in the over 60s. The history will resemble that of gastric ulcer, with anorexia and weight loss, though pain may be less prominent. Examination may reveal an epigastric mass and sometimes an enlarged left supraclavicular node of Virchow. Diagnosis is by gastroscopy and biopsy. Biopsy should be undertaken in every gastric ulcer, however benign in appearance.

If the ulcer is actively bleeding or shows SRH, biopsy may have to be deferred until the danger of rebleeding is receding after 48 hours, or until the mandatory follow-up endoscopy is carried out after a 4-week course of ulcer-healing treatment.

Gastro-oesophageal varices

The underlying portal hypertension is, in the majority of cases, due to cirrhosis of the liver with alcoholic cirrhosis a more common cause than postviral hepatic cirrhosis in the western world. There is a raised incidence of peptic ulcer in cirrhotics, especially in alcoholic and biliary cirrhosis. One must not therefore automatically attribute haematemesis to bleeding varices in a patient with cirrhosis.

Extrahepatic portal hypertension occurs rarely and is due to portal vein obstruction. This may date from infancy, following thrombosis of the portal vein due to umbilical sepsis, or be acquired as a result of malignant involvement from hepatoma or pancreatic carcinoma. Other causes are polycythaemia, cirrhosis itself, or portal pyaemia, for example due to an appendix abscess. Hepatic fibrosis due to schistosomiasis carries a better prognosis when bleeding occurs, because there is generally much better liver function. This is a major determinant in the outcome of variceal bleeding and is reflected in the different prognoses in the Child–Pugh grading (Table 11.2).

Haematemesis may be the first symptom in a cirrhotic patient, or there may be a history of chronic ill health, oedema, and ascites. Whatever the cause of the portal hypertension, the spleen will nearly always be enlarged and usually be palpable, and collateral vessels may be seen in the abdominal wall. The liver need not be enlarged and, indeed, is often small and fibrosed. Other signs of hepatocellular damage such as palmar erythema, leuconychia, spider naevi, gynaecomastia, testicular atrophy, parotid enlargement and Dupuytren's contractures may be present. Ascites and jaundice indicate a bad prognosis. Careful and repeated neuropsychiatric assessment must be made for signs of portosystemic encephalopathy. Hepatic fetor is frequently masked by the equally unpleasant smell of altered blood. Mechanisms initiating haemorrhage are not clearly understood. Immediate gastroscopy is essential to confirm this high-risk condition and initiate appropriate specific treatment (see below).

Rare causes of haemorrhage

Blood disorders such as thrombocytopenia, haemophilia and Von Willebrand's disease may present in this way. One should look for purpura, and for signs of increased capillary fragility as shown by Hess's test (see Ch. 29). Leukaemia can cause thrombocytopenia or portal vein thrombosis but may also cause gastric bleeding by infiltration and ulceration of the stomach. Inherited disorders include pseudoxanthoma elasticum, where the elastic tissue defect not only weakens vessel walls but is also responsible for the 'plucked chicken' appearance of the skin of the neck and angioid streaks in the retina. In the related Ehlers–Danlos syndrome there is a defect of supporting tissue which also predisposes to haemorrhage; there may be characteristic hyperextensibility of the skin with delayed recoil. Hereditary telangiectasia and multiple angiomas usually give rise to chronic blood loss. Similarly acute haemorrhage, except in children, is unusual in the Peutz–Jegher syndrome (intestinal polyposis associated with pigmentation of the lips). Diverticula of the gut rarely bleed massively with the exception of a Meckel's diverticulum, which may contain ectopic gastric mucosa which has ulcerated. Severe haemorrhage can occur in this condition and will present as melaena only.

FURTHER MANAGEMENT IN ACUTE AND CHRONIC ULCERS

Further management requires close collaboration with surgical colleagues who, in all but trivial bleeds, should see the patient jointly with the

Table 11.2 Child–Pugh grading of severity of cirrhosis at time of admission with variceal haemorrhage related to prognosis

	Score 1 pt	Score 2 pts	Score 3 pts
Bilirubin (μmol/l)	17–34	35–50	> 51
Prolongation prothrombin time (sec)	1–4	5–6	7+
Albumin (g/l)	> 35	28–34	< 33
Ascites	None	Mild	Moderate/ severe
Portosystemic encephalopathy (grade)	0	1–2	3–4

Grade A (5–6 points) carries a 5% mortality during an admission for acute variceal bleeding compared with 20% mortality in grade B (7–9 points) and over 40% mortality in grade C (10–15 points)

physician early on in his admission. Even though only a minority of patients will come to surgery (less than 20%) the surgeon will be able to make his baseline assessment before the patient has been resuscitated and sedated. Where the patient is over 60 and gives a clear past history of gastric or duodenal ulcer, with, perhaps, previous haemorrhage, SRH are present and transfusion exceeds 6 units, the case for surgery will be strong. It is preferable to operate electively after the bleeding has stopped, but the surgeon will also be prepared to go ahead if bleeding persists or recurs, especially if the patient's blood group makes further supplies of blood uncertain. In these circumstances when emergency surgery is indicated, delay and continuing massive transfusion increases the mortality. When similar situations arise in younger patients there is more reluctance to undertake surgery. However, though the vessels in the ulcer bed may not be as arteriosclerotic as in the elderly, scarring rather than healing is the best that is likely to occur, and there remains the likelihood that the patient may bleed again in the future.

The patient in whom there is not a clear-cut indication of the underlying pathology presents a problem should bleeding continue or recur. It is now common practice to gastroscope most patients with acute bleeding to try and make an early diagnosis. Gastroscopy is superior to radiology in that it is probably more accurate and the site of bleeding can be positively identified. It is particularly valuable when there is more than one possible source of blood loss and in detecting the sizeable number of bleeders who have gastric erosions in whom, in the past, radiology would have been negative. The need for surgery may be reduced by therapeutic endoscopy with laser, thermal or electrocoagulation of the bleeding point or its injection with adrenaline, to vasoconstrict, plus a sclerosant.

FURTHER MANAGEMENT IN BLEEDING VARICES

Apart from the basic problem of blood replacement there are two further objectives: stopping the bleeding and preventing hepatic coma.

The prothrombin time may be prolonged in cirrhosis and, although this is usually due to hepatocellular damage rather than to shortage of vitamin K, the latter should none the less be given parenterally. Vasopressin or balloon tamponade for not more than 24 hours, may temporarily arrest bleeding and 'buy time' to prepare for more definitive treatment of the varices by sclerotherapy if this is not used as a first measure.

Treatment and prevention of hepatic coma requires emptying of the bowel of blood by means of magnesium sulphate and perhaps suppression of colonic bacteria by lactulose or oral neomycin, and maintenance of both circulation and nutrition by transfusion and infusion of concentrated dextrose into a large vein.

CLINICAL PROBLEM

T	P	BP	R
36	130	90/60	34

Cold, pale, sweating

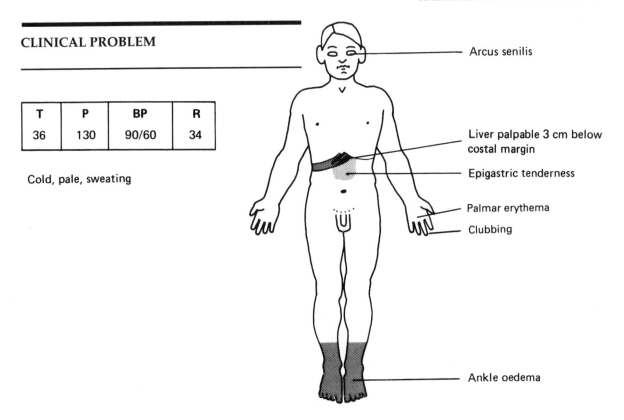

Arcus senilis

Liver palpable 3 cm below costal margin

Epigastric tenderness

Palmar erythema

Clubbing

Ankle oedema

An obese 55-year-old publican was admitted at 2 a.m. on a Saturday morning, having vomited a large quantity of fresh and altered blood 4 hours previously. He gave a history of increasingly severe epigastric pain over the previous 3 days. This occurred immediately after meals and on two occasions he had vomited his recent meal with relief of his pain.

For the previous 6 months he had had mild upper abdominal discomfort; his appetite had deteriorated and he had lost about 7 kg in weight. He denied excessive drinking although he agreed he was sociable! He smoked 30 cigarettes daily. He weighed 90 kg.

He had had winter bronchitis for the past 6 years. Four years previously he had been admitted to hospital with jaundice for 2 weeks and had been advised to reduce his alcohol consumption.

On examination, he was shocked, restless and pale. BP 105/70. Pulse 115/minute regular. There was a marked arcus senilis but no jaundice. The JVP was not raised, although he had moderate pitting oedema of both ankles. In the chest there were scattered rhonchi but no crepitations. He had early clubbing of the fingers and palmar erythema. The abdomen was markedly obese and the spleen could not be felt. The liver edge was palpable 3 cm below the costal margin, seemed smooth and regular in outline and was not

tender. There was diffuse tenderness in the epigastrium but no rebound tenderness. Ascites could not be detected. Melaena stool was present on rectal examination.

Haemoglobin was 9.6 g/dl and the film showed hypochromia and anisocytosis. He was sedated with 10 mg diazepam intravenously and was given 3 pints of blood over the next 6 hours. His pulse fell to 85/minute and his BP rose to 140/80.

One hour later the house physician was recalled to the ward because the patient had suddenly begun to complain of severe pain in the upper abdomen and lower chest. He now looked very ill, the skin being cold and pale. He was sweating profusely. The pulse was 130/minute, regular but thready. The BP was 90/60 and there was rapid shallow breathing. In the abdomen there was marked epigastric tenderness but bowel sounds were present.

QUESTIONS

1. What is the likely cause for his initial admission to hospital?
2. What might be the reason for his deterioration in hospital?
3. What other underlying diseases may be present?
4. How would you now manage the patient?

DISCUSSION

The gastrointestinal haemorrhage is most likely to have arisen from a simple gastric ulcer. The symptoms of anorexia, weight loss and post-prandial pain could also occur with gastric carcinoma but this is less likely to cause massive bleeding. The pattern of symptoms is not typical of a duodenal ulcer. An acute gastric erosion, as may occur after alcohol, could bleed in this way but is less likely in view of the 6-month history of symptoms. The low haemoglobin on admission might be due to recent massive blood loss but the presence of hypochromia and anisocytosis on the blood film suggests that there has also been chronic bleeding. His occupation, past history, hepatomegaly, clubbing and palmar erythema all suggest that he may have alcoholic cirrhosis. However, there are no signs of portal hypertension such as splenomegaly to suggest bleeding from oesophageal varices. The presence of cirrhosis would increase the likelihood of a peptic ulcer.

His further deterioration might be due to recurrence of bleeding. However, there has been no further haematemesis and the development of severe pain after haemorrhage would be most unusual. Indeed it should alert one to the possibility of perforation of an ulcer. Acute pancreatitis, perhaps precipitated by alcohol, can closely mimic ulcer perforation, but the pain frequently radiates to the back and is accompanied by vomiting. In either case, bowel sounds may continue to be heard or even be exaggerated until they disappear several hours later.

Myocardial infarction could also explain his later sudden collapse, and is a recognized complication of massive haemorrhage. Underlying coronary artery disease may be present but may have been previously asymptomatic. Although the pain of myocardial infarction may be poorly localized, the presence of epigastric tenderness is against this diagnosis. The clinical picture is compatible with massive pulmonary embolism but this is an unlikely complication at this stage, and there is no evidence of an underlying deep vein thrombosis.

The most likely diagnosis is a perforated and bleeding gastric ulcer which will require urgent surgical treatment. Investigation must therefore be immediately relevant and rapid. A straight X-ray of the abdomen is likely to be diagnostic by showing gas under the diaphragm. An ECG would probably be done even though it cannot exclude a myocardial infarction. The patient will require further intravenous fluid to resuscitate him sufficiently to allow surgery. In view of the pain which he has now developed, once the decision to undertake laparotomy had been made he would be given an analgesic such as diamorphine in place of further diazepam.

At laparotomy he was found to have bled from a lesser curve chronic benign gastric ulcer which had perforated into the lesser sac. He also had micronodular cirrhosis without evidence of portal hypertension. The ulcer was sutured but despite vigorous resuscitation he died 12 hours postoperatively.

12. Acute abdominal pain

The 'acute abdomen' does not always find its way to the surgical ward. Even when it does, it may be due to a cause not requiring surgery. None the less the problem of making an early diagnosis is sharpened by the knowledge that undue delay in removing a gangrenous appendix, suturing a perforated ulcer or relieving an obstructed bowel may seriously endanger the patient's life. Although delay in operating may be dangerous it can be equally harmful, for example in pancreatitis, to perform an unnecessary laparotomy.

The temptation to relieve what is often very distressing pain with opiates or other potent analgesics must also be resisted, until a diagnosis or the decision to perform a laparotomy has been made. Premature treatment in response to the patient's urgent appeals for relief of pain may irretrievably cloud the symptoms and signs on which a diagnosis can be made. Another treatment which may also modify the clinical picture is long-term steroid therapy.

Previous surgery may lead to unusual presentations of abdominal disease. Thus the pain of recurrent or stomal ulcer may have quite a different site and characteristics from that of the original peptic ulcer which was treated surgically. Other complications of previous surgery include intestinal obstruction from adhesions or the symptoms of dumping or afferent loop obstruction following partial gastrectomy.

A multiplicity of scars and a history of repeated emergency admissions in a man, who is often without job or family, should alert one to the Munchausen syndrome of malingering. Unless such a person can be positively identified, medicolegal considerations require that he is given the benefit of the doubt.

The more common categories of abdominal pain, and their causes, are discussed below.

COLIC

Colic is a true visceral pain arising from the affected viscus and created by tension or spasm of the smooth muscle in its wall. Because it is often an exaggeration of the inherent peristaltic activity of the organ it is often taught that colic frequently builds up to a peak, fades and then recurs in cycles. This is by no means always the case, especially when it is renal or biliary in origin. Pressure over the painful area sometimes gives a little relief and may be the basis for the patient's restlessness. He may draw his legs up, twist or even walk about. In all cases of colic – renal, biliary or intestinal – there is obstruction to pelvis or ureter, cystic or common bile duct, or the gut.

Renal colic

The commonest cause is a stone lodged either at the pelviureteric junction or, more usually, in the course of the ureter, especially near the vesicoureteric junction. If there is gross bleeding from a kidney into the pelvicalyceal system, blood clots may cause colic. It is said that obstruction of the pelviureteric junction can be caused by pressure from an aberrant renal artery, but it is usually due to an ill-understood neuromuscular abnormality resulting in spasm at this point. In this latter condition episodes of colic may occur during the diuresis that follows a large and rapidly ingested water load. ·

The characteristics of renal colic are distinctive. The pain begins in the loin and, if ureteric colic follows renal colic as it usually does, radiates round the flank into the groin, testicle or labia, and thigh. The patient is prostrated by the pain and may vomit, while there is often associated pallor, sweating and tachycardia. Depending on the cause there may be a residual dull ache in the loin between acute attacks, which can last several hours. The urine will usually show some abnormal constituents such as red cells, or sometimes pus cells or protein. In most cases of renal stone there is no underlying disease detectable, but one must always search for hyperparathyroidism or hypercalcaemia from some other cause. Some have idiopathic hypercalciuria. An emergency IVP is the most useful investigation, particularly to demonstrate pelviureteric obstruction, as this is usually intermittent. An acute attack of pyelonephritis often causes renal pain, but this is more constant and is associated with frequency, dysuria and pyuria, together with considerable constitutional disturbances such as high fever and rigors. Other conditions that may cause pain resembling renal colic are retrocaecal appendicitis, pancreatitis and gall-bladder disease.

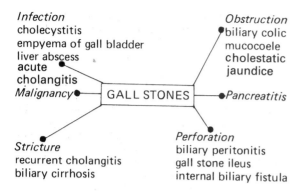

Fig. 12.1 The complications of gall stones

Biliary colic

This may be the first manifestation of the presence of gallstones. In an uncomplicated case a severe pain of sudden onset is felt in the epigastrium or under the right costal margin. It may follow a large meal but frequently there is no obvious cause. Nausea, vomiting and restlessness accompany it as it builds up over 10–40 minutes and there may be radiation of the pain to the right scapula. If the stone is not passed or does not drop back into the gallbladder from Hartman's pouch, where it is frequently lodged, infection of the retained bile may occur and acute cholecystitis supervenes (Fig. 12.1). There will then be fever, marked tenderness over the gallbladder, especially on inspira-

tion, and possibly pain in the shoulder tip. This pain is referred to this site because the inflamed overlying peritoneum is innervated by the phrenic nerve derived mainly from C4. A mild degree of obstructive jaundice may occur in half the patients where the stone reaches the common bile duct. The obstruction is not usually complete but if the stone is not passed, ascending cholangitis may supervene with a hectic fever and rigors. Back pressure of bile will then cause the liver to enlarge. Jaundice may also occur in acute cholecystitis. The cause is not clear but it is possible that the inflammatory mass may directly affect the adjacent liver or exert pressure on the hepatic or common bile ducts. Previous cholecystectomy by no means guarantees future freedom from further gallstones, colic, or jaundice, since stones may form in the stump of the divided cystic duct or in the hepatic ducts. When colic is accompanied by jaundice this is a valuable clue to its cause. In the absence of bilirubinuria or elevation of the serum bilirubin, other diagnoses must be considered – renal colic, pancreatitis, perforated peptic ulcer, myocardial infarction, appendicitis and upper intestinal colic for example. Plain X-ray of the abdomen is of limited value because only 10–15% of gallstones are opaque and abdominal ultrasound scanning is the most rewarding initial investigation (Fig. 12.2)

Intestinal colic

Intestinal colic is the cardinal symptom of intestinal obstruction. It is the pain that is most likely to be truly

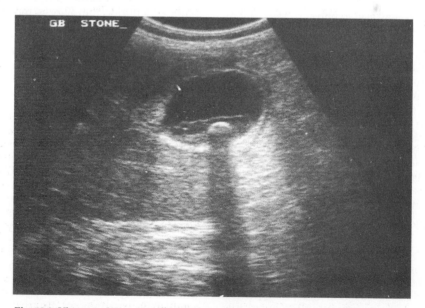

Fig. 12.2 Ultrasound scan of gallbladder showing gallstone within it casting a characteristic acoustic shadow. The gallbladder also contains 'sludge' and its wall is thickened, suggesting that episodes of cholecystitis have occurred. (Courtesy of Dr. Hakhamaneshi).

colicky in nature, with freedom from pain between bouts. When due to small bowel obstruction in a thin person, visible peristalsis may be seen to coincide with the colic and loud borborygmi are heard simultaneously. The pain is usually situated in the centre of the abdomen, or slightly lower in the case of large bowel obstruction. Although colicky at the outset it may become more constant, particularly if strangulation or infarction of the bowel supervenes. Vomiting is an early feature of small intestinal obstruction and it may later become faeculent. Although absolute constipation must ultimately occur it may be preceded by diarrhoea. Circulatory effects such as tachycardia, hypotension, dehydration and peripheral circulatory failure result from hypovolaemia, due to large volumes of fluid sequestered in the lumen of the obstructed bowel, and to absorbed toxins.

The many possible causes of mechanical obstruction must be considered when examining the usually distended abdomen. Any previous abdominal operation could be a source of adhesions. External hernial orifices must be carefully checked and particular attention paid to the femoral triangle. A femoral hernia occurs particularly in thin old women, and the tender lump below the inguinal ligament may either not be seen, due to prudery on the part of the patient matched by reticence in the doctor, or it may be misdiagnosed as a tender lymph node. Other internal mechanical causes may be confined to particular age groups. The commonest cause of intestinal obstruction in children is intussusception, the pathognomonic features being the sudden onset of pain with screaming, flexing of the thighs and vomiting, and the presence of a sausage-shaped tumour. Blood may be passed in the stool, or found on rectal examination. In the elderly intestinal obstruction may be caused by volvulus due to twisting of a long redundant pelvic colon on its mesentery. Initially the swelling may be localized to the left side of the abdomen. Strangulation of the obstructed loop progressing to gangrene is a dangerous complication.

Carcinoma of the distal colon may present acutely as large bowel obstruction without much previous history. Other causes of stricture such as Crohn's disease, tuberculosis or lymphoma, particularly when affecting the ileum, usually cause subacute obstruction over a period and are associated with other signs of the underlying disease. Obstruction from within the lumen is an unlikely event. Gallstone ileus appears in every list of differential diagnosis but rarely in reality. Following a gastrojejunostomy the possibility of bolus obstruction arises, for example by a segment of an orange.

Patients with underlying cardiovascular disease, such as rheumatic mitral stenosis with recent onset of atrial fibrillation, recent myocardial infarction with mural thrombus, or widespread atherosclerosis, are candidates for mesenteric artery occlusion by embolism or thrombus. Infarction of the bowel with signs of obstruction will occur. The pain is continuous rather than colicky, the patient is shocked and blood is passed per rectum. The most common site of occlusion is the superior mesenteric artery affecting the small bowel.

The most valuable investigation in making a diagnosis of intestinal obstruction is a straight X-ray of the abdomen. Taken in the erect position it should show fluid levels in the small intestine as well as gas. The gas shadow pattern may help to localize the site of the obstruction. The gas shadow caused by the most distal loop of obstructed bowel cannot always be identified with confidence.

Intestinal colic may be caused by a functional disturbance, such as spastic colon. The pain may be of sufficient severity to mimic other causes of acute abdominal pain.

Ischaemic colitis

Ischaemic colitis, affecting the region of the splenic flexure, which is the watershed area between the superior and inferior mesenteric artery, is a condition which is becoming more frequently recognized. In its most severe form there is large bowel obstruction due to infarction of the full thickness of the bowel with rapid deterioration and circulatory collapse due to toxaemia and septicaemia. Blood will be present in the stool. Plain abdominal X-ray may show evidence of obstruction together with a thumb-print or cobble stone appearance within the colonic lumen due to oedema of the mucosa. In less severe episodes, where the bowel muscle is preserved, shedding of the oedematous devitalized mucosa gives rise to acute bloody diarrhoea and pain, mimicking inflammatory or infective bowel disease; during healing the partly ischaemic muscle may be replaced by lengthy fibrous strictures, typically in the region of the splenic flexure.

Appendicitis

This is the commonest cause of acute abdominal pain. The classical textbook description is of central abdominal pain, often with colicky features, shifting after a few hours to the right iliac fossa. There is associated nausea, vomiting and slight rise in temperature. Initially there is localized tenderness with guarding in the right lower quadrant. When the overlying parietal peritoneum becomes inflamed, rebound tenderness can be elicited. Unfortunately less than half the patients present in such a characteristic fashion. Frequently the pain is right-sided from the outset. Depending on the position of the appendix, the signs may be most marked on rectal examination (pelvic appendix) or in the loin (retrocaecal appendix). Delay in diagnosis may result, and in a case of obstructive appendicitis where the lumen is blocked by a faecolith, perforation may occur as the rising intraluminal pressure leads to gangrene of the wall of the appendix. This will cause either local abscess formation, when a tender mass becomes palpable, or generalized peritonitis with abdominal pain, rigidity and distension, and loss of bowel sounds (Fig. 12.3).

Acute appendicitis has to be differentiated from right-sided pyelonephritis, renal colic, cholecystitis, or, in a woman, right-sided salpingitis or a twisted ovarian cyst. Some young children in whom laparotomy is performed have a normal appendix removed. There may be some enlargement of neighbouring lymph nodes and a diagnosis, in retrospect, of mesenteric adenitis is made. There is no sure way of making the diagnosis prospectively and avoiding operation.

There are no specific investigations which confirm the diagnosis of appendicitis, though a leucocytosis and a sterile pyuria may be present. Atypical presentations are particularly dangerous in the aged and young. The condition is less common at the extremes of age but when it does occur is more likely to be misdiagnosed and thus have a worse prognosis.

Diverticulitis

Colonic diverticula, particularly in the sigmoid colon, are found with increasing frequency after the age of 40. In the majority of patients they are asymptomatic,

the condition being termed diverticulosis. Some patients may have alternating diarrhoea and constipation with grumbling left-sided abdominal pain, this stage being designated diverticular disease. Other patients, either after a history of diverticular disease or having been symptom-free, develop acute diverticulitis. This has been likened to left-sided appendicitis with severe left iliac fossa pain, nausea, vomiting, fever and constipation. Local pericolic abscess formation may occur and blood and pus may be passed per rectum. Such abscesses, if they rupture, rarely cause generalized peritonitis as the local inflammatory reaction and neighbouring organs wall it off. This may result in fistulae to the bladder or vagina. Ischiorectal abscess may form and result in a fistula to the surface (Fig. 12.3).

Acute peritonitis

This may be a complication of acute infection such as acute appendicitis, diverticulitis or septic abortion. It will rarely be the first symptom in any of these situations. An important and common cause is perforation of a peptic ulcer. Often there will be a history of epigastric pain following food, sometimes making the patient afraid to eat, suggesting a gastric ulcer. Alteratively there may be hunger pain, pain between meals, and pain waking the patient in the early hours, suggesting a duodenal ulcer. However, with

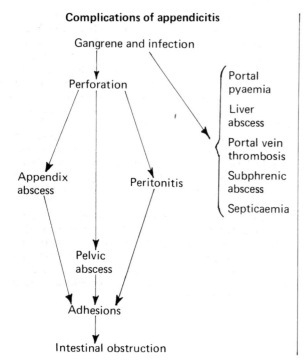

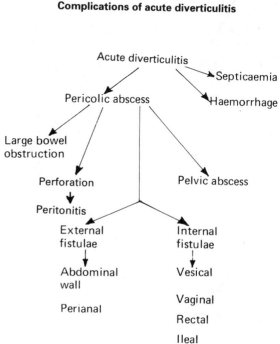

Fig. 12.3 The complications of appendicitis and acute diverticulitis

the increased use of non-steroidal anti-inflammatory drugs (NSAIDs) for arthritis, a patient may present with bleeding or perforation of an ulcer without any preceding symptoms to indicate its presence. The sudden onset of severe upper abdominal pain is accompanied by intense, 'board-like' rigidity of the abdominal wall and great reluctance by the patient to make any movement. Vomiting may occur and result in the patient being referred to hospital as a haematemesis. Although pain may precede bleeding it is most unusual for it to persist and if it does so, should raise the possibility of the dangerous, but fortunately rare, combination of bleeding and perforation (see Clinical Problem, Ch. 11). Following the initial pain and shock some patients may appear to improve over the next few hours, though signs of abdominal rigidity, tachypnoea and tachycardia persist. Generalized peritonitis will usually develop after

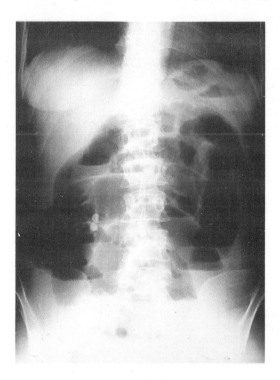

Fig. 12.4 Plain erect abdominal X-ray of a middle-aged woman presenting with acute central abdominal pain, distension and vomiting. Numerous fluid levels are seen in dilated loops of small intestine which was obstructed due to old adhesions. The dense opacities to the right of L4-5 were calcified lymph nodes. (Courtesy of Dr Hakhamaneshi.)

about 5 hours. Even though there may be little vomiting the patient will be dehydrated and haemoconcentrated due to the large outpouring of fluid into the peritoneal cavity. The resulting shock and hypotension may lead to the patient being nursed with the foot of the bed raised, which in turn will cause irritation of the diaphragm by the inflammatory exudate draining upwards. Signs of this will be shoulder-tip pain and often hiccups. A plain X-ray of the abdomen in the erect position (to show gas beneath the diaphragm) is the crucial investigation.

Various non-surgical conditions, like myocardial infarction, basal pneumonia, sickling crisis in HbS disease, diabetic ketoacidosis, tabetic crisis or acute porphyria, may enter the differential diagnosis in a less typical case, apart from many other of the causes of acute abdominal pain already discussed. One further condition that requires urgent surgery is a ruptured ectopic gestation. Shock may be great as rapid exsanguination can occur. There is often a tender mass in the pouch of Douglas on rectal examination and a blood-stained vaginal discharge. A history of a missed period may not always be forthcoming. A rare sign is of bluish discoloration around the umbilicus due to retroperitoneal tracking of blood from the retroperitoneal space (Cullen's sign).

Acute pancreatitis

This condition is characterized by severe upper abdominal pain which may radiate to the back. Although some fluid loss may occur due to vomiting, large internal losses from the acutely inflamed, and sometimes haemorrhagic, pancreas may occur. In addition there is release of vasoactive peptides into the circulation. A profound state of shock results.

On examination the abdomen is not as rigid and tender as in the peritonitis of a perforated ulcer – which is the main differential diagnosis. The bluish discoloration around the umbilicus or in the flanks due to retroperitoneal bleeding is rarely seen. Most identified cases in Britain are due to gallstones with alcohol the next most common cause; 20% of cases remain idiopathic.

An elevated serum amylase is the best diagnostic test available but has the limitation that it is also raised in many of the other causes of acute abdominal pain discussed above. The elevation may be transient but values above 1000 units are strongly suggestive of acute pancreatitis, the normal upper limit being 280 units.

CLINICAL PROBLEM

T	P	BP	R
39	130	100/60	30

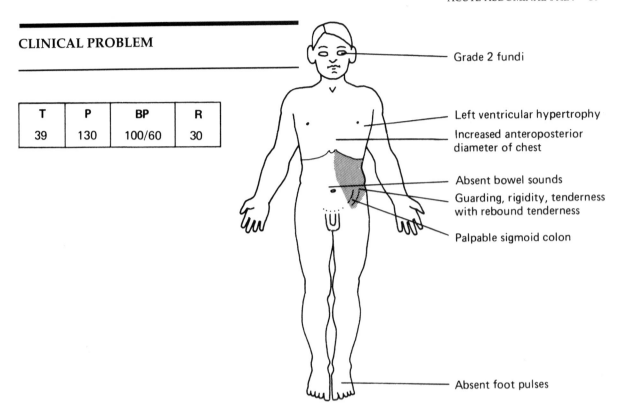

Grade 2 fundi

Left ventricular hypertrophy

Increased anteroposterior diameter of chest

Absent bowel sounds

Guarding, rigidity, tenderness with rebound tenderness

Palpable sigmoid colon

Absent foot pulses

A 73-year-old retired printer had lived alone for 2 years since the death of his wife. He was admitted to hospital complaining of left-sided abdominal pain, bloody diarrhoea and vomiting which had begun abruptly 6 hours previously. At first the pain had fluctuated but became constant later. The pain was not relieved when he vomited and the fluid contained bile, but no blood. He had passed a liquid stool containing fresh and altered blood.

He had had increasingly severe chronic bronchitis for some years, which now limited his exercise tolerance to one flight of stairs or 200 yards on the flat. With this amount of effort he would also develop constricting central chest pain. This followed a myocardial infarction 6 years previously. At the age of 28 he had had an appendicectomy.

He had been constipated for many years and had haemorrhoids which sometimes bled. During the last two years he had lost 4 kg in weight.

On examination he was febrile, sweating, and appeared dehydrated. T 39°C. In the cardiovascular system he had a BP of 100/60 and a tachycardia of 130/min regular with a poor volume pulse. The foot pulses and left popliteal pulse were not palpable.

The fundi showed AV nipping with narrowing and tortuosity of the arteries. There was left ventricular hypertrophy but no signs of heart failure. Examination of the chest showed evidence of emphysema, but there were no signs of acute infection. The abdomen was not distended but there was marked tenderness and rebound tenderness on the left side. Palpation was difficult because of localized guarding and rigidity. The sigmoid colon could be felt in the left iliac fossa but was only slightly tender. Bowel sounds were absent, and no bruits could be heard. The hernial orifices were clear. There was a midline lower abdominal scar. On rectal examination there were no masses or tenderness but there was both fresh and altered blood present without pus or mucus.

QUESTIONS

1. What is the probable cause of his presenting symptoms?
2. What immediate investigations would help in diagnosis and management?

DISCUSSION

The most likely causes of his abdominal symptoms are ischaemic colitis, acute diverticulitis or carcinoma of the colon, each causing large bowel obstruction. Ischaemic colitis is especially common in this age group and to support this diagnosis he has evidence of both peripheral vascular disease and coronary artery disease. In addition, although his present blood pressure is low, the presence of left ventricular hypertrophy and Grade II retinopathy indicate that he was previously hypertensive. The signs of fever, tenderness and bloody diarrhoea are all compatible with infarction of the bowel, and suggest that this is present in addition to obstruction. It is very likely that a constipated old man will have some degree of diverticular disease but the onset of his symptoms and the rapid deterioration argue against the diagnosis of acute diverticulitis. Carcinoma of the colon may present with large bowel obstruction, but the abrupt onset and marked tenderness with rebound are against this diagnosis. A sigmoid volvulus is common in old people, and strangulation may be present from the start, but rectal bleeding is not a feature. Furthermore, in this patient there is no abdominal distension such as would usually be present.

Other causes of bloody diarrhoea, such as ulcerative colitis or Crohn's disease, would not present for the first time with signs of peritonitis. Bacillary dysentery would not explain the peritonitis and there is no pus in the stool. Other causes of acute peritonitis such as a perforated peptic ulcer or diverticulum would not cause bloody diarrhoea.

A straight abdominal X-ray is likely to confirm the diagnosis of large bowel obstruction and may also show evidence of the mucosal oedema sometimes seen in ischaemic colitis, even on the plain film. Blood culture should be taken. An ECG is important as it may show a recent silent myocardial infarction which could be a source of systemic embolism. However, none of these measures should delay the immediate preparation of the patient for emergency laparotomy. This will include taking blood for grouping and cross-matching of at least 4 pints of blood. The haematocrit, urea and electrolytes would also be estimated. An intravenous infusion line would be set up and his dehydration treated with normal saline while the blood was awaited. In an elderly man with ischaemic heart disease it would be especially valuable to set up a central venous pressure line to control the rate of intravenous infusion and so prevent pulmonary oedema. Blood cultures should be taken before starting broad spectrum antibiotics (a combination of gentamycin, cloxacillin and metronidazole is widely used) and intravenous hydrocortisone could also be given (see Ch. 5 for treatment of septic shock).

> At laparotomy there was an extensive infarction of the transverse and descending colon with widespread thrombotic occlusions of the branches of the inferior mesenteric artery. Despite resection of the infarcted bowel he died 24 hours later.

13. Change in bowel habit

Many serious or unpleasant diseases vie for the title of the English Disease, but perhaps national pride prevents its application to constipation. There is no doubt that a morbid preoccupation with the bowels leading to injudicious and sometimes ferocious purgation can promote and perpetuate symptoms, thereby causing considerable anxiety or actual harm. As with most hobbies there is a large market to cater for the public's needs and indeed to encourage them with appeals for the need to achieve 'inner cleanliness'. Fact, as opposed to folklore, is hard to come by in establishing the norms of bowel habit. Surveys have shown that in 99% of normal people defaecation occurs between thrice daily and once every 3 days.

As with all presenting symptoms the patient's self-diagnosis of constipation or diarrhoea must not be accepted without a full description of his complaint being obtained. Much more significance should be attached to a recent change in bowel habit than to a very long history of diarrhoea or constipation. As always, the associated symptoms are vital in distinguishing between the various causes. Physical examination, including inspection of the stool, rectal examination, proctoscopy and sigmoidoscopy must always be undertaken before embarking on more detailed investigation. A malpractice which is still very common is to order a barium enema without prior sigmoidoscopy. A normal radiological appearance in no way excludes a carcinoma of the rectum, as the region proximal to the rectosigmoid junction cannot be confidently visualized radiographically. Rectal examination and sigmoidoscopy are therefore the means of establishing this diagnosis.

It is the functional nature of many bowel disorders that makes this particular symptom complex such a treacherous field. Unfortunately much teaching ignores this, so that the diagnosis of irritable bowel syndrome (IBS) is made by exclusion only. This can result in many unnecessary radiological examinations and other investigations which tend to reinforce the patient's view that there is some serious underlying cause. It may culminate in the rather negative reassurance that the clinician 'can find nothing wrong'. It is therefore important to make a positive diagnosis of a functional disorder, and to follow this by an explanation to the patient of the mechanism of the production of his symptoms. He can then be advised of the necessary modifications to his everyday life, and supportive drug therapy given if needed.

Since diarrhoea and constipation frequently coexist both in functional disorders, like the irritable bowel syndrome, and organic lesions, such as carcinoma of the sigmoid, the two symptoms will be dealt with together rather than separately. Furthermore, acute causes of diarrhoea, such as dysentery, gastroenteritis, food poisoning and cholera, and acute constipation, due to obstruction or dehydration, will not be specifically discussed here.

PATHOPHYSIOLOGY OF THE COLON

Steatorrhoea due to the various causes of malabsorption syndrome is dealt with in detail in Ch. 14. This group of disorders can usually be distinguished from other forms of diarrhoea by inspection of the stools. These are typically pale grey or putty-coloured, soft, bulky and greasy, or when associated with pancreatic disease, may contain oil droplets. They are offensive and tend to float in the lavatory pan, requiring repeated flushings. The patient invariably loses weight and has evidence of various nutritional deficiencies of which anaemia which may be megaloblastic, is the commonest. Some of the mechanisms responsible for steatorrhoea give insight into the functioning of the colon.

The prime activity of the colon is the absorption of water from the liquid contents entering the caecum, thereby creating the semisolid stool evacuated from the rectum. Absorption of water and electrolytes is not as effective or as rapid as in the small intestine. If the small intestine fails to reabsorb fully the daily 7 litres of gut secretions, and the products of digestion entering it, this will present an excessive load for the colon. The large bowel normally reabsorbs 500 ml and has a reserve capacity to reabsorb about 3 litres of water. The nature of the material entering the colon will also influence its function. Bile salts that have not been reabsorbed in the terminal ileum act as irritants, and indeed have been used therapeutically as purgatives. Unabsorbed sugars undergo fermentation to lactic acid by colonic bacteria. The lowered pH increases the frequency of defaecation and may promote a change in the bacterial flora to lactobacilli; this forms the rationale for the use of the non-absorbable sugar lactulose, as a laxative. Likewise the unabsorbed products of fat digestion have an irritant action on the bowel.

Mechanisms of transit through the colon are not clearly understood. The orderly onward peristalsis preceded by a wave of relaxation that occurs in the oesophagus (see Ch. 10) does not happen in the colon. Instead various non-progressive segmental contraction waves occur. The main propulsive act is called the mass movement: this occurs infrequently and an important initiating stimulus is eating. In man there is some doubt whether this is the same neural gastro-colic reflex shown in animal experiments. It seems more likely that it is humorally mediated by cholecystokinin (CCK) or a related peptide. There are many excitatory and inhibitory neural and chemical stimuli which exert their effect on the motility of the colon.

Defaecation occurs when the rectum has filled to a critical level so that stretch receptors in its wall are stimulated, giving rise to the desire to defaecate. At the same time reflex relaxation of the internal anal sphincter occurs, allowing rectal contents to stimulate the sensitive area of anal mucosa. This region alone can distinguish whether the contents of the rectum are solid, liquid or gas. Thus the final control of defaecation is voluntary and is brought about by relaxation of the external sphincter, fixation of the diaphragm and contraction of the abdominal and pelvic floor muscles. The acquisition of this voluntary control in childhood results in the change from the infant state of defaecation following most meals to the socially acceptable adult habit. However, if the urge to defaecate is repeatedly ignored, the rectum, like the bladder, relaxes to accommodate larger volumes without increase in pressure. Ultimately this results in infrequent defaecation from diminished rectal sensation. This illustrates how important an effect childhood toilet training can have on adult habits.

IRRITABLE BOWEL SYNDROME

This common condition is a cause of considerable misery to many young adults and presents a frequent diagnostic problem. The patients are usually tense and anxious, and concern about their symptoms creates further anxiety. They are often in situations at home or work which in other patients give rise to other psychosomatic syndromes such as palpitations or dyspepsia. There are probably inherited or acquired factors which determine which organ bears the brunt of the stress. Some patients give a history of previous migraine or bilious attacks. They may also have experienced the same bowel symptoms acutely before examinations or athletic events.

Two patterns are commonly seen. In the first, the minority, the complaint is of persistent painless diarrhoea, sometimes with mucus but never blood. There is no weight loss and general health is good. Interestingly the symptoms may date from a holiday abroad in which other members of the same party had the same attack of 'tourists' diarrhoea' but all except the patient made a full recovery. Bacteriological and virological studies are invariably negative at this stage, although it is particularly important to exclude amoebic giardia and salmonella infections. In the second group, which constitutes the majority, the patient experiences flatulence with diarrhoea, in which several loose motions are passed each morning or after meals. This alternates with constipation, which is associated with the passage of either small dry hard pellets or thin ribbon-like stools. Preceding defaecation there may be considerable abdominal pain. When this is located in the left iliac fossa and associated with a palpable and tender sigmoid colon there is little diagnostic difficulty.

Sigmoidoscopy shows a normal mucosa but can also be helpful in making a positive diagnosis. The bowel clamps down tight on the sigmoidoscope, and its passage, together with air insufflation, may accurately reproduce the pain. Pressure recordings from the colon have shown that there is an exaggerated response to various stimuli, including stressful interviews arousing hostility, entry of food into the stomach, and cholinergic drugs such as prostigmine. Indeed the patient may experience his pain during such a recorded contraction. This is in contrast to the diminished activity seen in the painless diarrhoea subgroup.

If the clinical picture is not sufficiently clear one may, despite normal blood count, ESR and negative stool occult bloods, feel it necessary to perform a barium enema to exclude organic disease of the colon. In such an unphysiological procedure one is hardly likely to detect what is essentially a physiological disturbance. There may be some evidence of spasm if the bowel has not been too vigorously prepared but an oral cologram (opacification of the stools by barium given by mouth) is more likely to give such positive findings. An oral cologram is not intended to demonstrate an organic lesion but may none the less, provide the patient with the necessary reassurance.

Diagnostic difficulty occurs if the pain arises from spasm of the splenic or hepatic flexure. This may mimic peptic ulcer or gallbladder disease (see Ch. 12).

In a small minority of patients a careful history supported by an elimination diet may incriminate certain dietary factors in the causation of diarrhoea. A relevant and perhaps overpublicized factor is intolerance to milk and milk products. This may be associated with a deficiency of lactase in the small intestinal epithelium. Lactose from milk therefore passes unsplit into the colon where lactobacilli convert it to lactic acid with consequent diarrhoea. Although lactase deficiency may occur secondary to other gut disorders such as gluten enteropathy, it is also present in many otherwise normal people. Certain ethnic groups such as Negroes and Cypriots show a high incidence of lactase deficiency but they are usually asymptomatic.

DIVERTICULAR DISEASE

This in some ways provides a bridge between the irritable colon syndrome and organic disorders since both a functional and structural abnormality are present. As in irritable colon it can be shown that there is a heightened response of colonic muscle to the same psychological, physiological and pharmacological stimuli. This occurs particularly in the sigmoid colon, the commonest site of diverticula, where pathological and radiological studies show thickening of the circular muscle. The point of interest is whether the irritable colon syndrome of the younger adults goes on to become the diverticular disease found in the over-40 age group. Certainly in the uncomplicated form the symptomatology is very similar, but diverticulosis without any symptoms is probably even more common and seems almost part of the ageing process.

The differential diagnosis from carcinoma of the colon is important in this age group, and a barium enema is an essential investigation. The symptoms of pain, tenderness in the left iliac fossa, and alternating diarrhoea and constipation are due to over activity of the circular muscle of the colon.

The diverticula may become inflamed causing acute diverticulitis, which has been called 'left-sided appendicitis'. It is usually associated with guarding, fever and leucocytosis. This may subside, but complications can occur of pericolitis and pericolic abscess formation may go on to a local peritonitis. There may be rupture to cause a generalized peritonitis. Perforation into the neighbouring organ such as bladder, vagina or another part of gut will cause fistula formation. Obstruction of the bowel and haemorrhage can also result, and clear differentiation from a sigmoid carcinoma may not be possible until after surgical resection (see Fig. 12.3, p. 86). The previous demonstration of colonic diverticulosis in such a patient must not induce temporizing optimism in the surgeon as there may be coexisting carcinoma (see Ch. 12).

CARCINOMA OF THE COLON AND RECTUM

Because of the fluid nature of the ileal contents which enter the caecum and the greater diameter of the ascending colon, disturbance of bowel habit is less likely to occur with right-sided growths. Passage of fresh or altered blood, and sometimes mucus, occurs with sigmoid and rectal lesions in contrast to the occult bleeding presenting as an iron deficiency anaemia that occurs from the right side.

With lesions of the ascending colon pain, often related to meals, may occur, and a mass may be palpable. In left-sided lesions pain due to partial obstruction is common and acute large bowel obstruction is a frequent presentation. Pain, however, is uncommon in rectal carcinoma although there may be a vague discomfort associated with a sensation of inadequate defaecation. Passage of mucus is particularly associated with carcinoma of the rectum. Early diagnosis by sigmoidoscopy followed by barium enema is particularly important in this group of cancers since radical surgery carries a relatively good prognosis.

ULCERATIVE COLITIS AND CROHN'S DISEASE

All age groups can be affected by either of these inflammatory disorders. In ulcerative colitis bloody diarrhoea is nearly always present, and the diagnosis is strongly supported by the presence of a granular proctitis on sigmoidoscopy. Although ulceration and pseudo polyps are not usually seen in the rectum, the appearance of the mucosa and the ease with which it bleeds on contact are characteristic. The disease spreads proximally in continuity and, if extensive, there may be systemic disturbances with fever, malaise, weight loss and anaemia. Rarer manifestations such as clubbing, erythema nodosum, pyoderma gangrenosum, and sacroiliitis may be of diagnostic value. Barium enema will confirm the diagnosis and indicates the extent of the disease (Fig. 13.1E).

In recent years a new entity has been delineated from ulcerative colitis in which the colon around the splenic flexure is mainly involved. Formerly called segmental colitis, it presents initially with pain as well as bloody diarrhoea and later barium enema may show a characteristic long length of stricture (Fig. 13.1A). It is now known to be of ischaemic aetiology, occurring in the watershed region of bowel between superior and inferior mesenteric artery territories. It occurs in elderly patients, often with other evidence of cardiovascular disease, and is due to occlusion or low flow in the inferior mesenteric artery (see Ch. 12).

In recent years it has also become apparent that Crohn's disease may not only involve the terminal ileum but the colon as well. In retrospect, cases had been misdiagnosed as atypical ulcerative colitis. Apart from the pathological differences of colitis being a superficial mucosal disorder, and Crohn's involving the full thickness of bowel wall with granuloma formation, there are important clinical differences (Table 13.1). Only half the patients with colonic Crohn's have rectal lesions seen on sigmoidoscopy. When present, these are patchy rather than uniform, with areas of oedema but not much bleeding. Deep fissuring ulcers may be seen and give a

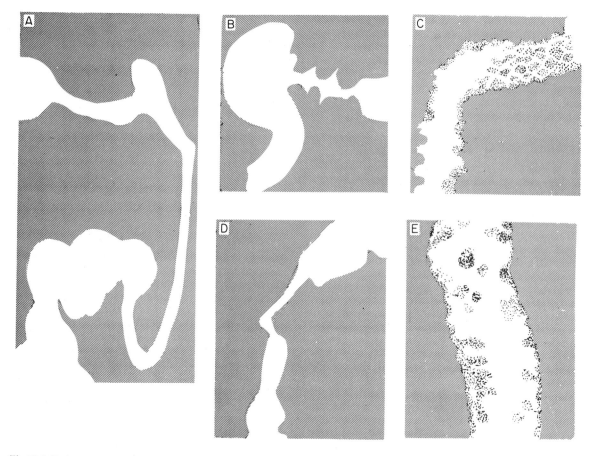

Fig 13.1 Barium enemas in colonic disease
A. Ischaemic stricture of splenic flexure and descending colon
B. Crohn's disease of transverse colon
C. Crohn's disease of colon showing 'cobblestone' appearance

D. Recurrent Crohn's disease causing a stricture at an ileocolic anastomosis
E. Ulcerative colitis of descending colon showing pseudopolyposis

characteristic 'rose thorn' appearance on barium enema (Fig. 13.1, B and C). The lesions are discontinuous. Perianal lesions are seen in over three-quarters of patients and include one or more painless anal fissures, associated with oedema, anal tags and discoloration of the adjacent skin. Perianal abscesses and fistulae are also common. Biopsy of these lesions may be of diagnostic value. Abdominal pain and the absence of blood from the diarrhoea are further differentiating points. Of course the more classical disease of the terminal ileum alone, or with colonic involvement, will cause diarrhoea; there may be colicky pain if a stricture is causing subacute obstruction and a mass may be palpable in the right iliac fossa (Fig. 13.1D). Small-bowel enema or barium follow-through will confirm the diagnosis. Scanning with

the patient's leucocytes labelled with indium can be used to detect and demonstrate the extent of inflammatory bowel disease and any complicating abscess.

SIMPLE CONSTIPATION

Two main categories occur and it is of importance to distinguish them since the approach to the treatment of each will be different. The condition called rectal dyschezia has been alluded to in the discussion of defaecation. These patients have normal colonic transit with delay occurring in rectal emptying. Large volumes of stool may be felt on rectal examination. In geriatric patients, actual faecal impaction with a spurious overflow diarrhoea may occur. Infirmity, confusion and similar disorders may render them

Table 13.1 Differential diagnoses of ulcerative colitis, colonic Crohn's disease and ischaemic colitis

	Ulcerative colitis	Crohn's disease	Ischaemic colitis
Age at diagnosis	20–40 years	0–50 years	Over 50 years
Symptoms			
Bleeding:	Very common	Unusual	Very common
Abdominal pain:	None	Common	Very common
Signs			
Abdominal tenderness	None	Sometimes	Very common
Abdominal mass	None	Sometimes	May develop over a few weeks
Anal lesions	Rarely, secondary to infection	Common, often painless May precede bowel disturbance	None
Sigmoidoscopy			
Rectal involvement	95%	50%	? 1%
Appearances	Uniform hyperaemia, granularity and contact bleeding	Discontinuous, oedematous and occasional ulceration	Very rarely engorgement of mucosa, oedema and bluish-purple discoloration
Radiology			
Distribution	Continuous with rectum	Often discontinuous with normal intervening colon	Left colon especially around splenic flexure
Internal fistulae	None	Sometimes	None
Strictures	Carcinomatous only	Common	May be lengthy and develop some weeks after onset
Mucosal lesions	Shallow granular ulceration and pseudo polyps	Fissuring ulcers with oedema in between ('cobblestones')	Mucosal oedema ('thumb-printing') and irregularity in early acute stage

immobile and unable to answer the call to stool, and are common contributory factors. In this condition the diet is often low in roughage and fluid content, while painful anal lesions such as haemorrhoids or fissures may further inhibit defaecation.

The second group of patients seem, by transit studies, to take an abnormally long time for caecal contents to reach the rectum, with the result that stools are hard and dry and may be painful to pass. The condition merges with the spastic variety of irritable colon. A variant of this type of constipation is the idiopathic megacolon. This differs from Hirschsprung's disease of children and Chagas's disease (infection with *Trypanosoma cruzei*) in that there is no evidence of destruction of ganglion cells.

Constipation is an important symptom of depression; a change in sleep pattern as well as bowel habit, often with early waking and inability to get back to sleep, may alert one to this diagnosis.

METABOLIC, ENDOCRINE AND DRUG CAUSES

Hypercalcaemia from any cause causes constipation, and is usually associated with nocturia, due to failure of renal concentration, lethargy, abdominal pain, nausea, vomiting, and mental disturbance even amounting to psychosis.

Thyrotoxicosis may be accompanied by diarrhoea whereas constipation is a common symptom of myxoedema.

The carcinoid syndrome, due to liver metastases from an argentaffinoma, is characterized by diarrhoea, flushing attacks, asthma and tricuspid and pulmonary valve disease.

A rare endocrine tumour causing diarrhoea is the non-beta islet cell pancreatic tumour giving rise to the Zollinger–Ellison syndrome. In most cases gross gastric hypersecretion of acid causes recurrent and multiple peptic ulceration with diarrhoea, attributable to inactivation of pancreatic and intestinal enzymes and conjugated bile salts by acid and the large volume of gastric fluid. Another pancreatic islet tumour causing profuse watery diarrhoea associated with hypokalaemia and achlorhydria is the VIPoma. The severity of the diarrhoea has led to the term pancreatic cholera and the diagnosis can be confirmed by measuring VIP (vasoactive intestinal polypeptide). In the rare medullary carcinoma of the thyroid there is diarrhoea in half of the patients.

A record of drugs is an essential part of history-taking. Opiates, codeine, aluminium hydroxide and ganglion-blocking agents are amongst constipating drugs whereas magnesium trisilicate, adrenergic blockers, and digoxin may cause diarrhoea.

CLINICAL PROBLEM

T	P	BP	R
38·2	90	130/90	22

Clinically anaemic

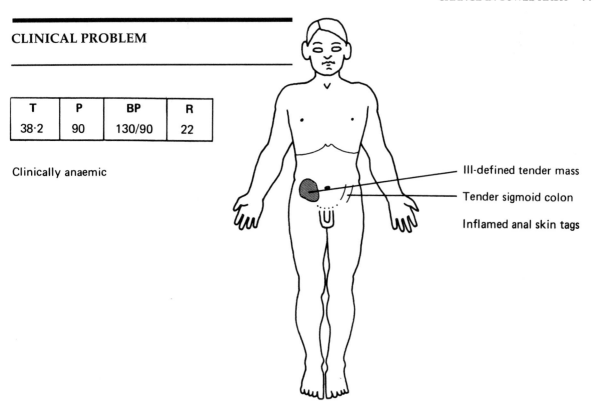

Ill-defined tender mass

Tender sigmoid colon

Inflamed anal skin tags

A 54-year-old market gardener was admitted to hospital for investigation. He complained that for 4-months he had had left-sided abdominal pain. At times the pain was colicky and was sometimes relieved by defaecation. During this period he had had alternating episodes of diarrhoea and consti-pation. He had also noticed streaks of blood in the stool which he had attributed to 'piles'. He had felt unwell with poor appetite and had lost 5 kg in weight.

For the previous 15 years he had had recurrent episodes of central and right-sided abdominal pain associated with diarrhoea but never constipation. The pain occurred about an hour after meals. His symptoms might persist for several months and his weight would fluctuate.

He had had two barium meal examinations 10 and 5 years previously, which were normal, except that on the second occasion a sliding hiatus hernia had been demonstrated. Two years previously he had had a sigmoidoscopy which was normal and a barium enema which showed a few sigmoid diverticula only.

On examination he was thin, clinically anaemic and appeared unwell. He was mildly febrile (T 38.2°C). The only abnormal findings were in the abdomen. He was tender in both lower quadrants. In the right iliac fossa there was an ill-defined tender rounded swel-ling in the region of the caecum. On the left side the sigmoid colon was palpable, tender and could be rolled under the fingers. On rectal examination no masses could be felt. Proctoscopy showed first degree internal haemorrhoids and there were also prominent and inflamed skin tags around the anus. Sigmoidoscopy to 20 cm was normal.

QUESTIONS

1. How would you account for his present symptoms?
2. What are the likely causes of his past symptoms?
3. What further investigations would you perform?

DISCUSSION

The illness leading to this patient's admission to hospital suggests a stenosing lesion of the left side of the colon. In this age group such a stenosis is very likely to be due to carcinoma, especially if it presents in a patient who was previously well. There are two situations however where previous illness might be associated with the development of cancer.

The risk of cancer in ulcerative colitis is related to the extent and duration of the colitis. It is probably only significant in patients with total colitis which has been present for 10 years. This patient's 15 year history is unlikely to be due to colitis for several reasons. The diarrhoea was never associated with blood loss until recently. Sigmoidoscopy in the past, and on admission, showed no evidence of procto-colitis which is invariably present and may extend any distance back towards the ileocaecal valve. Finally, barium enema 5 years previously showed no evidence of colitis.

Single and multiple colonic polyps are associated with carcinoma of the colon. When multiple the condition is usually inherited as a dominant charac-teristic and carries a particulary high risk of malig-nancy. The condition may be asymptomatic or cause diarrhoea and bleeding. In this patient the inter-mittency of the past symptoms, with pain as one of its features, and the absence of polyps on barium enema make their presence unlikely.

Diverticulosis of the colon, which has been radio-logically demonstrated in this patient, can give rise to large bowel obstruction if a pericolic abscess develops. The illness is more acute than in this patient. Diverti-cula in the absence of inflammation may give rise to symptoms indistinguishable from the irritable colon syndrome of either the spastic or simple diarrhoea variety. This patient's previous history does not fit easily into any of these categories as he has had recurrent episodes of diarrhoea and pain without constipation and they have been associated with loss of weight.

Stricture of the left side of the colon may follow some weeks after an episode of subacute ischaemic colitis. There is no such antecedent history in this patient and this diagnosis does not explain his past history.

Crohn's disease can affect the gut anywhere from mouth to anus, although the terminal ileum is the commonest site. Colonic lesions, in isolation or associated with those elsewhere, are well recognized. The clinical presentation in this patient shows many of the features of Crohn's disease. Recurrent episodes of diarrhoea, right-sided abdominal pain with a vague mass and weight loss and malaise over many years are a feature of involvement of the terminal ileum. Attention has been drawn to the long interval between the first symptoms and the establishment of the correct diagnosis in the past. If this patient's disease had been confined to the terminal ileum a barium meal without a follow-through examination of that area would have been negative. Likewise a barium enema can be negative though often the terminal ileum, and disease within it, is demon-strated. Unlike ulcerative colitis the rectum is fre-quently spared in colonic Crohn's disease but anal and perianal lesions are common. Considerable significance should be attached to the inflamed skin tags seen in this patient.

Further radiological studies must be undertaken, with a barium enema first. This will show the site of the presumed stenosis and may also provide a clue to the underlying disease. If Crohn's disease is present the lesion will be segmental with adjacent normal bowel. The mucosa may show a coarse cobblestone appearance and there may be deep ulcerating fissures, giving a spiky 'rose thorn' appearance. A stricture will probably be seen. A small-bowel enema of the small intestine, especially ileum, will be necessary. The detection and delineation of disease elsewhere in the gut is of importance in deciding the vexed question of the best treatment. Biopsy of the skin tags is of great help in establishing a histological diagnosis, as is colonoscopy, or, for left-sided lesions, flexible sigmoidoscopy.

> Barium studies confirmed the presence of strictures of the descending colon and terminal ileum. Biopsy of the skin tag showed non-caseating granulomata with giant cells. The diagnosis was Crohn's disease.

14. Steatorrhoea and malabsorption syndrome

The importance of steatorrhoea as a symptom is that it invariably indicates malabsorption not only of fat but also of other essential nutrients. The reverse may not always be true in that some patients with malabsorption may have seemingly normal bowel actions, though stool fat content is usually raised on analysis. Further, if digestion of fat is impaired for whatever reason, then, inevitably, it cannot be absorbed. Steatorrhoea has, therefore, been promoted from being synonymous with malabsorption to being the most important symptom and sign of malabsorption. Sometimes symptoms or signs associated with malabsorption of nutrients other than fat dominate the clinical picture, and may bring the patient to the haematologist, neurologist or dermatologist. For all these reasons the more comprehensive term of malabsorption is preferred.

PRESENTATION

A. Gastrointestinal symptoms

The patient with steatorrhoea usually complains of frequent passage of semi-formed stools. In place of a normal daily stool volume of 200 ml he may pass up to 2500 ml. In appearance, the stools are pale yellow or grey and are abnormally offensive. Sometimes they may appear greasy and, in the case of pancreatic steatorrhoea, oil droplets may be seen. In the absence of pancreatic lipase, fat digestion cannot even begin and the grossest steatorrhoea is often pancreatic in origin. When steatorrhoea is due to impairment of intestinal absorption of fat, oil droplets are not usually seen in the stool as some degree of fat digestion will have taken place. The stools are often lighter than water and float; characteristically, the patient will say that he has to flush the toilet repeatedly. Frequent inspection and weighing or measurement of stool volume is a good guide to response to treatment.

Abdominal distension is a common finding which may be accentuated by loss of muscle and fat in the rest of the body. It is particularly prominent in children with gluten enteropathy but can occur in all forms of malabsorption syndrome. It may be associated with discomfort and flatulence. Various factors contribute, including muscular weakness due to muscle wasting and hypokalaemia, and gas, due to fermentation of the bulky stools in transit.

Abdominal pain is an uncommon feature confined to patients with pancreatitis and those with strictures causing subacute intestinal obstruction, of which the commonest cause is Crohn's disease. However, some patients with coeliac disease remark on the disappearance of abdominal discomfort when a gluten-free diet is instituted.

Vomiting is unusual, occurring chiefly in children with coeliac disease.

Change in appetite is an important symptom which may be overlooked. In a minority of patients, for example with a 'mechanical' cause such as resection of the ileum for mesenteric infarction, there may be an increased or ravenous appetite associated with weight loss resembling uncontrolled diabetes or thyrotoxicosis. In many other intestinal causes such as gluten enteropathy, however, there is marked anorexia. The resultant diminution in calorie intake contributes significantly to the weight loss in addition to the calorie wastage in the stools due to the malabsorption.

B. Nutritional symptoms

Weight loss is a prominent symptom which can only in part be attributed to the increased faecal loss of long-chain fatty acids, lactic acid and nitrogen due to malabsorption of fat, carbohydrate and protein respectively. The accumulation of oedema as a result of hypoproteinaemia may mask the loss of weight. In some cases the calorie loss is compensated for by an increase in appetite. In other patients, with less severe malabsorption, weight may be maintained although other deficiencies may still be present.

Anaemia is common, and is sometimes the only presenting symptom. Iron deficiency occurs commonly but is frequently associated with a macrocytic megaloblastic anaemia, giving rise to a dimorphic blood film. It is therefore important to measure the serum iron in patients with malabsorption even though red cell indices do not suggest iron deficiency. Malabsorption of folic acid is the commonest cause of megaloblastic anaemia. When vitamin B_{12} deficiency is present it suggests that the cause of the malabsorption is either disease of the terminal ileum, which is the site of its absorption, or the contaminated bowel syndrome where the dietary vitamin B_{12} is utilized by bacteria in the small intestine.

Failure to grow will only be apparent in childhood. The limbs are affected more than the trunk and in an adult with presumed adult coeliac disease comparison of the crown–pubis with pubis–heel, or half-the-span, dimensions, may show the trunk measurements to be more than one inch (2.5 cm) greater in addition to an overall reduction in height. Additional evidence from the greater heights of siblings or parents and a vague history of abdominal symptoms dating back to childhood often suggest that adult coeliac disease has been present for longer than suspected.

Metabolic bone disease may cause changes in height due to vertebral collapse, or, in children, bowing of the legs due to rickets. Malabsorption of vitamin D and calcium causes rickets in children and osteomalacia in adults, whereas protein deficiency predisposes to osteoporosis. When these develop acutely, bone pain can be a distressing symptom. Apart from obvious radiological changes, pseudo fractures are characteristic (Looser zones). These may be painless. They involve only the cortex of the bone, particularly in the scapulae and pelvis. Long-standing untreated osteomalacia may induce a compensatory or secondary hyperparathyroidism which may further complicate both the clinical and radiological picture. Bone biopsy may be necessary to disentangle the situation.

Tetany may develop acutely due to the great loss of calcium, which combines with fat in the stools. Calcium loss can very easily exceed the average daily intake of 1000 mg when it is remembered that normally 400 mg is secreted in saliva, bile, pancreatic juice and succus entericus, and may fail to be reabsorbed. Obvious bone disease may not be present. The role of coexistent magnesium deficiency contributing to tetany has become apparent in recent years with the interesting observation that correction of magnesium deficiency alone may raise the serum calcium and relieve tetany in some cases. Trousseau's and Chvostek's signs should be looked for to detect latent tetany.

Peripheral neuropathy occurs rarely and is usually due to vitamin B_{12} deficiency when amyelopathy may also be present, giving subacute combined degeneration of the cord. In contaminated bowel syndrome these changes may be marked, for not only is there vitamin B_{12} deficiency but the responsible intestinal bacteria may also synthesize folic acid, giving rise to supranormal blood levels. Nature thus commits the cardinal therapeutic error of treating vitamin B_{12} deficiency with folic acid! Thiamine deficiency may be responsible for a pellagra-like

peripheral neuropathy in rare cases. Mental changes such as depression and irritability are relatively frequent but often tend to be overlooked or underestimated and only appreciated in retrospect by patient and physician.

Oedema is due to hypoalbuminaemia which has several causes. Not only is there failure of absorption of ingested protein but there is often an increased loss of protein into the gut lumen and failure of hepatic synthesis.

Keratitis and impaired dark adaptation or night blindness may be caused by vitamin A deficiency.

A wide variety of skin changes which seem secondary to malabsorption in that they improve when the malabsorption is corrected, are recognized. The commonest skin lesion is a nondescript eczema of patchy distribution which may be associated with itching. Sometimes a more characteristic psoriasiform eczema accompanied by pigmentation is seen. A gluten enteropathy is the usual cause of the underlying malabsorption and both gut and skin respond to gluten withdrawal from the diet. Protein depletion may cause fissuring of the keratin layer, giving rise to a crackled skin appearance. Oral lesions including glossitis, angular stomatitis, cheilosis and buccal ulcers may occur due to deficiencies of riboflavin, nicotinic acid, folic acid and other unidentified deficiencies. Bleeding gums, due to scurvy from ascorbic acid deficiency, and skin purpura from vitamin K deficiency may also be seen.

In dermatitis herpetiformis, where bullous lesions occur symmetrically over the extensor aspect of the limbs, buttocks and shoulders, over three quarters of patients have some degree of villous atrophy of the small bowel. This is rarely associated with clinical malabsorption, and usually there is only a mild anaemia due to deficiency of iron or folate. These deficiencies respond to gluten withdrawal; in over 70% of patients the skin will also improve, so that after about 2 years, dapsone, a specific remedy for the skin lesions, can be withdrawn.

CONFIRMATION OF MALABSORPTION

Normally about 93% of the dietary intake of fat is absorbed. Demonstration of increased faecal fat excretion remains the 'gold standard' test in demonstrating the presence of malabsorption, despite inaccuracies in adequate stool collection and the unpleasantness of the laboratory procedure. Attempts have been made to circumvent it by measuring absorption of radioactive fatty acids (palmitic or oleic acid). The passive absorption of the non-metabolized carbohydrate D-xylose, measured by its subsequent urinary excretion and sometimes blood levels, is usually abnormal in mucosal disease (and normal in maldigestion). It is relatively easy to perform but subject to error if there is delayed gastric emptying or renal impairment, but may be used to monitor response to treatment, for example in children with gluten enteropathy.

ASSESSMENT OF EXTENT OF DEFICIENCIES

The further battery of tests usually undertaken serves several purposes. Firstly, treatment of the patient can be planned to replace the deficient substances. Secondly, demonstration of these deficiencies lends further support to the diagnosis of malabsorption syndrome. Thirdly, the pattern or profile of these deficiencies may give strong clues as to the underlying cause of malabsorption in a particular patient; for example, steatorrhoea with impaired vitamin B_{12} absorption and high, rather than low, folate levels would suggest terminal ileal disease or contaminated bowel syndrome. It will already be obvious from the many ways in which the syndrome presents that a wide range of tests will be necessary.

DIAGNOSIS OF THE UNDERLYING CAUSE

Intestinal biopsy is invariably required and is now much more easily undertaken by multiple low duodenal sampling at gastroscopy, which is replacing the more cumbersome jejunal biopsy by Crosby capsule. However, the abnormalities seen may be relatively non-specific, because any disease process affecting the division and migration from the crypts to the tips of the villi of the intestinal mucosal cells will produce much the same effect. In place of the normal finger-like villi there may be leaves, ridges or convolutions. This is called partial villous atrophy. This is accompanied by an increased cellular infiltrate of the lamina propria. These findings occur in gluten enteropathy, tropical sprue and other mucosal disorders. A balder appearance of flat cobblestones is called subtotal villous atrophy and is virtually pathognomonic of gluten enteropathy. Only in such rare disorders as Whipple's disease, intestinal lymphangiectasia, amyloid, and some cases of intestinal lymphoma may there be characteristic diagnostic findings. Intestinal biopsy may often therefore confirm the presence of malabsorption rather than clearly indicate its cause. However, when repeated after a period of specific treatment such as a gluten-free diet in coeliac disease, broad-spectrum antibiotics and folic acid in tropical sprue, or broad-spectrum antibiotics in Whipple's disease, improvement may be seen which, in conjunction with clinical and biochemical improvement, helps to clinch the diagnosis.

Where a structural abnormality such as diverticula, fistulae or previous surgery is the suspected cause, small bowel contrast radiography will be indicated. A small-bowel enema by intubation is replacing the older barium follow-through in most instances. A plain abdominal radiograph is generally unhelpful unless looking for the calcification sometimes found in chronic pancreatitis

CAUSES OF MALABSORPTION SYNDROME

Other diagnostic procedures will be mentioned below in the discussion of individual causes. Although one particular disease may exert its effect by several mechanisms (e.g. Crohn's disease) a simple classification based on the disorders of intestinal function is instructive.

Inadequate digestion

(a) Pancreatic insufficiency – mucoviscidosis, chronic pancreatitis.
(b) Inactivation of pancreatic enzymes – gastric acid hypersecretion (Zollinger–Ellison syndrome).
(c) Inadequate mixing of chyle, bile and pancreatic enzymes – Polya gastrectomy.
(d) Bile salt deficiency – biliary obstruction, ileal resection, bacterial deconjugation in contaminated bowel syndrome.

Mucosal cell disorders

(a) Gluten enteropathy (coeliac disease).
(b) Tropical sprue.
(c) Whipple's disease.
(d) Amyloidosis.
(e) Intestinal ischaemia.
(f) Intestinal lymphoma.

Inadequate digestion

Pancreatic disease. The confirmation of pancreatic insufficiency will involve tests stimulating pancreatic function such as the secretin–pancreozymin or Lundh test. Pancreatitis of sufficient severity to cause steatorrhoea will always be associated with abnormal ducts visualized by ERCP (endoscopic retrograde cholangiopancreatography).

Gastric disease. Hypersecretion of hydrochloric acid of sufficient degree to inactivate pancreatic enzymes in the lumen of the intestine occurs in the rare Zollinger–Ellison syndrome due to a pancreatic tumour secreting gastrin.

One of the several mechanisms whereby partial gastrectomy combined with gastrojejunostomy gives rise to malabsorption, is the mechanically obvious one where chyle rapidly enters the jejunum 'missing' the bile and pancreatic juices secreted into the afferent loop.

Disorders of bile salt metabolism. (See Fig. 14.1). Conjugated bile salts are essential to the emulsification of fat, which is a prerequisite of its digestion by lipases. They also facilitate the absorption of the products of fat digestion in the jejunum by forming micelles with them. After fulfilling this

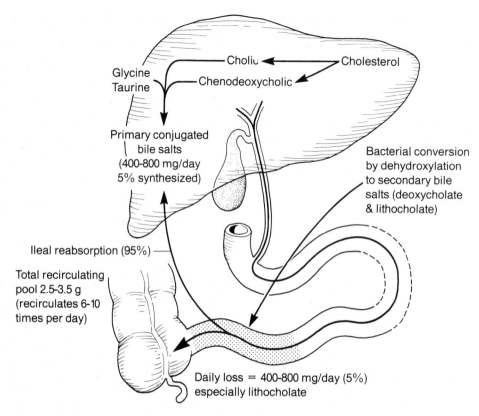

Fig 14.1   The pathways of metabolism of bile salts

function in the jejunum 95% of bile salts are reabsorbed and return to the liver. The site of reabsorption is largely by a specific transport mechanism confined to the ileum, i.e. distal to the site of fat absorption. The liver is therefore required to supplement this enterohepatic circulation by producing about 5% of the body's bile salt pool daily. The maximum bile salt production of which it is capable is probably 20% of the total body bile salt pool. Steatorrhoea due to conjugated bile salt deficiency may therefore be due to failure of hepatic synthesis, due to chronic liver disease; obstruction to flow of bile, as in biliary cirrhosis; failure of ileal reabsorption, usually due to ileal resection; increased deconjugation of bile salts as in contaminated bowel syndrome.

Contaminated bowel syndrome. Primary bile salts (cholic and chenodeoxycholic acid) are conjugated in the liver with glycine and taurine. In this form they are highly dissociated at the normal intestinal pH giving them their detergent properties of being both water- and fat-soluble. Deconjugation can be brought about by bacteria and the deconjugated salts are very much less dissociated and therefore less effective. Furthermore, the specific ileal reabsorption mechanism is for the conjugated form. These factors are important in producing contaminated bowel syn-

drome which occurs in conditions associated with stasis in the small intestine. This may be due to strictures (congenital, tuberculous, Crohn's disease or following radiotherapy); diverticula of jejunum or duodenum; blind loops, such as the afferent loop of a Polya gastrectomy; or disturbances of motility, such as muscle degeneration in systemic sclerosis or autonomic neuropathy in diabetes mellitus. Bacteria, normally confined to the colon, will then multiply in the small intestine producing significant counts greater than 1 million/ml. Another means whereby infection may be introduced is through a fistula (jejunocolic due to a stomal ulcer, colonic diverticulitis or Crohn's disease), or by resection of the ileocaecal valve. Reduced gastric secretion and impaired humoral or cellular immunity may also sometimes be contributory factors.

E. coli and anaerobes including *Bacteroides* are the most commonly found organisms. The latter seem more important since they will cause deconjugation of the bile salts and hence steatorrhoea. In addition these bacteria utilize vitamin B_{12} and may synthesize folic acid as mentioned above. The resultant vitamin B_{12} malabsorption can be confirmed by the Schilling test and will not be corrected by intrinsic factor as in pernicious anaemia. Urinary indican excretion may be raised due to excess bacterial activity, but intestinal aspiration and culture is the definitive test. The ^{14}C glycocholate breath test depends on bacterial deconjugation of the radioactive glycine, allowing its absorption and metabolism to $^{14}CO_2$ as shown by the estimation of exhaled radioactive carbon dioxide. In a normal subject the conjugated glycine remains attached to cholic acid in its enterohepatic circulation, with no ensuing radioactivity in the breath. Furthermore, whatever the cause of the contaminated bowel syndrome, nearly all cases will show at least a temporary improvement when given broad spectrum antibiotics.

Mucosal disorders

Coeliac disease and coeliac syndrome. Coeliac disease in children, responding rapidly to withdrawal of gluten from the diet, does not usually present any diagnostic difficulties. There was semantic confusion regarding its presentation in the adult before it was appreciated that one could often trace symptoms back to childhood, however mild they might have been. The adult disease was formerly called idiopathic steatorrhoea. As only 70% of cases may show a complete mucosal response to gluten withdrawal (and even then, more slowly than in children), some prefer to call it primary coeliac syndrome, rather than adult coeliac disease as this implies that it is due to gluten sensitivity. Another reason for the introduction of the term coeliac syndrome was to embrace the large number of conditions in which a secondary, and often transient, malabsorption syndrome was demonstrable. Secondary coeliac syndrome may occur in a wide variety of conditions in which damage to the rapidly dividing intestinal mucosal cells occurs. Such a situation will occur during the use of the cytotoxic drugs. Other drugs have also been incriminated, such as neomycin and phenindione. Severe protein malnutrition (Kwashiorkor) and exten-sive skin disease such as psoriasis and eczema affecting more than 60% of the body surface, may also be responsible (dermatogenic enteropathy). Several debilitating diseases such as infectious hepatitis, ulcerative colitis or disseminated malignancy, may give rise to secondary coeliac syndrome. Although impaired xylose absorption, partial villous atrophy, and sometimes steatorrhoea occurs, thereby resembling coeliac disease, there is not usually a response to gluten withdrawal, but the condition resolves with successful treatment of the underlying cause. In most instances malabsorption is not clinically significant.

The relationship of malignancy and malabsorption is of great interest. Lymphoma, usually affecting the distal jejunum and ileum, should always be considered when malabsorption presents for the first time in middle or late life. Of greater interest still is the finding of localized areas of lymphoma in the jejunum (an unusual site) or small bowel carcinomas (even more unusual) in association with long-standing coeliac disease, particularly when it has not been treated by gluten withdrawal. This possibility should always be considered if there is a sudden unexplained deterioration in a previously well-controlled patient with long-standing coeliac disease. It also suggests that all such patients should be treated with a gluten-free diet however mild their symptoms may be. Infections superimposed on underlying mucosal disease like latent gluten enteropathy may bring it to clinical notice or may in their own right cause diarrhoea with malabsorption. Giardiasis has for long been such an agent. The increasing number of immuno-compromised patients as a result of HIV infection or cytotoxic treatment may allow other pathogens to flourish, such as the protozoa *Cryptosporidium* or *Isospora belli* and *Mycobacterium avium intracellulare*. Despite a high index of suspicion it is frequently impossible to identify the presumed pathogen in AIDS patients and treatment is accordingly very difficult.

CLINICAL PROBLEM

T	P	BP	R
37·2	90	90/40	22

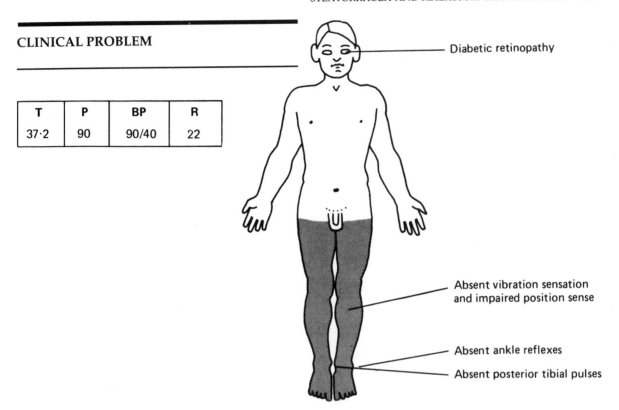

Diabetic retinopathy

Absent vibration sensation
and impaired position sense

Absent ankle reflexes

Absent posterior tibial pulses

A 42-year-old accountant was admitted from the diabetic clinic for investigation. In the previous 3 months he had become impotent and had also noticed dizziness on getting out of bed. He had been very happily married for 15 years. There had been no previous sexual problems and he had had intercourse once or twice weekly over the previous 10 years. He had also recently experienced episodes of diarrhoea, which began suddenly, often at night, and lasted for 3 to 4 days.

For the past year he had complained of epigastric discomfort, distension and nausea after food, which had responded to an alkali mixture from his GP. During this time he had also had episodes of angina, which usually occurred when he was hurrying for his morning train. Although he had not altered his diet he had recently lost 4 kg in weight. He had found his diabetes more difficult to control, having experienced hypoglycaemic episodes in the early morning, while he had noticed occasional heavy glycosuria after meals.

He had developed diabetes 14 years previously at the age of 28. For most of this time he had taken 16 units soluble and 32 units protamine zinc insulin each morning. There was no family history of diabetes. He had healthy twin sons aged 12.

His only other past illness had been an attack of mumps parotitis at the age of 26. This had been an unpleasant attack associated with right-sided orchitis, and severe epigastric pain. There had later been atrophy of the affected testis.

His job was a secure one, and he enjoyed his work. He was financially very successful and he had had no recent domestic worries.

On examination he had a pulse of 90/min, regular. The posterior tibial pulses were absent in both legs, the skin of the legs being cool and dry to the touch. The blood pressure was 110/60 lying and 90/40 standing. The fundi showed bilateral blot haemorrhages, while hard exudates were seen at the periphery. In the nervous system the ankle reflexes were absent, and the plantar responses were flexor. There was loss of vibration sense below the hips, with some impairment of position sense in the feet.

Urinanalysis showed 2% glucose and 200 mg/l albumin. The stools were unformed, clay-coloured and greasy. Laboratory analysis of a 3-day collection taken shortly after a recent episode of diarrhoea showed a faecal fat loss of 10.5 g/day.

QUESTIONS

1. What is the likely cause for his symptoms over the past three months?
2. What is the relevance of his past history of mumps to his present illness?
3. What further investigations would you undertake?
4. What treatment would you recommend?

DISCUSSION

Not all of this man's symptoms can be attributed to malabsorption, some being due to the underlying diabetes. There are several clues as to the cause of the steatorrhoea.

If a patient has diabetes this suggests he may have disease of the pancreas. If steatorrhoea is also present then the exocrine as well as the endocrine function may well be affected. The usual sequence of events is nearly always that malabsorption develops some time before the diabetes. Furthermore, a history of chronic pancreatitis, often presenting with acute recurrent attacks, is usually obtained, though cases of painless chronic pancreatitis are described. In this patient diabetes antedated steatorrhoea by nearly 14 years.

This patient's history strongly suggests that during an attack of mumps 16 years ago he suffered from acute pancreatitis. Although pancreatitis due to mumps may be associated with transient glycosuria it is very doubtful whether it is ever a cause of chronic pancreatitis, with the development of permanent exocrine and endocrine deficiencies. Sterility, which should not be confused with impotence, may occur with bilateral orchitis but this was not the case here. His past history of mumps is therefore not relevant to his present illness.

This patient, like many diabetics, has evidence of accelerated vascular disease in his symptom of angina and the finding of absent foot pulses. It is becoming increasingly recognized that mesenteric ischaemia may occur in such a setting. This is an important condition to detect as in a proportion of patients the state of chronic insufficiency is a prelude to the more catastrophic and lethal small bowel infarction. Post-prandial discomfort with repeatedly negative barium meal examinations of the stomach and duodenum often occurs in this syndrome. The patient learns by experience that smaller meals cause less pain, and as a result may consequently lose weight. Sometimes the mesenteric ischaemia causes malabsorption, but this is usually not gross. It would not, however, explain the episodic and nocturnal nature of this patient's diarrhoea.

With evidence of retinopathy and nephropathy it is very likely that neuropathy, the remaining member of the triad of diabetic complications, is present. Peripheral nerve involvement would explain his absent ankle reflexes and loss of vibration and position sense, while autonomic neuropathy would explain his impotence, his postural hypotension (the cause of his dizziness), and his cold dry legs.

There is a well-recognized association between autonomic neuropathy and diarrhoea. The diarrhoea frequently occurs episodically and, for ill-understood reasons, nocturnally. It has been shown that gut motility is impaired by the autonomic neuropathy, giving rise to stagnation in the small intestine and its colonization by bacteria. This in turn gives rise to the contaminated bowel syndrome described above. Gastric atony with delay in emptying and vomiting may also occur. In the presence of a diabetic peripheral neuropathy it would be unnecessary to invoke vitamin B_{12} deficiency as a cause for this patient's signs in the legs but it should, none the less, be excluded.

Despite further investigations it may not be possible to make the diagnosis of contaminated bowel with absolute certainty. The autonomic neuropathy could be confirmed by the lack of response of pulse and blood pressure to Valsalva's manoeuvre. Barium meal and follow-through might show evidence of stasis and dilatation of loops of small intestine and possibly of the stomach. Aspiration and culture of small intestinal contents is a difficult procedure and the screening test of urinary indican estimation is frequently within normal limits. A vitamin B_{12} absorption test and a serum folic acid should be done.

The response to therapy would also be of diagnostic value. Improvement in the symptoms and steatorrhoea after a 5-day course of a broad-spectrum antibiotic such as tetracycline would be expected.

> The presence of an autonomic neuropathy was confirmed. He was able to curtail subsequent episodes of diarrhoea by courses of antibiotics.

15. Jaundice

The differential diagnosis of jaundice embraces the whole of liver disease. The majority of patients who present with jaundice can usually be placed into the categories of obstructive, hepatocellular or haemolytic jaundice on the basis of history, examination and bedside tests of urine and stools. More sophisticated tests may be necessary to diagnose the precise cause within these categories, but the greatest problem is the minority of jaundiced patients whose illness obstinately refuses to follow textbook descriptions. In the production of jaundice more than one mechanism may be responsible. The 'pharmaceutical explosion' of recent years has produced its own considerable problems, since drugs can produce nearly all the different patterns of jaundice, and probably account for at least 10% of patients presenting to hospital with jaundice.

BILIRUBIN METABOLISM

The correct clinical approach to jaundice must be based on an understanding of bilirubin metabolism (see Figs. 15.1 and 15.2).

The first step in the production of bilirubin is the breakdown of red blood cells by the reticulo-endothelial system to release haem and produce unconjugated (prehepatic) bilirubin. This is relatively water insoluble and when estimated in the serum requires the addition of alcohol as a solvent before it will react with the diazo dye used in the van den Bergh reaction. This addition of alcohol is the basis of the indirect van den Bergh reaction. Any cause of increased haemolysis may cause jaundice but because of its water insolubility, unconjugated bilirubin will

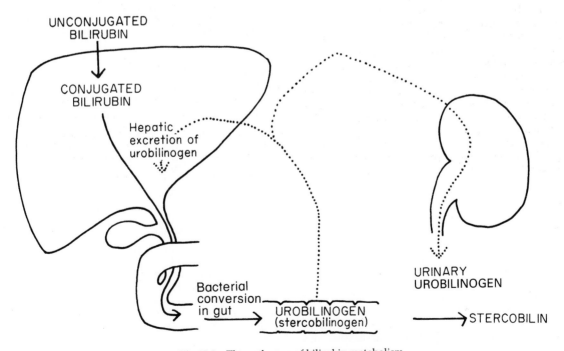

Fig.15.1 The pathways of bilirubin metabolism

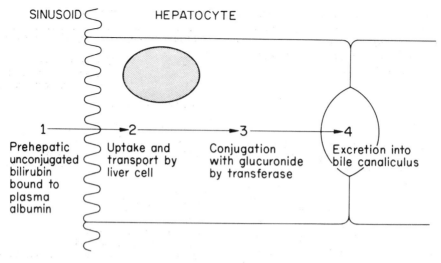

Fig. 15.2   The metabolism of bilirubin in the liver cell

not appear in the urine and haemolytic jaundice is therefore termed acholuric. Conjugated bilirubin on the other hand is water soluble and therefore will react directly with the dye in the van den Bergh test and will appear in the urine. Conjugated hyperbilirubinaemia occurs in all forms of obstructive jaundice.

The unconjugated bilirubin is transported in the blood bound to the plasma proteins, especially albumin. If it is displaced from its protein binding sites it has an affinity for lipids and may be taken up by the brain. Certain drugs such as sulphonamides and salicylates may interfere with protein binding. In the newborn, where a 'physiological' jaundice may occur due to immaturity of the conjugating enzymes of the liver, administration of these drugs may sometimes precipitate or exacerbate such jaundice and cause kernicterus.

The next steps are uptake of bilirubin by the liver cells and transportation to the endoplasmic reticulum, which is the site of the enzyme glucuronyl transferase. Here bilirubin is conjugated with glucuronide to form conjugated, water-soluble (post-hepatic) bilirubin. Defects in these steps occur in the congenital hyperbilirubinaemias, of which the commonest is Gilbert's disease. Inheritance of this condition is by an autosomal dominant character. The defect is chiefly one of uptake of unconjugated bilirubin by the liver cell but occasionally conjugation itself is impaired. When this is the case, production of the enzyme glucuronyl transferase can be induced by phenobarbitone. Male fern, once used in the treatment of tapeworm infestation, may interfere with transport of bilirubin to the endoplasmic reticulum, and novobiocin with its conjugation and cause jaundice.

The conjugated bilirubin is then concentrated in the liver cell and excreted into the canaliculus and thence into the larger branches of the biliary tree. The

hereditary defect associated with failure of excretion is the Dubin–Johnson type of hyperbilirubinaemia characterized by brownish-black pigmentation of the liver, probably due to melanin. Cholecystographic media compete with conjugated bilirubin and therefore will not be concentrated in the presence of excess bilirubin or, conversely, may precipitate jaundice. Methyl testosterone jaundice (and that due to other oral C 17 alkyl-substituted testosterone compounds) is due to impaired canalicular excretion of bilirubin. This is a dose-related phenomenon unlike the hypersensitivity type of intrahepatic cholestasis seen in susceptible patients taking phenothiazines.

Virtually all the conjugated bilirubin is excreted into the gut, where it is converted to stercobilinogen and then to stercobilin. Some of the former is reabsorbed from the gut and mostly re-excreted into the bile, while a small amount is excreted into the urine as urinary urobilinogen. The inability of the liver cell to re-excrete sterobilinogen, with its appearance as excess urinary urobilinogen, is a simple but sensitive test of liver function. It is also of considerable diagnostic value in jaundice. In the presence of total obstruction from whatever cause, urobilinogen must disappear from the urine since no bile is passing into the gut. In viral hepatitis there may be excess urinary urobilinogen in the early stage, due to liver cell damage. If, in viral hepatitis, a phase of intrahepatic cholestasis supervenes, urobilinogen will disappear from the urine and reappear when the cholestasis subsides. In obstructive jaundice pale stools are due to the absence of bile pigments, whereas they may be darker than usual with the excess production of sterobilinogen in haemolytic jaundice. Continuing complete obstruction with prolonged absence of urinary urobilinogen suggests a carcinoma of the head of the pancreas, since a stone impacted in the common bile duct will usually allow some bile to escape into the gut. Daily examination and recording of the stool appearance and urine urobilinogen are therefore simple but important measures in both the diagnosis and prognosis of jaundice.

TYPES OF JAUNDICE

Cholestatic jaundice

The differential diagnosis between extra- and intra-hepatic causes of cholestasis is greatly facilitated by early upper abdominal ultrasound imaging looking for evidence of dilatation of intra- and extrahepatic bile ducts (remembering that it takes a few days after the appearance of jaundice for this to occur).

A. Extrahepatic. Not every patient with gallstones will be fat, female, fair, fertile and forty. A family history of cholelithiasis may be obtained. A preceding history of flatulent dyspepsia may culminate in an attack of central abdominal pain, not always colicky, or right upper quadrant pain radiating to the scapula. Vomiting is a common feature. Fever is not invariable and, if pronounced, may indicate cholangitis. With the jaundice there is often pruritus due to retention of bile salts (see Fig. 14.1, page 102). Examination usually reveals tenderness in the epigastrium and over the gallbladder. Dark urine and pale stools are the hallmark of obstructive jaundice. A neutrophil leucocytosis and raised sedimentation rate are due to the associated cholangitis. Apart from the raised direct-reacting bilirubin, the serum alkaline phosphatase will be disproportionately raised with respect to the transaminase which may indeed be normal.

If the obstruction were not relieved, biliary cirrhosis might eventually develop. An earlier complication is acute cholangitis due to ascending infection of the bile ducts. This renders the mucosa oedematous, making the obstruction complete. Bouts of fever with rigors ensure and septicaemia, usually due to *E. coli*, may occur. This syndrome of Charcot's intermittent biliary fever is more likely to occur after previous biliary tract surgery, when it may be due either to stricture formation or to residual calculi.

Carcinoma of the head of the pancreas is a rather loose term embracing carcinoma of the ampulla of Vater, the lower end of the bile duct, or of the acini of the pancreas. In its diagnosis and differentiation from gallstone obstruction there are several helpful pointers and investigations:

1. Patients are more often male and over 50 years old.

2. Onset is insidious, often with weight loss and malaise preceding the onset of jaundice. The jaundice progresses steadily, compared with the more acute and intermittent pattern seen with gallstones.

3. Contrary to older textbook description, pain is a common feature and is often felt in the back; it may result in the patient adopting a hunched position or

Table 15.1   Causes of jaundice

Prehepatic unconjugated hyperbilirubinaemia
Haemolysis
Congenital defects: Gilbert's syndrome
(uptake/conjugation defect)
Crigler– Najar (conjugation defect)

Hepatocellular jaundice
Acute
Viral hepatitis A, B, C, D NANB
Other viruses: glandular fever, cytomegalovirus
Drugs – dose-dependent, e.g. paracetamol
– idiosyncratic: numerous, e.g. halothane
Toxins
Autoimmune hepatitis
Alcoholic 'hepatitis'

Chronic
Chronic viral hepatitis (B, C)
Chronic autoimmune hepatitis
End-stage liver disease : cirrhosis of any cause
alcoholic
hepatitis B/C
autoimmune
haemochromatosis
Wilson's disease

Cholestatic jaundice
A Extrahepatic obstruction of biliary tree
Gallstones
Carcinoma of head of pancreas
Benign (usually postoperative) stricture
Carcinoma of ampulla of Vater or bile ducts
Sclerosing cholangitis

B Intrahepatic
Drugs: numerous, e.g. chlopromazine
Primary biliary cirrhosis
Cholestatic phase of viral hepatitis
Alcohol: acute fatty infiltration–'alcoholic' hepatitis
Primary and secondary cancer
Lymphoma
Pregnancy

sitting bent over the bed. The pain is not colicky. Pruritus may occur.

4. Examination may reveal an enlarged gallbladder in half the patients, although present at laparotomy in three-quarters.

5. An associated thrombophlebitis may occur in the adjacent splenic vein, resulting in congestive splenomegaly. A remote effect is the occurrence of thrombophlebitis elsewhere in the body.

6. There may be evidence of metastases such as an enlarged left supraclavicular gland of Virchow.

7. Stools may contain occult blood, in addition to showing pallor due to obstruction. Their fat content may be raised although clinical steatorrhoea is uncommon and most of the patient's weight loss is attributable to the cancer.

8. In addition to the persistent absence of urinary urobilinogen, glycosuria may be present.

9. Pancreatic scanning by ultrasound or CT scan may show a mass in the head of the pancreas rather than gallstones, as well as confirming the presence of dilated bile ducts. It may also reveal liver metastases.

10. Contrast radiology includes ERCP (endoscopic retrograde cholangiopancreatography) in which the pancreatic ducts may be visualized and be distorted by tumour, and the common bile duct, if visualized, may enable a distinction to be made between tumour and gallstones. The endoscopic examination will show a carcinoma of the ampulla of Vater. Percutaneous transhepatic cholangiography is more hazardous but is more likely to visualize the biliary tract.

With these diagnostic advances it is unusual to have to perform a laparotomy to make a diagnosis.

B. Intrahepatic As the causes of intrahepatic cholestasis are often initially obscure even after history, examination and simple tests, it is sometimes desirable to perform liver biopsy. Provided duct dilatation has been excluded by ultrasound, clotting is normal, or has been corrected by parenteral vitamin K, the platelet count is greater than 50 000 and the patient can cooperate in breath-holding, the procedure should be safe. A typical biopsy appearance of intrahepatic cholestasis with an eosinophilic and mononuclear portal zone reaction and some liver cell degeneration may be due to drug hypersensitivity, and could prevent an unnecessary laparotomy.

Hypersensitivity to phenothiazine, chlorpropamide, thiouracil, or phenylbutazone is the commonest cause of intrahepatic cholestatis. It can occur several weeks after stopping the drug and even after a single dose. There may be a rash, fever and eosinophilia accompanying the obstructive jaundice. Though usually self-limiting, obstructive features may persist for months or even years, closely resembling primary biliary cirrhosis. Hypercholesterolaemia, xanthoma formation and secondary malabsorption from bile salt deficiency could than develop, and histological differentiation may be impossible. The mitochondrial immunofluorescence test (where the antibody is directed against pyruvate dehydrogenase in the mitochondrial membrane) could then be positive in most patients with primary biliary cirrhosis and will differentiate it from prolonged drug cholestasis. Apart from the cholestatic phase of viral hepatitis and acute alcoholic hepatitis mentioned below, the other rare causes of intrahepatic cholestasis are cholangiocarcinoma and sclerosing cholangitis when confined to the intrahepatic bile ducts.

Hepatocellular jaundice

Viral hepatitis is the commonest cause. The clinical presentation of types A and B is very similar. Glandular fever and cytomegalovirus (CMV) may also cause hepatitis. A history of recent contacts of injections of any type must always be sought as well as sexual contacts and transfusion of blood or blood products. In all forms of hepatitis, the presenting symptoms are similar with a flu-like illness, fever, sore throat, malaise, depression, loss of libido and taste for alcohol and tobacco. The disappearance of fever heralds the arrival of jaundice which rapidly deepens. Bilirubinuria, which may have preceded overt jaundice, increases, but urobilinogen may disappear from the urine if cholestatis develops. The stools initially are not pale. Liver tenderness and slight enlargement is a common finding but spontaneous pain does not occur. The spleen may be moderately enlarged.

If, instead of the usual pattern of recovery beginning in the second week of the illness, jaundice, pyurexia, and malaise persist, the illness may be entering the phase of chronic hepatitis. This carries a bad prognosis, for as liver cell failure progresses, splenomegaly appears and either cirrhosis develops, sometimes with portal hypertension, or death occurs from liver failure. All these complicated forms of hepatitis are more commonly seen with type B hepatitis and in middle-aged women, in whom the prognosis must therefore always be guarded. Laboratory investigations usually give strong support to the diagnosis. There is no leucocytosis, but a relative lymphocytosis with atypical morphology (viral lymphocytes) is seen. Alkaline phosphatase is usually only slightly raised whereas the transaminase is markedly elevated. The gamma globulins rise and, if the illness is prolonged, the albumin falls.

Diagnostic difficulty also arises if the complication of cholestasis develops, with the stool and urine changes previously mentioned, together with equivocal biochemical tests. The possibility is that an atypical painless cause of 'surgical' extrahepatic obstruction responsible for the jaundice is being missed. Ultrasound examination would be the next step, preceding either liver biopsy or visualization of the biliary tract by contrast radiography as discussed above. Serological tests for hepatitis B and C are helpful, though hepatitis A never progresses to chronic hepatitis or cirrhosis.

The most dangerous dose-related drug cause of hepatocellular jaundice is paracetamol poisoning. When presentation is delayed, preventing the use of acetylcysteine as antidote, the condition may progress to fulminant hepatic failure and death.

Drug hypersensitivity may cause a hepatitis indistinguishable from the viral type. The hydrazine derivatives such as the monoamine oxidase inhibitors used in the treatment of depression are notorious in this respect and have resulted in fatalities. The incidence is, fortunately, low. The anti-TB drugs isoniazid and pyrazinamide (which are also hydrazines), ethionamide and anaesthetic halothane are other idiosyncratic causes.

Direct hepatotoxicity related to dose occurs with carbon tetrachloride, this having been extensively studied in experimental animals. Other causes include cytotoxic drugs, large doses of tetracycline, especially in pregnancy, and overdoses of metals such as iron.

Cirrhosis is only accompanied by jaundice as a late and serious manifestation of the disease. An exception is primary biliary cirrhosis where jaundice is present before advanced liver failure. In cirrhosis the presence of jaundice indicates that there is little hepatic reserve and is therefore usually found in conjunction with other signs of liver failure: ascites and oedema, hepatic precoma or chronic encephalopathy, and portal hypertension. There may be an acute cause for the deterioration of liver function such as gastrointestinal haemorrhage from a peptic ulcer or varices, a drinking bout in an alcoholic, or injudicious drug therapy.

Acute alcoholic hepatitis typically occurs in an alcoholic without previous symptoms of liver disease, who suddenly develops a large tender liver, jaundice, and ascites. Although the liver shows fatty infiltration, the damage is reversible and need not progress to cirrhosis. The jaundice, curiously, may have the features of obstructive rather than hepatocellular jaundice.

Chronic active hepatitis occurs in young, often obese and hirsute women, and may progress imperceptibly to cirrhosis over months or several years. It is characterized by gross elevation of gamma globulin (above 40 g/l). The involvement of other systems such as skin, joints, pleura and, rarely, kidneys suggests an autoimmune mechanism. These features do not however warrant the misleading name of lupoid hepatitis. Smooth muscle antibodies and ANF are usually present.

Haemolytic jaundice

The presenting symptom is rarely jaundice. Symptoms are due more often to the underlying cause, the rate of haemolysis, or the degree of anaemia. The degree of haemolysis may vary from the lemon yellow tinge of an elderly patient presenting with pernicious anaemia, to a severe haemolytic crisis precipitated by drugs or broad beans (favism) in a patient with an inherited red cell deficiency of glucose-6-phosphate dehydrogenase (G6PD). In these more severe episodes there may be malaise, fever, headache, aching pains in the limbs, and sometimes, collapse. If the haemolytic process is chronic there may be splenomegaly and pigment stones in the gallbladder, which might give rise to the further complication of obstructive jaundice. The stools are dark, due to excess stercobilin, but the urine, although containing excess urobilinogen, is normal macroscopically. Rarely, haemolysis is so great that haemoglobinuria occurs, darkening the urine (as in blackwater fever due to falciparum malaria). Apart from the raised indirect reacting bilirubin, other liver function tests may be normal. The blood picture shows a normocytic normochromic anaemia with reticulocytosis and immature red blood cells.

Important hereditary causes include hereditary spherocytosis, G6PD deficiency, and haemoglobin disorders such as sickle cell disease and thalasaemia.

Acquired causes include the idiopathic autoimmune type of haemolytic anaemia and that associated with collagen diseases and chronic lymphatic leukaemia. Rhesus incompatibility in the newborn and mismatched transfusion at any age can produce severe jaundice. Drugs such as phenylhydrazine may have a direct lytic effect. Others such as methyl dopa may initiate an autoimmune reaction, while primaquine may expose an underlying G6PD deficiency, a condition particularly common in Negroes.

CLINICAL PROBLEM

T	P	BP	R
38·4	64	120/70	24

Jaundice

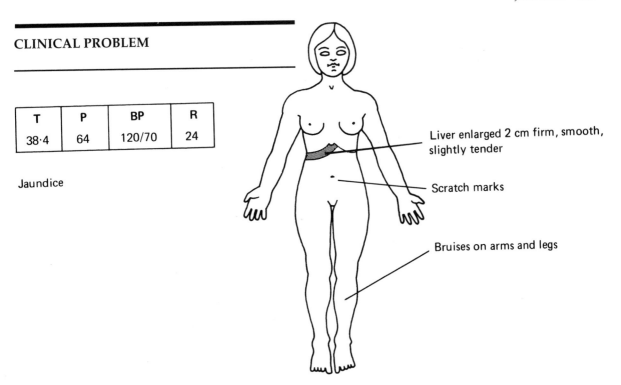

Liver enlarged 2 cm firm, smooth, slightly tender

Scratch marks

Bruises on arms and legs

A 55-year-old divorced secretary was admitted to hospital with a history of increasing jaundice for 4 weeks. She had noticed that her urine had become darker and that her stools had become pale during this time. Over the past 3 months she had had a poor appetite and had lost 7 kg in weight. Apart from some flatulent dyspepsia, especially after fatty food, she had not had any abdominal pain. There had been no fever.

She had a long history of psychiatric problems since the age of 30. She had suffered from depression and anxiety with bouts of heavy drinking. She had had two admissions to psychiatric hospitals and also had been admitted to a general hospital after an overdose of barbiturates. She had been treated with a variety of psychotropic drugs in the past and for the last 4 months had been prescribed phenelzine and trifluoperazine for agitated depression. She smoked 30 cigarettes per day.

On examination she was jaundiced and had obviously lost weight. The skin showed scratch marks on the trunk and several bruises over the arms and legs for which she could not account. No lymph nodes were palpable and the respiratory, cardiovascular and central nervous systems were normal. In the abdomen the liver could be felt 2 cm below the right costal margin. It was firm and smooth with a regular edge and only slightly tender. The spleen and gallbladder were not palpable and ascites could not be detected. Pelvic examination was normal. The urine contained bilirubin but urobilinogen was absent.

QUESTIONS

1. What are the likely diagnoses?
2. What investigations would you undertake to establish the diagnosis?
3. What would be your further management?

DISCUSSION

The patient has the features of obstructive jaundice with bilirubin but no urobilinogen in the urine, and pale stools. The presence of scratch marks, even though the patient has not complained of itching, is in keeping with cholestasis.

The insidious painless onset and steady progression together with the preceding ill-health is unlike the history of gallstone obstruction of the common bile duct. Various other causes of extrahepatic and intrahepatic cholestasis must be considered. Carcinoma of the head of the pancreas is a likely cause and would account for the preceding weight loss. Other forms of cancer may cause obstructive jaundice due to metastases in the lymph nodes of the porta hepatis pressing on the main hepatic ducts, or to secondary deposits within the liver. The latter would probably result in greater, more irregular, and possibly more painful enlargement of the liver than is present here. Primary sites to be considered would be stomach, bowel, bronchus or breast. In Western Europeans hepatomas invariably occur only after a lengthy history of cirrhosis. Although there is a history of alcoholism in this patient there are no stigmata of chronic liver disease (spider naevi, palmar erythema, parotid swelling or Dupuytren's contracture) to suggest cirrhosis. Furthermore, obstructive jaundice is not a common early feature in the development of a hepatoma. Carcinoma of the bile duct is rare but presents in much the same way as a carcinoma of the head of the pancreas.

The drug history of this patient could be relevant. Phenelzine is a monoamine oxidase inhibitor which may cause jaundice; this however is hepatocellular rather than obstructive. Trifluoperazine is a phenothiazine and may cause intrahepatic cholestasis. The illness preceding the jaundice makes drug cholestasis unlikely. The duration and progression of the jaundice seen here is not usual in phenothiazine jaundice but can occur and lead to difficulty in distinguishing it from primary biliary cirrhosis. This latter condition occurs particularly in middle-aged women and is characterized by intense pruritus, xanthomata of skin and tendons, and pigmentation of the skin in addition to jaundice.

Infective hepatitis may take a complicated course in middle-aged women and a cholestatic phase may develop. A prodromal illness of 2 months before the appearance of jaundice is rather lengthy.

The purpose of investigation is first to confirm that the jaundice is primarily obstructive rather than hepatocellular and then to establish the site of obstruction. When jaundice has been present for 4 weeks the biochemical pattern may not be clear-cut, as hepatocellular damage can supervene as a result of obstruction. However, if the liver alkaline phosphatase is proportionally more raised than the transaminase, the jaundice is more likely to be obstructive. The gamma glutamyl transpeptidase will also be raised in obstructive jaundice and more elevated than the alkaline phosphatase if the jaundice is due to alcoholic liver disease. The prothrombin time will also be prolonged but should be correctable with parenteral vitamin K if there is no significant hepatocellular damage. Hepatitis B should be excluded by looking for the surface antigen (HB_sAg). Mitochondrial antibodies and other non-organ specific antibodies might be found in primary biliary cirrhosis or the less likely autoimmune chronic active hepatitis and a high titre of alpha-fetoprotein would suggest a hepatoma.

A chest X-ray should always be done to look for bronchial carcinoma and bone secondaries. The next investigation should be ultrasound scanning of the liver, pancreas and biliary tree; alternatively a CT scan would serve a similar purpose but is less readily available and more expensive. These tests should determine whether the cholestasis is extrahepatic. If the biliary tree is not dilated the cause is likely to be intrahepatic and liver biopsy to determine its cause will be a relatively safe procedure. If the ultrasound shows dilated bile ducts it may also suggest the cause of extrahepatic cholestasis by revealing gallstones or an abnormal pancreas. Contrast radiology either by ERCP or transhepatic percutaneous cholangiography would be the next and, probably, final step before laparotomy. An alternative palliative treatment to be considered in a carcinoma of the head of pancreas would be the endoscopic placement of a stent through the obstructed lower common bile duct.

The patient came to laparotomy and was found to have a carcinoma of the head of the pancreas. Adjacent lymph nodes were involved and a liver secondary was present. A choledochojejunostomy and gastrojejunostomy were performed.

16. Swelling of the abdomen

Many patients who present with the complaint of abdominal distension are describing a symptom rather than a visible or measurable physical sign. Such a feeling of bloatedness is a common feature in the acid–ulcer–dyspepsia syndrome and in irritable bowel syndrome (IBS). The patient has a great desire to belch which may give him a certain amount of relief. Sometimes he will swallow air repeatedly to provoke eructation in the hope of achieving this. However, there is little evidence that distension of the stomach by gas is the true cause of the discomfort experienced. Although it is rightly unfashionable to attribute too many symptoms to spasm, this would none the less seem to be the relevant factor. The patient's insistence that his abdomen visibly swells after meals, necessitating loosening of garments, is not usually confirmed by examination. The associated symptoms of pain, relieved by food or antacids, and perhaps heart burn, should help to eliminate this as a cause of the symptom of abdominal distension.

Paradoxically, many patients exhibiting the physical signs of abdominal swelling may have few symptoms directly caused by it. Unless the swelling is great or rapid they may not even be aware of it.

Whilst the old adage of swelling of the abdomen being due to fat, fluid, fetus, faeces, or flatus provides a starting point in differential diagnosis, it will be necessary to consider the causes and their differentiation in greater detail. The need for careful examination of the abdomen under ideal conditions of relaxation in the fully flat position cannot be sufficiently emphasized. This must be combined with a full general examination which may reveal important clues to the underlying causes – for example anaemia, jaundice, lymphadenopathy or congestive cardiac failure. A well known diagnostic trap is the patient with constrictive pericarditis. This is insidious in its onset and may present with abdominal swelling due to ascites. The jugular venous pressure may be so greatly elevated that its upper border is lost behind the angle of the jaw and it is therefore overlooked.

Gaseous distension

Having previously discussed the symptom of distension, one must consider it as a physical sign.

Whatever the cause of gaseous distension there is usually swelling of the whole abdomen. In thin people loops of bowel may be discerned and percussion of the abdomen will give a resonant note.

In malabsorption syndrome, particularly coeliac disease (gluten enteropathy) in children, a pot belly appearance is characteristic. This is pronounced when standing, probably because associated protein malnutrition and, perhaps, electrolyte deficiency, cause weakness and hypotonia of the abdominal wall musculature. The similar appearance in starvation and Kwashiorkor is an all too familiar appearance when famine strikes in an underdeveloped country. As discussed in Ch.14 – Steatorrhoea and Malabsorption Syndrome – there will be other important clues in a patient with malabsorption syndrome, such as a history of frequent, soft, bulky, pale, greasy offensive stools and weight loss, together with such deficiency disorders as anaemia or metabolic bone disease.

Distension of the abdomen due to obstruction of large or small bowel is an acute surgical emergency and will be dominated by other symptoms of pain, vomiting and absence of stool or flatus. If diagnosis is delayed, signs of localized or generalized peritonitis develop. The various causes will be revealed by the ensuing laparotomy. Plain abdominal X-rays in erect and supine positions will confirm the presence of gas and fluid levels. Intestinal obstruction should always be considered in the elderly patient with gaseous abdominal distension, even if the other features are not prominent.

Fat

Excess adipose tissue both in the subcutaneous layers of the abdominal wall and in the mesentery does not require detailed description. The dependent Falstaffian paunch is an all too common feature of overfed western society. Sometimes fat is deposited selectively in the trunk and abdomen as in Cushing's syndrome or in patients receiving long-term steroid therapy. Such abdominal swelling associated with a moon face is in contrast with the spindly limbs caused by muscle wasting as a result of enhanced protein catabolism. Rapid fat deposition leads to stretching of the skin with the appearance of striae in flanks and thighs. When due to steroids the striae are livid or pigmented, whereas this is not the case in simple obesity. Additional physical signs of steroid excess such as acne, hirsutism, dorsal fat pad giving a buffalo hump, osteoporosis perhaps causing vertebral collapse, and kyphosis will support the diagnosis.

The main problem presented by fat is that it may be confused with other causes of abdominal swelling. The sheer amount of fat present makes percussion of the abdomen unreliable and palpation uncertain.

Solid swellings

Every pathological museum contains some tumours impressive for their size alone. In life these rarely present great diagnostic problems. Large solid swellings are usually due to enlargement of an organ which is normally present and will conform to the physical signs associated with that organ.

Gross splenomegaly may present as a dragging sensation in the left half of the abdomen with a superficial mass moving downwards and medially on inspiration. Palpation confirms the presence of a firm mass with sharp borders and a notch on the medial aspect. The upper border cannot be defined. It will be dull to percussion. Because of its size it may, unlike a moderately enlarged spleen, be palpable bimanually, sharing this sign with an enlarged kidney. Gross splenomegaly in the UK is usually due to the myeloproliferative disorders – myelosclerosis (myelofibrosis) and chronic myeloid leukemia. A blood count will be the next important step, showing a leuco-erythroblastic anaemia in the case of myelosclerosis or an anaemia with neutrophil leucocytosis with some immature cells in chronic myeloid leukemia. Disorders of the reticuloendothelial system, particularly giant follicular lymphoma and less commonly Hodgkin's disease, may cause similar gross enlargement of the spleen. Here there will usually be associated lymph node enlargement and biopsy of one of these will be necessary to establish the diagnosis. In tropical countries additional causes such as kala-azar and chronic malaria would have to be considered. The latter is probably the cause of big spleen disease described in Africa, where there may be considerable difficulty in demonstrating the parasite in the peripheral blood.

Gross hepatomegaly will be confirmed by percussion and palpation. A malignant cause due to secondary or primary cancer is most likely. The latter, a hepatoma, is found increasingly as a terminal complication of cirrhosis of all aetiologies. The coexistent cirrhosis may, in turn, give rise to signs of hepatocellular dysfunction. These include palmar erythema, leuconychia, spider naevi, skin pigmentation, gynaecomastia and testicular atrophy, parotid swelling and Dupuytren's contractures. Hepatomas may rapidly

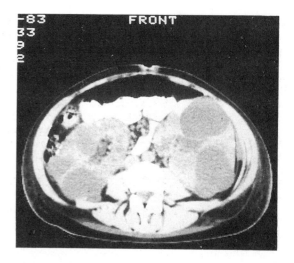

Fig. 16.1 Transverse CT scan of lower abdomen with oral contrast showing grossly enlarged kidneys with rounded areas of different attenuation. The diagnosis was polycystic disease. (Courtesy of Dr Hakhamaneshi).

reach a large size, giving rise to pain, tenderness and modular enlargement of the liver. The same blood and reticuloendothelial disorders as cause gross splenomegaly may similarly affect the liver.

The commonest cause of uterine enlargement is, of course, pregnancy. The history of amenorrhoea may have been withheld, but the associated breast changes cannot be suppressed. The swelling will arise from the pelvis and should be confirmed by vaginal examination. Fibroids may assume huge proportions, and are then prone to develop complications of torsion or haemorrhage. Menorrhagia is a frequent accompaniment. Again bimanual pelvic examination should confirm the diagnosis.

The only likely cause of huge kidneys presenting as abdominal swelling is polycystic disease. Although both kidneys are involved they are frequently asymmetrical (Fig. 16.1). They are bimanually palpable, move downwards on inspiration and may be resonant to percussion because of overlying bowel.

Rarely, large retroperitoneal tumours such as dermoids, sometimes undergoing sarcomatous change, cause swelling of the abdomen. Retroperitoneal lymph node enlargement due to lymphosarcoma, may present similarly. It is particularly important to examine the testes for a primary site of a tumour giving rise to retroperitoneal metastases.

Fluid swellings

This category resolves itself into the differentiation of fluid-containing swellings, such as an enlarged bladder, ovarian or pancreatic cyst, from fluid in the peritoneal cavity. Having detected ascites, its cause must then be determined.

Cystic swellings, as they enlarge, will tend to adopt a central abdominal position irrespective of their site of origin. The two common sites are ovarian and pancreatic. Ovarian cysts can assume large sizes without causing symptoms and are first noticed by the patient because of increasing lower abdominal swelling. Frequently they are found accidentally on routine examination. They rise out of the pelvis, are rounded in outline and do not usually exhibit a fluid thrill or shifting dullness. They may be bimanually palpable on pelvic examination. Diagnostic confusion may be created by a distended bladder. Painless retention with overflow characteristically occurs in males with a long-standing obstruction due to prostatic enlargement. It may rarely occur in women with a neurogenic bladder due to tabes dorsalis or spina bifida.

Cysts of the pancreas most commonly occur as a complication of pancreatitis. They are usually lesser sac pseudocysts, the walls of which are formed by adjacent structures as a reaction to the released pancreatic enzymes. The development of a palpable abdominal mass some days or weeks after an attack of acute pancreatitis, sometimes associated with a re-elevation of the serum amylase or a continuing elevation of the urinary amylase, suggests the diagnosis. Abscess formation can also occur in this situation, but the patient is usually more ill and has a persistent fever and neutrophil leucocytosis. True pancreatic cysts and mesenteric cysts are much rarer and do not follow any clear-cut illness. All these pancreatic swellings occur, of course, in the upper abdomen.

The physical signs leading to a diagnosis of ascites will depend on the amount of fluid present in the peritoneal cavity. Gross ascites will cause generalized abdominal distension with bulging of the flanks and eversion of the umbilicus. There will be generalized dullness to percussion, a fluid thrill can be elicited, and the liver and spleen, even if enlarged, may not be palpable, or, perhaps, only ballotable. Abdominal wall veins may be prominent, but are not necessarily diagnostic of the underlying cause. Thus, branches of the inferior epigastric system draining normally towards the groin are often prominent. If flow is in the opposite direction it suggests the development of a collateral circulation between branches of the inferior and superior vena cavae. This is usually due to the pressure of the ascitic fluid on the IVC rather than thrombosis, since venous flow returns to normal with disappearance of the ascites. When portal hypertension is present a collateral circulation between portal and systemic venous system may develop. The veins involved are in the ligamentum teres and appear as a caput medusa; that is veins radiating from the umbilicus, or as veins in the flanks. When less ascitic fluid is present the area of dullness may be horseshoe shaped, i.e. the centre of the abdomen is resonant and the dullness can be shown to shift on turning the patient from side to side.

The differential diagnosis of abdominal swellings has been greatly aided by modern imaging techniques, particularly ultrasound scanning, which is relatively inexpensive and effective.

Causes of ascites

Ascitic fluid may be an exudate or a transudate and this is usually reflected in the protein content. Exudates may be due to malignancy, or infections due in turn to tuberculosis, E. coli or pneumococcus. Transudates are usually due to a combination of raised portal venous pressure (portal hypertension) and lowered plasma colloid osmotic pressure due to hypoalbuminaemia. Portal hypertension will usually lead to splenomegaly, but whether the liver is enlarged will depend on the underlying cause. Other mechanisms involved in the formation of a transudate are an associated increased hepatic lymph flow and sodium and water retention by the kidneys due to a hyperaldosteronism and increased antidiuretic hormone (ADH) activity. Although large amounts of fluid may be present in the abdomen, the circulating plasma volume may be low due to hypoalbuminaemia, resulting in lowered colloid osmotic pressure allowing loss of salt and water from the intravascular compartment. This will reduce renal blood flow and glomerular filtration. This, together with stimulation of postulated volume receptors, resulting in aldosterone secretion, causes sodium and water retention and potassium loss (see Ch. 3 – Oedema). Furthermore if liver function is impaired, the hepatic inactivation of aldosterone, ADH and other steroids such as oestrogens may be reduced.

The causes of transudates include:

1. Hepatic causes of portal hypertension. In the majority of cases this is due to cirrhosis of any aetiology, or fibrosis, as in schistosomiasis. An additional factor is that hepatic albumin synthesis is reduced. The liver may be shrunken (e.g. post-necrotic cirrhosis), enlarged (e.g. alcoholic portal cirrhosis) or normal sized.

2. Extrahepatic portal hypertension due to thrombosis of the portal vein. This may be due to adjacent or remote malignancy, infection, such as an ascending pyelophlebitis from an appendix abscess, or a thrombotic tendency such as in polycythaemia. The liver need not be enlarged.

3. Thrombosis of the hepatic vein (Budd–Chiari syndrome) or of its intrahepatic branches, as in veno-occlusive disease associated with drinking bush teas, first described in the West Indies. The liver will be enlarged and tender, and the patient usually jaundiced.

4. Raised systemic venous pressure transmitted back to the portal venous system. This may occur in

severe congestive cardiac failure of long standing whatever the cause. The liver will be enlarged, tender and may be pulsatile if tricuspid regurgitation is present. Constrictive pericarditis is another cause.

5. Gross hypoalbuminaemia from other causes. This is usually due to excess urinary or gut loss of protein, of which nephrotic syndrome is the most frequent cause.

Ascites with the features of an exudate can result from bacterial infection of a pre-existing transudate. The possibility of an infection is one reason for always performing a diagnostic paracentesis of 100 ml or more of fluid. The protein content of the fluid will be above 25 g/l in an exudate, and below this figure in a transudate. A transudate will usually appear clear whereas an exudate may be cloudy, turbid or blood-stained, depending on the cause. Culture for tuberculosis and pyogenic organisms should be undertaken, together with examination of the centrifuged deposit. Malignant cells may be difficult to distinguish from the normally shed peritoneal cells, but should none the less be sought. A raised white cell count in the fluid should suggest infection, and needle biopsy of the peritoneum has been shown to improve the accuracy of diagnosis of tuberculosis.

CLINICAL PROBLEM

T	P	BP	R
38·9	104	120/80	28

Spider naevi

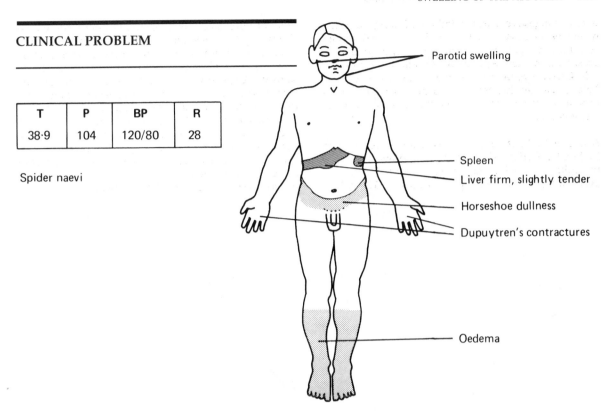

Parotid swelling

Spleen

Liver firm, slightly tender

Horseshoe dullness

Dupuytren's contractures

Oedema

A 54-year-old freelance journalist was admitted from the outpatients clinic. He was complaining of swelling of the abdomen and pain in the right upper quadrant which had come on rapidly over the previous 10 days. For the past few months, he had felt unwell, with poor appetite and a lack of desire to smoke or drink. He had also lost nearly 12 kg in weight.

He had been attending hospital intermittently for the preceding 16 years, having initially presented with jaundice and a tender enlarged liver following a prolonged alcoholic bout. He had only been partially successful in controlling his alcohol problem, and every few years would break loose with several weeks of continuous drinking. This had resulted in two further hospital admissions with jaundice, malaise and tender enlargement of the liver, which improved while in hospital. His wife had, despairingly, left him two and a half years previously. He had never before had oedema, ascites or splenomegaly. He had been gaining weight steadily over the years until at the time of his separation he weighed 89 kg. He smoked 40 cigarettes daily, and for the past 2 years some cough had been constantly present. His stools and urine appeared normal to him.

On examination, he looked ill and had a temperature of 38.9°C. This fever persisted during his hospital admission. He was not visibly jaundiced. He had bilateral ankle oedema, and there were numerous spider naevi present on the arms and chest. He had bilateral Dupuytren's contractures and parotid swelling. In the abdomen, there was ascites, as shown by swelling of the flanks with a horseshoe area of dullness. There was generalized, firm, smooth, slightly tender enlargement of the liver, the left lobe was palpated with difficulty through the rectus sheath but contained an irregular hard tender area. The spleen was felt 2 cm below the left costal margin.

Initial investigations showed HB. 12.8 g/dl with normal indices and normal appearance of red cells on the film. WBC $7.4 \times 10^9/l$ with normal differential. ESR 37 mm. Platelets: $330 \times 10^9/l$. Prothrombin time: 19 sec (control 12 sec). Serum bilirubin: 34 μmol/l. AST: 42 i.u./l (normal 2–20). Alkaline phosphatase: 300 i.u./l (normal 30–100). Serum albumin: 21 g/l. Serum globulin: 49 g/l. Electrophoretic strip showed decreased albumin and an increase in alpha-2 and gamma globulin.

QUESTIONS

1. What are the likely causes for the recent deterioration in this patient?
2. What are the possible causes of the ascites?
3. What further investigations should be performed?

DISCUSSION

There is little doubt from the history, examination and investigations that this patient has cirrhosis. The strong history of alcoholism with earlier episodes suggestive of acute alcoholic hepatitis, makes alcohol the most likely cause and the presence of Dupuytren's contractures and parotid swelling supports this diagnosis.

When deterioration in health occurs in a cirrhotic patient, the first causes to be considered are whether the cirrhosis has progressed to the stage of decompensation and whether portal hypertension has developed. Weight loss, anorexia and malaise are common, though not very specific, symptoms of advanced cirrhosis. Likewise, low grade pyrexia may be associated with decompensation. Spider naevi indicate active liver disease. A falling serum albumin concentration with rising bilirubin and transaminase levels are signs of a poor prognosis.

Two features in this patient suggest that there is more than decompensation. Abdominal pain and liver tenderness do not occur in simple cirrhosis and suggest the complication of hepatoma. The disproportionate elevation of alkaline phosphatase, in the absence of obstructive jaundice, also suggests an expanding intrahepatic lesion. Hepatoma is an increasingly common terminal event in all forms of cirrhosis, though its incidence is greatest in the relatively rare form associated with haemochromatosis.

The development of splenomegaly and ascites in a patient with cirrhosis is invariably due to portal hypertension and associated hypoalbuminaemia. Portal hypertension more commonly occurs in the macronodular type of cryptogenic or post-hepatitic (post-necrotic) cirrhosis than in the micronodular type associated with alcohol. The late development of the signs of portal hypertension in this patient, coinciding with the suspicion of a hepatoma, suggests that the block may be extrahepatic due to portal vein thrombosis, which can complicate hepatoma.

Ascites can result from a primary infective peritonitis due, for example, to tuberculosis which is more common in alcoholics. A more probable complication is secondary tuberculous infection of pre-existing ascites caused by portal hypertension. Similarly, secondary infection of ascitic fluid with Gram-negative bacteria can also occur and give rise to pyrexia. Secondary deposits in the peritoneum from either a hepatoma or a carcinoma of the bronchus, stomach or pancreas may cause malignant ascites and a tender nodular liver.

Other diseases occur more commonly in patients with cirrhosis. Pain suggests the possibility of peptic ulcer but would not explain the other features present. Gallstones are found more frequently in cirrhotics but this patient has not had biliary colic, does not have obstructive jaundice and is tender over the left lobe of the liver rather than the gallbladder. Pancreatitis is associated with alcoholism; however, this patient has not been drinking recently and although he is losing weight he does not have steatorrhoea.

Investigation is unlikely to provide much further evidence for cirrhosis since this diagnosis has already been reasonably well established. The hepatic origin of the elevated alkaline phosphatase could be confirmed by electrophoretic fractionation or by estimation of the 5-nucleotidase; the retention of bromsulphthalein will be increased and the urine will contain excess urobilinogen. Liver biopsy is the only means of making a certain diagnosis of cirrhosis, but is precluded by the prolonged prothrombin time.

The main purpose of investigation in this patient is to establish the cause of his deterioration in the hope that it may be treatable. The most direct way of diagnosing hepatoma by biopsy is also excluded by the prolonged prothrombin time. An ultrasound or CT scan would confirm a cirrhotic pattern with an area of different density corresponding to the suspected hepatoma. The presence of high levels of alpha fetoprotein in the blood is highly specific in suspected hepatoma. The ascitic fluid must be examined for its protein content, to distinguish transudate from exudate, and for malignant cells; it must also be cultured for tuberculosis and other bacteria. It would also be reasonable to perform blood cultures to exclude Gram-negative bacteraemia. At the time of diagnostic paracentesis, a peritoneal biopsy should be performed to look for TB or malignant deposits.

A chest X-ray might show either a bronchial carcinoma or tuberculosis. A gastroscopy or barium meal would probably be undertaken to look for oesophageal varices, gastric cancer or peptic ulcer.

Liver ultrasound scan confirmed the presence of a large uniform density in the left lobe of the liver; the rest of the scan was compatible with the diagnosis of cirrhosis. Alphafetoprotein was present. The ascitic fluid contained 40 g/l protein and highly atypical cells suggestive of malignancy were seen. He rapidly deteriorated over the next 5 weeks, his ascites failing to respond to treatment. A hepatoma with peritoneal involvement arising from a micronodular cirrhotic liver was found at postmortem.

17. Loss of weight

Patients often present with vague and non-specific symptoms which provide the physician with no immediate indication as to the underlying disease. The difficulty may be increased by the fact that some symptoms can often occur as a result of a purely psychological disturbance. Among such symptoms is loss of weight. In children, an equivalent abnormality is a failure to gain weight at the usual rate. It is a routine in medical history-taking to ask what the weight is, to confirm this oneself, and to assess its significance against the height and build of the patient. Even more important is to enquire whether there has been any recent change in weight. Any loss of more than 5% of the normal body weight should be considered significant and a reason sought for its occurrence. Weight loss of less than this can usually be ignored. Sometimes the patient's account of weight loss seems at variance with his appearance and it is then important to carry out regular weighings over a few weeks to confirm that progressive weight loss is actually occurring.

THE CLINICAL ASSESSMENT

Apart from the amount of weight lost it is important to know how rapidly the loss has occurred. The more rapid the loss, the more likely it is to be due to organic disease. The weight of most people, whether normal or not, remains remarkably constant at its usual level over very long periods, although in women there is commonly some fluctuation in weight with the menstrual cycle. With middle age, both men and women tend to gain weight and this is often marked in women after the menopause. Loss of weight is widely recognized as a common symptom of disease, so that even if the patient regards loss of weight as beneficial, other members of the family will regard it more seriously. This latter situation may occur in young girls, who for cosmetic reasons want to lose weight, and who may be unwilling to recognize when the weight loss has passed acceptable bounds.

In the evaluation of weight loss the most important variable to consider is appetite. If one does not eat, weight loss is inevitable – a fact some patients are unwilling to believe! Thus sometimes loss of weight can be adequately explained by a primary alteration in intake. Assessment of how much a patient is eating can, however, be difficult without an independent witness such as a spouse or parent, and on occasions even this is not sufficient. Indeed some patients will require admission to hospital and elaborate observation simply to establish how much food they are actually consuming. If the appetite has declined one should always try to relate this temporally to the alteration in weight, the situation being obviously more straightforward where the loss of appetite come first.

In a small contrasting group of patients the striking feature is the presence of an excellent or even increased appetite and intake of food, with weight loss. The diagnosis here is usually obvious, diabetes mellitus and thyrotoxicosis being the commonest diseases which produce this pattern although there are, of course a number of others, such as pancreatic steatorrhoea (see Ch. 13).

In perhaps the largest group of patients, weight loss will seem to be excessive in response to an intake of food which is said to be normal or only slightly depressed. Here the range of possible diagnoses is widest, including the possibilities mentioned earlier. If the patient has some other presenting symptom this will usually allow further enquiry to be made along appropriate lines. If no other complaint is made, systematic questioning will be needed, bearing in mind the more likely diagnoses. Two conditions commonly associated with serious causes of weight loss are anaemia and fever, and these must always be specifically excluded both clinically and by appropriate investigation. The diseases one is most concerned with will be a number of endocrine disorders, the various malabsorption states, gastrointestinal malignancies and chronic infections. Disseminated malignancy arising from any site, or multifocally as in the lymphomas, may also be responsible. In most of these patients the diagnosis will already have been established. The many abnormalities such as opportunistic infections, lymphoma and Kaposi sarcoma complicating the immunosuppressed state created by HIV infection, may present in non-specific ways such as weight loss and malaise. Finally, there is depressive mood change with anxiety, perhaps the commonest reason of all for weight loss.

Routine enquiry for the common respiratory symptoms of cough, sputum, haemoptysis, chest pain or shortness of breath, may be valuable. In the previous century in Britain, and even today in many other parts of the world, weight loss in a young adult always raised the possibility of pulmonary tuberculosis, the other early symptoms being cough, haemoptysis and night sweats with fever. Today, a patient with weight loss and haemoptysis will be more likely to have carcinoma of the bronchus, particularly if he is a cigarette smoker. In this condition widespread dissemination can occur even though the primary remains occult. Some patients with bronchiectasis may produce very large quantities of sputum, and if this is associated with poor appetite, some degree of weight loss easily ensues. This diagnosis will be suggested by the large volume of sputum, the production of which is often related to the posture of the patient. It is often purulent and foul-smelling in character, and usually results in halitosis. In emphysema weight loss can be marked, and this diagnosis should be considered if breathlessness is the main complaint.

Polyuria occurs commonly with diabetes mellitus, and is often marked, the patient being also aware of the associated polydipsia. In uraemia there may be some degree of cachexia and there is a characteristic loss of the diurnal rhythm of urine secretion with resulting nocturia. In the treatment of uraemia a low protein diet may exacerbate the weight loss. Blood in the urine is always abnormal, whether macroscopic or microscopic, and may be the only indication of an underlying hypernephroma.

Weight loss due to heart disease is described — cardiac cachexia. It is, however, uncommon, and a reflection of severe heart disease, with a low cardiac output and congestive failure resulting in impaired perfusion and nutrition of the tissues. The other symptoms of heart disease will usually be present, and the diagnosis will not be in doubt. Infective endocarditis should always be considered in patients with minimal cardiac lesions.

IMPORTANT CAUSES OF WEIGHT LOSS

Endocrine disorders

The two most important conditions are diabetes mellitus and thyrotoxicosis. The diabetic who presents with weight loss will usually be young and turn out to be insulin dependent. The other typical symptoms of polyuria and polydipsia will normally be present and indeed the initial presentation is often with ketoacidosis. Even if these features are absent, the diagnosis will rarely be missed if the urine is always tested for sugar.

Hyperthyroidism is usually associated with weight loss, and although in a young woman the clinical picture will often be typical and the diagnosis straightforward, in an elderly male it is much more easily missed. Important confirmatory symptoms will be an excellent appetite despite the weight loss, heart intolerance, sweating, diarrhoea, shortness of breath on exertion, palpitation, undue fatiguability at all times together with a general motor overactivity and nervousness. In the elderly, however, the symptoms of cardiovascular disease often dominate and the patient may present with angina pectoris, or congestive heart failure which is usually high output in type. Atrial fibrillation is also common and may be either paroxysmal or permanent. There can be difficulty in distinguishing between the thyrotoxicosis and anxiety states, where weight loss is also common. In general an increase in appetite with a marked loss of weight will suggest thyroid overactivity rather than a psychoneurotic disturbance.

In adrenal insufficiency weight loss is a feature. The clinical severity and rate of progression may be variable and may be exacerbated by any form of stress. The symptoms are often very non-specific, and include tiredness, lassitude, and vague gastrointestinal complaints such as nausea and vomiting. They are all too easily put down to psychological inadequacy. Depression and other psychoses may occur secondarily and will respond only to adequate steroid replacement therapy. Pigmentation is perhaps the single most helpful sign in leading to the diagnosis and in some patients may be associated with vitiligo. Dizziness and faints can result from the postural hypotension which may occur in addition to the overall lowering of the blood pressure. Loss of body hair may be marked, especially in women, and be a source of complaint, but sexual functions are otherwise unaffected and amenorrhoea is unusual.

Patients with hypopituitarism are usually of normal weight. In some, however, loss of weight with reduction in subcutaneous fat does occur, but this is rarely extreme. Very marked emaciation is more likely to indicate a diagnosis of anorexia nervosa. Failure of anterior pituitary secretion leads to a fineness and wrinkling of the skin. Libido is reduced and body hair lost. The genitalia show atrophy, and there is usually oligo- or amenorrhoea. Any or all of the features of hypothyroidism can be present. Pigmentation of the skin is generally reduced, as is the pigmentary response to sunlight. So-called pituitary cachexia, however, only occurs if the pituitary destruction has been caused by a wasting disease such as tuberculosis or secondary carcinoma.

Gastrointestinal causes

Simple failure to eat enough food in mentally normal individuals is an uncommon cause of weight loss in developed countries. While many people, either because of ignorance or poverty, have a poor diet, the total number of calories consumed is usually reasonable, for the cheaper foods usually have a high carbohydrate content. In the elderly, lack of money may be combined with lack of drive and a loss of interest in food, together perhaps with ill-fitting and painful false teeth. Weight loss is an inevitable result. Vomiting or diarrhoea for any reason will rapidly lead to loss of weight, which in the more acute and severe cases will be mainly due to dehydration. Long-continued vomiting always suggests some mechanical obstruction of the upper bowel, a common cause being pyloric stenosis following on a long-standing duodenal ulcer. Gastric cancer may also cause vomiting but here the anorexia will be more marked and the whole history shorter and of more rapid progression. Retching and vomiting, particularly in the mornings, is common in the chronic alcoholic, but weight loss occurs later, probably because of the high calorific value of the alcohol consumed. Very marked emaciation results from obstruction of the oesophagus, the cause being usually a carcinoma, when dysphagia rather than vomiting will be the major complaint.

Many patients who in the past have been treated for their peptic ulcer by partial gastrectomy will have found that they lost weight and that regaining weight postoperatively proved difficult. The causes of this are several and include some degree of malabsorption due to gastrointestinal hurry, together with reduced intake because of the small gastric remnant. Their simple loss of weight rarely requires treatment even though more specific deficiencies may require attention.

Any inflammatory cause of chronic diarrhoea particularly if due to disease of the small bowel will usually lead to weight loss – for example Crohn's disease and ulcerative colitis. Weight loss will also occur with the steatorrhoeas and here it may at times be difficult to arrive at the diagnosis. Diarrhoea is by no means obligatory, nor may the stools show the classical steatorrhoeic appearance. This is particularly so in some cases of coeliac disease. In those patients suffering primarily from pancreatic disease the steatorrhoea is usually more obvious. Tuberculous disease of the small bowel is now very rare, as is amyloid disease. Lymphoma of the gut is increasingly being recognized and may present in this way. Tropical sprue will usually be suggested by the history of past residence in the tropics, and is an important diagnosis to make, as the response to treatment is normally good. Previous surgery resulting in excessive reduction in absorptive area, blind loops, or fistulae, will again be suggested by the history (see Ch. 13).

Malignant disease of the large bowel may cause weight loss, but this is a less striking feature than with carcinoma of the stomach. The major associated symptoms will be of alteration in bowel habit, blood in the stool with left-sided lesions, whereas carcinoma of the caecum and ascending colon present with anaemia or a palpable mass.

The chronic infections

These are not now a common cause, as far as Northern Europe is concerned with the exception of HIV and AIDS mentioned above and in Ch. 30. Tuberculosis must be considered, but is usually easily excluded by chest X-ray. Miliary tuberculosis can still be a difficult diagnosis, but the presentation is unlikely to be that of a simple loss of weight. Some cases of infective endocarditis may progress only very slowly, with general debility, weight loss and fever as major features. There will usually be some pointer to a cardiac lesion and ultimately of course embolic phenomena will develop. Blood cultures are the essential investigation in infective endocarditis, and microscopic haematuria is often present. Weight loss is a common feature in chronic brucellosis, and here serological tests will help in the diagnosis. (For further investigation of PUO see Ch. 30).

Malignant disease

It has already been emphasized that weight loss is an important feature in most gastrointestinal malignancies, particularly carcinoma of the stomach. It also occurs in the majority of cancers when the tumour is extensive, and may also occasionally occur for reasons which are not clear at an early stage when the tumour is small. In some cases it may be because of infection and fever associated with the primary tumour, but if marked must always suggest dissemination of the cancer. In the lymphomas weight loss may also occur early on, and lymph adenopathy, anaemia, purpura and bone pain may all be present.

Psychiatric causes

Weight loss is a common feature of both anxiety and depressive states and is usually proportional to the severity of the disturbance. In depression the loss of appetite may be almost complete and the loss of weight correspondingly severe. In some cases of depression the presence of other somatic symptoms such as loss of libido, early waking and constipation will aid in the diagnosis. The depression and accompanying weight loss will often respond to antidepressants or, failing that, ECT.

Anxiety states may occasionally prove difficult to differentiate clinically from thyrotoxicosis but this should no longer be a serious problem with the ready availability of thyroid function tests.

Some schizophrenics may show disinterest in food and lose weight, and patients in a phase of manic excitement may also fail to eat adequately as a result of their restlessness and easy distractability. In neither case is the diagnosis likely to prove difficult.

Anorexia nervosa is increasingly common, and occurs predominantly in young females. It consists of a gradual and progressive reduction in food intake so that finally gross emaciation occurs which can be fatal. In contrast to the physical state they characteristically remain very active and restless. Amenorrhoea is almost invariable and a number of other minor physical changes occur, such as lanugo. Some patients have a history of obesity, for which they have dieted vigorously, and anorexia nervosa has supervened, perhaps interspersed with or preceded by bulimia (binge eating and self-induced vomiting). There is, however, invariably a deeper disturbance of personality, mood and family background. Despite the apparent wellbeing professed by the patients, they are seriously ill and must be admitted to hospital for treatment. Management is difficult and is made more so by the lengths to which the patient will go to hide food or to induce vomiting surreptitiously. Patients will also be unreliable in taking any prescribed medication. The main differential diagnosis is hypopituitarism. Anorexia nervosa can itself cause endocrine disturbances through the hypothalamic–pituitary axis. Unlike organic causes of hypopituitarism, hypothyroidism is a relatively early feature.

CLINICAL PROBLEM

T	P	BP	R
37·2	100	110/70	22

Anaemic

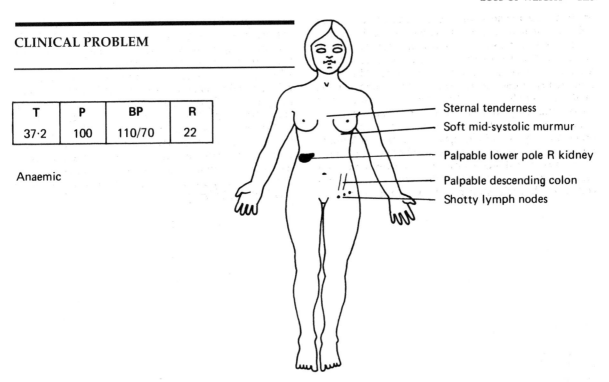

- Sternal tenderness
- Soft mid-systolic murmur
- Palpable lower pole R kidney
- Palpable descending colon
- Shotty lymph nodes

A 52-year-old woman was referred to the out-patients clinic. She was Indian and spoke little English, although she had been in the UK 5 years. The history given by the husband was that over the last 8 months she had lost a great deal of weight and had now become very thin. He denied that she had been attempting to diet and said that he had never objected to her previous weight. Her appetite had never been good, but had been worse recently. For the previous few months she had felt increasingly tired and had found difficulty in coping with her domestic responsibilities. She was very concerned about this, as she felt she was not caring adequately for her family. Over this time her sleep had been poor, but there had been no early waking. She also complained of occasional dyspepsia for some years, and of some generalized aching in her limbs more recently.

Previously she had been well except for malaria as a child and typhoid when she was 14. She did not smoke or drink alcohol. Her periods had been scanty for the last 8 months, but previously had been heavy and lasted about 8 days. Her parents were dead and she had seven siblings alive and well. She had four healthy children, two of whom were still at home.

On examination, she seemed quiet and withdrawn, and had obviously lost weight. Height 158 cm, weight 45 kg. She was a little pale, but there was no abnormal bruising or bleeding. The pulse was 100/min regular and the blood pressure 110/70. No abnormality was present in the cardiovascular system except for a soft mid-systolic murmur, best heard just internal to the apex. No abnormal signs were present in the lungs, but pressure over the sternum elicited a little tenderness. The descending colon was palpable and slightly tender and the lower pole of the right kidney could be felt. Rectal examination was normal. A few shotty lymph nodes could be felt in both groins. Neurological examination revealed no abnormality. Urine examination was normal.

QUESTIONS

1. What are the most probable diagnoses?
2. What investigations would be of value?

DISCUSSION

Although psychiatric causes of weight loss are common, organic disease must be first excluded and then, of the patients still remaining, the majority will probably be found to be suffering from a depressive illness. Carcinomatosis could be responsible for this woman's loss of weight, but after 8 months it is a little surprising that no symptoms or signs have developed pointing towards the primary growth. A palpable right kidney is common in thin people and its significance uncertain since the urine is normal on routine examination. Sternal tenderness always suggests marrow infiltration with tumour or leukaemia. However, a good history could not be obtained because of language difficulties and under such circumstances one is commonly forced to rely on a battery of screening investigations. A depressive illness is a possibility, and may be occurring as a reaction to the disruption of old ties and the social isolation which many immigrant wives experience. Against this is the tachycardia and systolic murmur, which suggests anaemia, and also the body pains. Anaemia, however, is never a sufficient diagnosis in itself and one must always find the underlying cause. Lymphoma is not a common cause of this clinical picture, but could certainly explain this patient's illness. Tuberculosis must always be considered as a cause of loss of weight, especially in patients from India, who are prone to the extrapulmonary forms of the disease.

Management at this stage must be by further investigation and not by any therapeutic trial, whether of haematinics or of psychotropic drugs. A blood picture is mandatory, not only for the haemoglobin but also for the white cell count and differential, and an examination of the stained film. The ESR is also a valuable screening investigation. Chest X-ray will always be part of the routine work-up of such a patient. It may show pulmonary tuberculosis, primary or secondary carcinoma and bony deposits. Sternal secondaries are not easily identified on routine chest films and spine views must be obtained. A bone scan will be more sensitive than radiology in the demonstration of bone lesions. A marrow examination, especially from the tender area, may give the diagnosis.

Investigation of this patient showed a normochromic normocytic anaemia of 8 g/dl. The ESR was very high at 95 mm. CXR revealed scattered osteolytic lesions in the ribs, and bone marrow examination established a diagnosis of secondary carcinoma. An IVP showed a left-sided hypernephroma.

18.   Confusion and dementia

A wide variety of organic brain syndromes occur in which psychiatric symptoms are prominent and may constitute the initial presentation. It is usual to divide them into acute and chronic syndromes, but this is by no means a sharp distinction and there is very considerable overlap.

Acute brain syndromes develop quickly and are usually associated with clouding of consciousness and impairment of orientation. Memory is affected, there is often marked distractability and as a result concentration is poor. The severity of the condition varies greatly, from delirium to coma. Frequently the syndrome is completely reversible. An example is delirium tremens due to alcoholism.

In contrast the term chronic brain syndrome is used very similarly to the older diagnosis of dementia. Here the onset is more gradual, and the clinical course usually more steadily progressive. There is much less clouding of consciousness and confusion, and orientation may be reasonably good. Memory impairment is variable, but is usually present and particularly affects recent memory. In chronic brain syndrome or dementia, it is intellectual failure which predominates. In the past this diagnosis was commonly thought to imply an irreversible deterioration in mental function, but this is not now an essential part of the definition, even though it is still true in the majority of cases. As a result of advances in treatment considerable improvement may be obtained in some dementias, for example those due to neurosphilis, vitamin B_{12} deficiency and low-pressure hydrocephalus.

An important differential diagnosis is between dementia and depression. These two conditions are both common and increase in frequency with advancing years. They constitute therefore an increasingly frequent problem in diagnosis and management. In their early stages both are easily missed. Although both are often regarded as psychiatric diagnoses, their very frequency and the multitudinous guises under which they can present, means that all clinicians must be expert in establishing an initial diagnosis, even if the later management is more specialized.

In practice many mistakes are made because early in the disease the conventional medical history and physical examination often fail to suggest any abnormality. Only by a conscious evaluation of the mental state of the patient both directly and on the basis of information from friends, relatives and employers, will a diagnosis be reached. This analysis of the mental state must be done formally, as is the examination of the various visceral systems, otherwise no meaningful assessment will be arrived at. It cannot be emphasized too strongly that to rely on simple social conversation and the patient's spontaneous complaints is, in the majority of cases, totally inadequate. Tests should include recent and past memory, abstract reasoning and calculation, assessment of affect, insight and orientation. There may be physical signs of a frontoparietal lesion such as a grasp reflex.

In dementia the very nature of the condition, with its progressive loss of intellectual capacity, often results in loss of insight, so that the patient commonly is unaware of his own deterioration and remains well satisfied by the level of his performance. This is the reason for the sound aphorism of the neurologist – 'always suspect dementia in the patient who has no complaints.'

In the future, computerized psychometric testing may form part of screening protocols for the elderly, allowing semi-automatic recognition of early cognitive failure.

THE PRESENTATION

In the confusional states any history will, at best, be fragmentary and unreliable. This is usually immediately obviously and every effort must be made to obtain an account of the patient's illness from some reliable informant. Without this information it may well be impossible to establish the reason for a confusional episode in some cases. The circumstances under which the patient has been found may be suggestive of the cause, and the police and social agencies can be of considerable help on occasion. The patient's belongings should be carefully searched, particularly for evidence of drugs. He may carry a card or bracelet if he suffers from a common disease such as diabetes mellitus in which hypoglycaemia can often present as confusion, from a rare disease such as porphyria, where neuro-psychiatric syndromes are not infrequent, or from epilepsy where post-ictal confusion is common.

Dementia is characterized by the development of significant intellectual failure, in the presence of clear consciousness, in someone of previously normal intelligence. The main defects will be in memory, in calculation, and in the power of abstract thought. More subtle changes commonly occur in social, moral and ethical standards. These may show themselves in a wide variety of ways, such as deterioration in dress, in table manners, in sexual manners, in musical appreciation, and in religious feeling. In contrast, early in the illness, other aspects of mental functioning are usually well preserved, the mood is normal, there are no hallucinations or delusions, and thought content is not abnormal.

Commonly in dementia the patient attends his doctor only at the request of others. In the case of a man this will frequently be an employer, concerned at the deterioration of his work, although it is striking how long those in higher executive and professional positions may conceal their decay. Sometimes the disappearance of moral control leads to uninhibited sexual behaviour and so to a request for a medical opinion from the courts. Rarely, delusional symptoms develop. The grandiose beliefs of those with General Paralysis of the Insane are still seen occasionally, although today most cases present as a simple dementia. In women, a loss of interest in their appearance is often a significant sign, followed perhaps by increasing incompetence in household management.

MEDICAL HISTORY

This can be of considerable importance and should be taken in as much detail as is possible. Recurrent episodes of confusion may occur due to hypoglycaemia, either iatrogenic from insulin therapy or due to an islet cell tumour. Porphyria also may cause repeated attacks of neuropsychiatric disturbance. Episodes of mental clouding are frequently seen in chronic liver disease with extensive portocaval anastomoses and may be precipitated by dietary indiscretions. Drugs are an important cause of confusion. In middle-aged housewives, benzodiazepine addiction and intoxication is not uncommon, while in younger people cannabis, amphetamines, heroin and LSD must all be considered. Industrial exposure to hazards such as lead, mercury and manganese can also be responsible for acute brain syndromes, so that an occupational history should be obtained in any difficult case.

There are not many features in the past history which are significant in the diagnosis of dementia. Repeated head injury such as occurs in professional boxes may lead later to the 'punch drunk' syndrome of which dementia is a part. Any severe infection of the brain will lead to some permanent damage and this may be associated with overt deterioration later on in life. Whether a long-standing history of epilepsy may predispose to a later dementia remains controversial. It is probable that the repeated anoxia of frequent grand mal fits does produce some permanent damage to the brain. Histologically this is similar to the changes produced by recurrent hypoglycaemia.

A history of alcoholism must always be sought. A wide variety of neuropsychiatric syndromes can occur in the alcoholic, and the underlying alcoholism may be more easily missed in a patient with dementia, than it is in a patient presenting with delirium tremens. The possible role of the newer drugs of habituation and addiction in causing dementia is not yet clear. A history of thyroid, gastric or terminal ileal surgery should arouse suspicion of thyroid or vitamin B_{12} deficiency. The slowing of mental processes in myxoedema can be confused with dementia; indeed, in some patients actual intellectual failure may be present. Vitamin B_{12} deficiency is well known to present on occasion as dementia alone. A variety of neuropsychiatric disturbances can also occur with disorders of calcium metabolism. Involvement of the central nervous system is a well-recognized feature of AIDS and many patients will ultimately show features of intellectual failure.

A history of coronary heart disease, peripheral vascular disease, or of hypertension will increase the likelihood of there being cerebrovascular disease. Both confusional states and dementia due to this cause are extremely common, but are not usually a source of diagnostic difficulty. There will usually be a history of strokes or transient ischaemic attacks (TIAs) in the past and obvious evidence of this on present physical examination. Sometimes, however, progressive intellectual failure occurs on the basis of multiple small vessel occlusions or haemorrhages without there having been any major episodes of infarction. This is a pattern more often seen in association with hypertension. The family history may also be of importance. Huntington's chorea is inherited as a simple Mendelian dominant and cases in earlier generations of the family may have become incarcerated in a mental hospital because of dementia or psychosis before the striking choreiform movements developed. The only history obtainable may then be of some severe and rather non-specific psychiatric illness which led to permanent admission to hospital. The other presenile dementias such as Pick's and Alzheimer's diseases may sometimes show a familial tendency. Tuberose sclerosis is inherited as an autosomal dominant, but partial forms are common and the mutation rate is high.

EXAMINATION

In the acutely confused patient there may be obvious motor restlessness and distractibility. Indeed the overactivity can be so marked as to constitute a major problem in management. Sometimes hallucinations are prominent and if present these are often visual in nature. A typical example are the small animals commonly seen in delirium tremens. Such experiences merge into those of an illusionary nature, and sensory misinterpretations are particularly likely if the lighting is poor, as occurs at night. The presence of confusion and agitation may make any systematic examination very difficult, and certain aspects such as neurological sensory testing will usually be impossible.

Many general medical conditions can produce a chronic confusional state and this is a common feature of terminal liver and renal failure. It may also be seen in severe cardiac and respiratory failure. However, consciousness is usually impaired and there is not usually any diagnostic difficulty.

In dementia, physical examination is commonly normal. It is important to look for the signs of vascular disease, both arteriosclerotic and hypertensive, paying particular attention to the fundi. Bilateral cerebrovascular disease may be evident in the form of pseudobulbar palsy with emotional lability, difficulty in swallowing, dysarthria, jaw jerk and bilateral pyramidal signs. Evidence of a primary neoplasm should be sought, as multiple cerebral secondaries may first present with a rapidly developing dementia. Occasionally, such dementia may turn out to be a non-metastatic complication of malignancy. Usually the primary neoplasm will be a carcinoma of the bronchus, while occasionally multifocal leucoencephalopathy may occur with a lymphoma. The presence of adenoma sebaceum will lead to a diagnosis of tuberose sclerosis, in which the mental deterioration can occur quite late on in childhood, after a period of normal or even high intelligence.

Chronic alcoholism may be suspected if there are signs of peripheral neuropathy or portal cirrhosis. Severe dementia may occur in hepatolenticular degeneration (Wilson's disease). The presence of a Kayser – Fleischer ring is pathognomonic, and there may be choreiform movements and cirrhosis.

In the central nervous system there may be focal signs indicating vascular disease or tumour. The presence of papilloedema will indicate raised intracranial pressure, which may have been completely unsuspected. The visual fields must always be tested and they may provide the first evidence of a tumour such as basal meningioma. The signs of vitamin deficiency, which may present great diagnostic difficulty, are important. In our society the deficiency most likely to cause dementia is vitamin B_{12}. The picture of subacute combined degeneration of the cord is often very typical but early on the signs may be minimal (see Ch. 25). There is usually an associated peripheral neuropathy, and a combination which must always arouse suspicion is paraesthesiae with depression of the ankle jerks and extensor plantar responses.

The association of dementia with evidence of damage in the pyramidal, extrapyramidal, or lower motor neurones will suggest the possibility of a presenile dementia, a group of disorders consisting of Pick's, Alzheimer's and Jakob–Creutzfeld's diseases.

INVESTIGATION

In dementia, a major problem was how vigorous one should be in searching for a remediable cause. Neuroradiological examination by arteriography or air encephalography was unpleasant, time-consuming, expensive, with a very real morbidity, and, in the older age groups, some mortality. However, the advent of isotope and then CT scanning has transformed investigation, rendering it essentially non-invasive. In the majority of patients the ultimate diagnosis will be of cerebral arteriosclerosis or a senile dementia.

Haemoglobin indices, blood film, thyroxine, calcium, urea and electrolytes, and serum B_{12} must always be done. In the elderly, or in those where malabsorption is suspected, it may be reasonable to add a serum folate even though neurological complications are rare in folate deficiency. Serological tests for syphilis remain mandatory as so often it is impossible even to suspect, let alone establish, the diagnosis on clinical grounds. Ideally, these should be done on both blood and CSF. Chest X-ray will help to diagnose carcinoma of the bronchus. A skull X-ray is occasionally of value, showing signs of raised intracranial pressure, or abnormal calcification in a tumour or associated with an angioma, or shift of a calcified pineal gland due to a space-occupying lesion. Serology for HIV infection is essential in any patient coming from one of the established 'at risk' groups.

An EEG may show the generalized abnormality of the metabolically induced chronic confusional state. It can also indicate local space-occupying lesions, and malignant gliomas and abscesses often cause marked abnormalities. More specific changes have been claimed in the presenile dementias, but in the main these are not of great value. Radioisotope scan is helpful as a straightforward screening test for localized abnormality, whether tumour, subdural haematoma or angioma. SPECT (Single Photon Emission Computerized Tomography) isotope imaging of cerebral blood flow using HMPAO (Ceretec) is becoming more widely available and allows one to obtain a clear-cut picture of brain perfusion at the moment of injection of the radiopharmaceutical.

Characteristic patterns may be seen in both Alzheimer's and arteriosclerotic dementia, commonly allowing their differentiation.

CT is of the greatest value in demonstrating the presence of infarct, oedema, haematoma or tumour. The size, shape and location of the lesion will usually be clearly shown, and whether it is single or multiple. Distortion of the ventricular system will also be easily seen, together with evidence of the cortical thinning and ventricular dilatation of cerebral atrophy. There has been recent interest in dementia developing in association with, and secondary to low pressure hydrocephalus. Here, isotope encephalography is indicated and some of the cases so diagnosed have improved on ventricular shunting. The condition remains ill-understood.

Carotid angiography is now rarely performed as part of the investigation of dementia. It is particularly helpful in further delineating vascular anomalies such as aneurysm and angioma, and will also show stenotic lesions of major vessels. It can demonstrate indirectly many space-occupying lesions by the distortion of the arteries and veins they produce and can sometimes suggest the presence of ventricular dilatation if this is marked.

In some specialized centres, help in distinguishing organic brain disease from a psychiatric illness such as depression may be available from the clinical psychologist. Usually this will take the form of psychometric testing to elicit the overall pattern of the patient's ability. A discrepancy between the level of performance in relation to the patient's previous achievements will be the main sign of organic deterioration with tests of language function showing less impairment than those of visuospatial performance and of logical analysis. Some psychologists also use various forms of projective tests such as the Rorschach and the thematic apperception test (TAT). These are claimed, probably with some validity, to be of value in diagnosing the various types of psychiatric disturbance in a more positive way and not simply by exclusion of the organic.

Depression is a common disease and the diagnosis can easily be missed, particularly in the elderly where all deterioration is readily put down to senility. Previously the only treatment available was ECT, which commonly makes any associated organic brain disease worse. Now, with numerous effective antidepressant drugs available, appropriate treatment should always be given. If the differential diagnosis between depression and dementia is in doubt, a course of antidepressants is safe and should always be tried.

In the dementias, the physician's main task is to diagnose early those cases where there is a treatable cause without exposing the majority of patients, for whom little help is available, to excessive investigation. New drugs are however becoming available, as Alzheimer's disease is now a major research area. The future for therapy may therefore be less gloomy than in the past.

CLINICAL PROBLEM

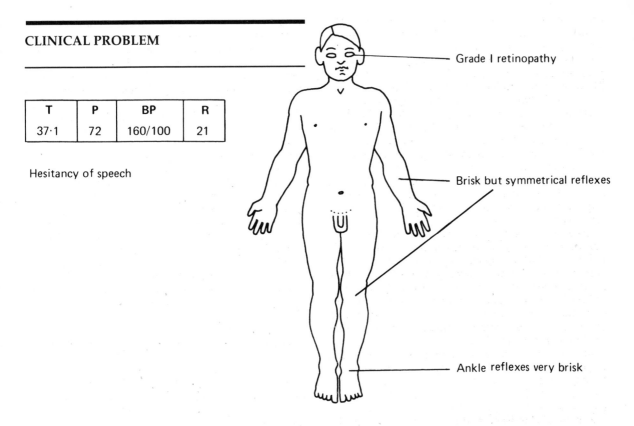

T	P	BP	R
37·1	72	160/100	21

Hesitancy of speech

Grade I retinopathy

Brisk but symmetrical reflexes

Ankle reflexes very brisk

A 50-year-old accountant was seen in the outpatients' clinic at the request of his general practitioner. The patient had originally consulted his doctor only because of the anxiety of his wife, who felt that his health had deteriorated recently. She complained that for the past 6 months he had seemed nervous and a little depressed. He had increasingly brought work home from the office to complete and she believed that there had been some dissatisfaction with him in his firm. He had worked in his present job for the last 12 years and had always appeared to cope in the past without difficulty. He had not been especially successful in his career, and his present post was not one of very great responsibility. The patient had told the GP that he thought his wife was being unreasonably concerned. He felt perfectly fit, although he admitted that he had been under some pressure recently in his job. He explained this by the greatly increased volume of work which had developed over the last few years.

He had been found to be moderately hypertensive (170/110) at a routine insurance examination 3 years previously, and had been taking a small dose of a diuretic regularly ever since. Otherwise he had been well except for an inguinal hernia that had been successfully repaired 2 years earlier. There was no relevant family history.

The GP found no abnormality except that his blood pressure was still raised at 170/105 but he referred the patient to hospital mainly to reassure the wife.

On direct questioning the patient did say that one thing had bothered him recently. For the last few months he had had some difficulty with his walking and on several occasions had tripped and fallen. He tended to catch the toe of his right shoe particularly on the edges of carpets and kerb stones.

On examination there was a slight hesitancy of speech. His fundi showed Grade I changes and the BP was a little raised at 160/100. He was right-handed. The cranial nerves were normal, but in the limbs it was noted that all the tendon reflexes were very brisk. While taking the history and talking to the patient no abnormality was apparent in his appearance, personality or in his use of language. Simple tests of mental arithmetic such as serial 7s revealed, however, a surprising number of mistakes for a man of his occupation and background.

QUESTIONS

1. What are the main diagnoses that must be considered?
2. What investigations should be done immediately?

DISCUSSION

The diagnosis in this man is uncertain at this stage. He has no complaints, and the explanation he offers of his recent behaviour is rational and may well be true. There are, however, a number of disturbing points. Until recently he had always been able to cope with his responsibilities and his job is apparently not especially arduous. He has had difficulty in walking, and its nature raises the possibility of a pyramidal lesion involving particularly the right leg. His hesitancy of speech may also have an organic basis. He is known to be hypertensive, and this must increase the likelihood that cerebrovascular disease is present.

An alternative explanation which would also be reasonable would be a psychiatric one. He is a man never of outstanding talent and of mediocre achievement. He is now aged 50, a time when depressive illnesses become increasingly common. There may well be more work than he can comfortably cope with and this may have triggered a depressive reaction. Depression is commonly associated with some degree of anxiety and agitation, and in itself will impair his work performance, thus putting increasing stress upon him. Any affective disturbance is often denied by the patient, who may have no insight into his condition. Anxiety is the commonest cause of increased tendon reflexes, and there are no unequivocally abnormal signs present on examination. The impaired concentration so often produced by emotional distress could also explain his poor performance on tests of arithmetic ability.

At this point, therefore, the two main alternative diagnoses are of a mixed anxiety depressive state, or some diffuse organic disease of the nervous system, as yet in an early stage of development, but already impairing higher mental functions, speech and gait.

If there is the possibility of an affective illness it is always worthwhile trying the effect of an anti-depressant such as imipramine. This will not influence organic disease but may completely reverse any depressive mood change. In the past when the only effective treatment available for depression was ECT, such a diagnostic trial was not possible, for ECT may produce considerable deterioration in the presence of organic brain disease.

Immediate investigation need only be quite simple. The chest should be X-rayed, mainly to exclude a carcinoma of the bronchus, dementia being a feature of cerebral metastases or of the much rarer non-metastatic complications of this tumour. Examination of the blood will reveal any anaemia, which may be a reflection of some other underlying disease such as carcinoma of the stomach or vitamin B_{12} deficiency. At the same time a normal blood picture in no way removes the necessity to estimate the serum B_{12}, as dementia can occur without either anaemia or the typical findings of subacute combined degeneration of the cord. Syphilis is rare, but it would still be wise to check the WR, even though a negative blood WR does not completely exclude this diagnosis. If neurosyphilis is ever seriously suspected a lumbar puncture must be done and the serology of the CSF examined. Straight X-rays of the skull are a simple investigation although they are unlikely to provide much useful information. If the pineal is calcified, a midline shift might be detected, while a rise in intracranial pressure might show itself by erosion of the clinoid processes. Some cerebral tumours, such as craniopharyngiomas and oligodendrogliomas, may be calcified and thus reveal themselves. In the past a very common screening test at this stage was an EEG. This has now been replaced in this clinical context by one or other of the various imaging techniques.

Planar isotope scan is a simple, relatively cheap and effective screening procedure for many space-occupying lesions. X-ray CT scan is a more powerful investigation in this situation and can give additional information concerning ventricular dilatation and cortical atrophy. If available, SPECT scanning to visualize blood flow may allow even more diagnostic information; patients with Alzheimer's typically show symmetrical bilateral reduction in flow to both parietal and frontal lobes, even at a stage when the X-ray CT scan is still normal. All these investigations except SPECT were done in this patient and revealed no abnormality. Cerebral biopsy was considered, but rejected as being unlikely to show any treatable abnormality.

> Over the next 2 years he showed continued intellectual deterioration to the level of profound dementia. His speech difficulty increased and he became completely mute. Over this time the tendon reflexes became more exaggerated, and ankle clonus with extensor plantar reflexes developed. His walking difficulty increased and on examination both upper and lower limbs showed generalized wasting with widespread fasciculation. At no time was there evidence of any sensory loss and there were never any cerebellar signs. Autopsy revealed generalized depletion of neurones in the cerebral cortex, with degeneration of both upper and lower motor neurones. A diagnosis had been made in life of Jakob–Creutzfeldt syndrome and a subsequent CT scan showed ventricular dilatation and diffuse cerebral atrophy. This was confirmed by the histological findings.

19. Fits and faints

The patient who complains of a transient disturbance of consciousness is a common problem. He may describe this in a variety of ways, and the words he uses often confuse rather than clarify the situation. Although often the complaint is of blackouts, these may also be described as episodes of dizziness or weakness. The history may be of recurrent falls, or of peculiar 'turns' the nature of which the patient is unable to describe. In unravelling this type of problem the clinical history is of the greatest importance. In many patients both the physical examination and the special investigations will add nothing further to one's knowledge, and all decisions as to diagnosis and management will have to be based simply on the patient's story. This is commonly the case in idiopathic grand mal epilepsy. The patient will rarely provide his physician with the opportunity of observing one of his attacks. During them he may have little idea himself of what is occurring, and a reliable eye-witness is therefore of the greatest value. The pattern of an attack can be complex. For example, what starts as a syncopal episode may precipitate and merge into an anoxic convulsion.

Usually one is dealing with some variety of fit or faint.

Fainting reflects the absolute dependence of the brain upon a continuous supply of oxygen and glucose, deprivation of either rapidly leading to alteration or loss of consciousness. The usual reason for this will be a failure in cerebral perfusion for cardiac or vascular reasons, but rarely there may be recurrent hypoglycaemia alone.

Patients suffering from a psychiatric illness, usually of an affective nature, may experience recurrent feelings of depersonalization or unreality. These states are difficult to describe, and the history may be suggestive of some form of temporal lobe fit. It is important to be aware of this possible difficulty and always consciously to evaluate the mental state and the background personal and social factors against which the present symptoms have developed. One should aim always to make a psychiatric diagnosis on positive evidence, and not simply by exclusion of the organic. One must ask the patient whether he feels depressed or anxious, and seek the common accompanying somatic features.

Recurrent blackouts even when due to some relatively minor physical cause may greatly alarm the patient, and he may well have his own, often inaccurate views as to their significance. It is important to ask after these, and if necessary to reassure him that he does not have a cerebral tumour – a common fear.

PRECIPITATING FACTORS

The individual features of an attack must be analysed if possible in considerable detail: when and how often they occur, whether the onset is abrupt, as is usually the case in epilepsy, or more gradual as is usual in syncope. Injury, aura, incontinence, tongue-biting and abnormal movements all suggest epilepsy. The circumstances under which the attacks occur are often of the greatest help in arriving at the diagnosis. One should ask exactly what the patient was doing at the time he lost consciousness. Syncope due to vagal slowing of the heart precipitated by emotion or pain remains by far the commonest cause of loss of consciousness, although most patients will not seek medical advice. In some patients epileptic fits can be provoked or rendered more frequent by emotional distress. A relationship to the menstrual cycle may be present with either fits or faints and this is therefore not a point of great value in diagnosis. Recurrent fainting is not uncommon in the early months of pregnancy. Prolonged standing, particularly in young asthenic individuals, and especially in warm weather, is a frequent cause of fainting, but does not often cause any problem in diagnosis.

Alcohol withdrawal may precipitate fits in those with a low convulsive threshold. Iatrogenic hypotension, when severe, may cause recurrent faints. Usually the cause is overvigorous treatment of hypertension, with an excessive fall in blood pressure either on standing or exercise. This is much less frequently seen with newer hypotensive drugs such as the beta blockers. Other drugs may however produce hypotension as a side-effect, the most important being the phenothiazines. Fortunately fits do not usually occur because of the patient's treatment, although some drugs like chlorpromazine may increase the frequency of fits in known epileptics. The sudden cessation of long-standing treatment with barbiturates may precipitate fits, even in those not known to be epileptic.

EPILEPSY

The usual difficulty in this field is the tendency to regard all recurrent disturbance of consciousness as epileptic. The reverse error is much less common. The major clinical forms of fit do not usually cause any confusion in diagnosis. The grand mal and petit mal attack are both typical in the majority of patients, and the correct diagnosis is quickly arrived at.

The psychomotor attack of temporal lobe epilepsy may however cause diagnostic difficulty. Here consciousness may not be lost, and the discharging focus can give rise to recurrent episodes which are easily regarded as psychiatric rather than epileptic. The initial aura may be very complex, and a wide variety of hallucinations can be experienced. In most people the sequence is repeated very precisely in each recurrent attack, and this stereotypy is of help in reaching the correct diagnosis. Clinical states very similar to those found in schizophrenia can occur, although there may in addition be some clouding of consciousness. In the investigation of these patients EEG examination is of great importance, and sphenoidal leads may well be needed if such a temporal lobe focus is suspected.

A most important rule is that although an abnormal EEG tracing will often support the diagnosis of epilepsy, a normal record does not disprove a diagnosis which has been made on clinical grounds.

As in cardiology, ambulatory recording of the EEG over 24 hours may be of real value in selected patients, if diagnostic abnormalities are captured.

CEREBROVASCULAR DISEASE

Cerebrovascular disease is very common, and when it involves the vertebrobasilar system it may give rise to recurrent attacks of brain-stem ischaemia in which for a brief moment consciousness is impaired or lost. There are usually other symptoms which will indicate the site of ischaemia, such as visual disturbance, diplopia, vertigo, facial paraesthesiae and drop attacks. There is often evidence of arteriosclerosis elsewhere. Cervical spondylosis is commonly present and in certain positions of the head and neck, the vertebral arteries may be compressed, producing brain-stem ischaemia. Another common reason for the effects of vascular disease becoming manifest is the development of anaemia, and with correction of the anaemia, there is often cessation of the attacks.

Transient ischaemic attacks (TIAs) seem often to occur in a cluster over a period of months, with spontaneous improvement. The difficulty lies in recognizing the subgroup of patients in whom the TIAs are the forerunners of a major stroke. Fortunately this sequence does not occur as frequently with vertebrobasilar attacks as with TIAs in the carotid territory. In the past, although their dependence on underlying cerebrovascular disease was recognized, the occurrence of only transient symptoms was explained by postulating a temporary fall in blood pressure. In the majority of patients this is now recognized as not being the causal factor. There is increasing evidence that platelet micro-emboli arising from atheromatous plaques in the extracranial vessels can be responsible. One uncommon syndrome which has aroused interest, and where active treatment is possible, is the subclavian steal syndrome. Here there is a stenosis of the subclavian artery proximal to the origin of the vertebral artery. Exercise of the arm on that side will lead to a reduction in peripheral vascular resistance locally so that there is a further fall in pressure beyond the stenosis. As a result there is reversal of flow in the vertebral artery of that side and blood from the contralateral vertebral artery is used to supply the arm rather than the brain stem. The relation of symptoms to exercise and the lower blood pressure on the side of the stenosis should suggest the diagnosis and indicate the need for arteriographic investigation.

In elderly hypertensive patients there is often widespread arteriosclerosis of the major cerebral blood vessels, and scattered areas of cerebral infarction, haemorrhage and ischaemia may be present even in the absence of any history of a major stroke. These damaged regions may be electrically unstable, and can give rise to epileptic attacks. Such fits may occur spontaneously, but can also be triggered by the temporarily reduced cerebral perfusion associated with syncope.

Migraine is a very common disorder and in the past an association with idiopathic epilepsy was commonly assumed, although there is little evidence to support this. A particular variant of migraine has been described in which the vascular spasm involves particularly the vertebrobasilar system. The teichopsia are often especially vivid, vision may be impaired or lost, and there can be dysarthria, tinnitus and ataxia. There is frequently occurrence of loss of consciousness, which may last for up to half an hour. However, unlike epilepsy, the loss of consciousness is usually gradual and the patients are not completely unrousable. This is an important condition to be aware of, as the majority of patients are young women, and the mistaken diagnosis of idiopathic epilepsy is easily made. Although the attacks respond only poorly to treatment, they usually stop spontaneously within a few years.

SYNCOPE

Micturition syncope is not uncommon and must not be confused with nocturnal epilepsy. It usually affects elderly men, when they get up at night from a warm bed to empty their bladders. The exact mechanism is unclear, but is probably a combination of postural hypotension from venous pooling, together with a mild Valsalva manoeuvre associated with straining to micturate. A related syndrome is cough syncope, in which prolonged or severe coughing may cause faintness or actual loss of consciousness. The treatment in both these conditions is self-evident once the diagnosis has been made. Again, as the patient may have forgotten the actual circumstances of his attack, it may be necessary to have an eyewitness account before the diagnosis can be made.

Autonomic control of the peripheral vasculature may be impaired in a number of diseases and on occasion gives rise to troublesome fainting, due to postural hypotension. This can occur in a number of forms of neuropathy, and is well recognized in diabetes. It is also seen sometimes in tabes dorsalis, syringomyelia and Parkinsonism. Another rare cause is the infiltration of the sympathetic ganglia that is sometimes seen in amyloidosis. Control of symptoms in these conditions can sometimes be very difficult.

Fainting can be caused by an abrupt fall in cardiac output. This may be due to acute myocardial infarction, but is more often the result of change in cardiac rhythm. A failure to maintain cerebral perfusion in the face of a falling cardiac output is much more common in the elderly, where compensatory reflexes are less effective. A very slow or a very fast heart rate will both lead to a fall in output and fainting may follow, especially at the onset of the arrhythmia. Fast arrhythmias are more likely to occur paroxysmally, and so give rise to recurrent attacks. The episode may begin with palpitation but this is often forgotten by the patient. Diagnosis can be difficult unless the pulse is felt or an ECG obtained during an attack. The heart rate will change abruptly at the beginning and end of the arrhythmia. The paroxysm is due to control of the heart by a new pacemaker in the atria or ventricles. The commonest type is atrial tachycardia, although atrial flutter and fibrillation may also be responsible. Recurrent bouts of ventricular tachycardia may also occur and then the prognosis is much more serious as the arrhythmia may proceed to cardiac arrest and ventricular fibrillation. The separation of these conditions is clinically difficult, although it can be done to some extent by their varying response to carotid pressure. For certain diagnosis an ECG is essential (see Ch. 1), and the use of 24-hour ambulatory monitoring using small tape or solid state recorders has transformed the problems of diagnosis in these patients. For those with less frequent arrhythmias event recorders can be used, but these typically will require the cooperation of the patient or companion at the onset of the attack.

In paraoxysmal atrial tachycardia the rate is regular at around 200/min. The heart sounds are similarly very constant in quality and loudness, being unaffected by respiration, changes in position, and exercise. This precise regularity no matter how long an attack lasts is very characteristic. The period of syncope occurs at the commencement of an attack and is usually short-lived in relation to the length of the arrhythmia. Some patients notice that sudden movements of the head, severe exercise, or emotional distress precipitate attacks, but in the majority of cases they occur for no obvious reason. There is usually no permanent harm done, but sometimes heart failure can be induced if there is underlying heart disease. Rarely, because of the marked reduction in cardiac output, cerebral infarction may occur.

Pressure on the carotid sinus may itself rarely give rise to spontaneous symptoms of faintness or loss of consciousness. Most patients are elderly and have evidence of arteriopathy. Over-reaction of the carotid sinus occurs on quite normal neck movement, and it is assumed that in some way the sinus has become 'irritable'. If the condition is suspected, massage of the sinus should produce an excessive bradycardia and fall in blood pressure. In the past the diagnosis of carotid sinus syncope has been made despite the absence of any change in pulse or pressure, and reflex changes in the cerebral circulation were postulated. These patients, who undoubtedly suffered fainting when they turned their heads, were probably suffering from vertebral artery compression from the osteophytes of cervical spondylosis. Some cases of increased sensitivity of the carotid sinus are due to the infiltration of the area by tumour, and this will usually be evident on clinical examination. In treatment one must explain the condition to the patient and advise him against tight collars and sudden neck movements.

Syncopal attacks are a common feature of complete heart block. They may occur at the onset of the block before the idioventricular rhythm establishes itself, and also in unstable situations where the rhythm is varying between partial and complete block. When complete block is established, Stoke–Adams attacks may occur due to ventricular asystole, or if the rate falls below 20/min, or if ventricular tachycardia or fibrillation occur. A constant ventricular rate of 30 or above does not normally cause fainting. The duration of unconsciousness will depend on the length of the period of asystole. If it is more than 30–60 seconds, then an anoxic convulsion, which can be local or generalized, may occur. The clinical diagnosis of complete heart block is usually obvious once the pulse has been felt. Additional clinical signs which are pathognomonic are the changing intensity and quality of the first sound, and cannon waves in the JVP, which occur as a result of the varying relationship between atrial and ventricular systole which results in the atrium sometimes contracting when the tricuspid valve is closed. A generalized flush at the end of the attack is also characteristic. The diagnosis can still be difficult as a considerable number of patients may have attacks due to temporary periods of complete block, the rhythm in between being quite normal, both clinically and on the ECG. They will usually progress over a period of months to complete block, when the attacks usually stop, but the diagnosis becomes evident! Again, ambulatory monitoring is of the greatest value.

Another cause of recurrent episodes of faintness is following head injury. This is usually self-evident, but on occasion the patient may go on for weeks or months after the accident suffering blackouts, and the differential diagnosis from post-traumatic epilepsy becomes a problem. Medicolegal complications are commonly present and the management of these patients is often difficult until any question of compensation has been settled. Other features of the post-traumatic state such as headache, failure of concentration, and dizziness are usually present and will help in the diagnosis.

HYPOGLYCAEMIA

Hypoglycaemia can prove difficult (Table 19.1). In the known diabetic the situation is straightforward, but recurrent hypoglycaemia may occur at the stage of prediabetes. Hypoglycaemia in the diabetic does not only occur in the patient receiving insulin but is a well-recognized hazard with the long-acting sulphonyl ureas, particularly in the elderly patient with cerebral arteriosclerosis. Another common cause of hypoglycaemia is the condition of functional reactive hypoglycaemia, where there is thought to be an excessive insulin response to a glucose load. The hypoglycaemia comes on some 3 hours after a meal, but is not usually severe enough to cause loss of consciousness. A similar syndrome can occur after partial gastrectomy. In both situations the glucose tolerance curve shows a lag storage pattern. Treatment is by reducing the carbohydrate content of the diet. A very important, though rare, cause is an insulinoma of the pancreas. The majority of these tumours are benign, only 10% being malignant. Most occur in late middle age and about a quarter of patients give a family history of diabetes. Presentation is very varied and may be bizarre. Recurrent loss of consciousness, recurrent

Table 19.1 Causes of hypoglycaemia

Insulinoma
Large non-pancreatic tumours; retroperitoneal sarcoma, hepatoma
Hypopituitarism
Hypoadrenalism
Liver disease: inherited glycogen storage disorders, cirrhosis, acute liver failure, alcohol
Drugs: insulin, sulphonylureas
Reactive hypoglycaemia (only occurring after a meal), prediabetes, thyrotoxicosis, post-gastrectomy, anxiety

fits both local and general, and recurrent psychiatric disturbances are all common, and frequently occur before breakfast as a result of the overnight fast. In the investigation of this group of patients the prolonged glucose tolerance test (6 h) and the prolonged fast test (up to 72 h) are of value. Every effort should also be made to obtain a blood glucose during an attack. The plasma glucose measurement is of greater value if it can be related to simultaneous plasma insulin levels. A low plasma glucose will, in a patient with insulinoma, be associated with an inappropriately high plasma insulin level.

Certain other diseases have also to be considered when investigating the cause of recurrent blackouts. Tetany, due to a low ionized calcium, does not usually present much difficulty. Paraesthesiae and carpopedal spasm may occur, and Chvostek's and Trousseau's signs should be looked for. An important cause of transient lowering of the ionized calcium is hysterical hyperventilation which can be confused with epilepsy.

Narcolepsy is uncommon and often missed. It may be confused with epilepsy, fainting, and psychiatric disturbance. This is particularly unfortunate as simple and effective treatment is available. The sleepiness of narcolepsy is in every way comparable with normal sleep except that it is excessive and occurs under inappropriate circumstances. The patient can always be easily awakened, and the response to amphetamine is usually good. The frequent association with cataplexy, sleep paralysis and hypnogogic hallucinations is often of help in the diagnosis.

CLINICAL PROBLEM

T	P	BP	R
37	92	160/80	22

Anaemic

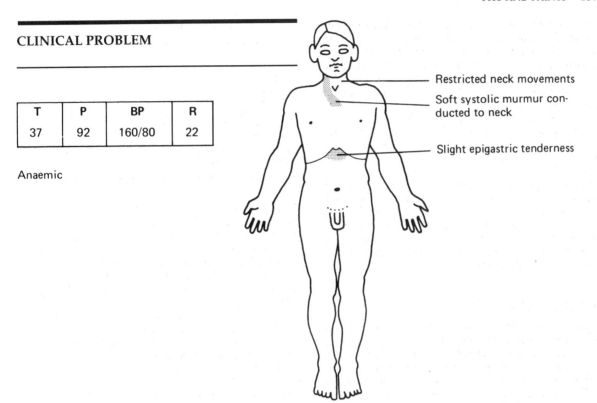

Restricted neck movements

Soft systolic murmur conducted to neck

Slight epigastric tenderness

A 63-year-old male porter presented with the complaint of recurrent blackouts over a period of 3 months. These had occurred mainly during the day while he was at work in the market carrying carcasses of meat, but several had occurred in the evening after he had stood up following an evening's television. The attacks had become more frequent, but had not otherwise altered. He usually had no warning that an attack was going to occur, but on two occasions felt briefly unwell so that he was able to sit down before the blackout occurred. He would become unconscious for a variable period of time, but usually for about 3 minutes. On one occasion only he was incontinent of urine, but had never injured himself. Afterwards he would feel a little weak, though usually able to carry on working following a short rest.

He had smoked 20 cigarettes daily for many years, and for 5 years had had attacks of bronchitis each winter. For 12 months he had suffered occasional rather vague epigastric discomfort and excessive belching, indefinitely related to meals. This had sometimes troubled him in bed at night and occasionally when bending to pick up a carcass. For the same period of time he had felt increasingly tired and had become somewhat depressed. He was a regular beer drinker, usually taking 3–4 pints each night. No-one in his family had suffered from epilepsy although his son had had teething convulsions as a child.

On examination he looked older than his stated age and was a little pale. He was moderately obese. Pulse 92 regular, large volume. Blood pressure 160/80. In the cardiovascular system a soft systolic murmur could be heard over the precordium and was best heard in the aortic area. It could also be heard in the neck. There was no thrill and no signs of heart failure, and the lungs were clear except for the occasional rhonchus. The fundi were normal. Neck movements seemed a little limited and both extension and rotation to the right were painful. No abnormal signs were present in the nervous system. In the abdomen there was minimal epigastric tenderness. Rectal examination was normal and there was no blood evident on the glove.

QUESTIONS

1. What investigations should be done initially on this man?
2. What are the probable diagnoses?

DISCUSSION

The story this man gives of recurrent blackouts is more suggestive of syncopal attacks than epilepsy, but either could account for his symptoms. Examination shows a slightly raised pulse rate and an increased pulse pressure. He is pale, and has signs compatible with bronchitis and mild cervical spondylosis. The aortic systolic murmur is unlikely to be due to aortic stenosis because of the wide pulse pressure. It is probably due to increased blood flow over a roughened aortic valve: aortic sclerosis. At the same time it should be evaluated by cardiac ultrasound, ideally with Doppler quantification if any significant lesion is present. The epigastric tenderness is difficult to evaluate and might well be of no significance for it is a common finding. Vertebrobasilar ischaemia is the likeliest diagnosis, with the attacks clearly related to head movements and changes in posture. There are features suggestive of anaemia which may have precipitated symptoms of vertebrobasilar insufficiency. Full investigation is needed, as a wide variety of disease could be responsible for his symptoms. In the initial investigation of this type of case, a full blood picture must be obtained, as the clinical assessment of anaemia is extremely inaccurate. With this type of history, symptomatic epilepsy is a possibility, and therefore both chest and skull X-ray are indicated. Carcinoma of the bronchus is one of the commonest causes of cerebral tumour, and usually the chest X-ray is abnormal. Skull X-ray may show signs of raised intracranial pressure; there may be shift of the pineal, or even pathological calcification.

Further neuroradiology would depend on the outcome of the initial tests. If these suggested a cerebral lesion then an isotope or CT scan would be indicated, the choice depending on local circumstances. In any patient suffering from recurrent alteration of consciousness an EEG should be obtained, even though in most cases it will be normal. Lumbar puncture would not be a necessary test.

In any smoker, carcinoma of the bronchus must be considered as a possible diagnosis, and cerebral metastases may not give rise to clear-cut epileptic attacks. Furthermore, it is not uncommon for patients to present with cerebral symptoms while their chest X-ray still appears normal with no evidence of the primary tumour. Idiopathic epilepsy is very unlikely to present for the first time at this age.

The diagnosis in this man proved to be transient ischaemic attacks arising in the vertebrobasilar territory, provoked by a severe anaemia due to a bleeding gastric ulcer. On the day after admission he passed a large melaena stool. With treatment of his anaemia no further attacks occurred.

20. Coma

It is common to be confronted with a patient in coma, where the cause is not immediately obvious (Table 20.1). A similar, though by no means identical, problem is presented by the patient who is confused or stuporose.

HISTORY

In this clinical situation, where the usual history is lacking, it is essential to gather as much information as possible from ancillary sources. Relatives and friends must be questioned and the patient's belongings searched. The exact circumstances under which he was found must be carefully elicited. It is of particular importance to know if self-poisoning is a likely cause, and if so what drug or chemical could be involved. The empty bottle or suicide note may give this information.

Table 20.1 Causes of coma

Trauma (concussion and contusion)
Post-ictal
Drugs and alcohol
Vascular:
 cerebral haemorrhage
 subarachnoid haemorrhage
 cerebral infarction
 extradural and subdural haematoma
 hypertensive encephalopathy
Cerebral tumour, primary and secondary
Cerebral infections:
 meningitis
 encephalitis
 abscess
 cerebral malaria
Metabolic causes:
 hypoglycaemia
 hypothyroidism
 hypothermia
 diabetic hyperglycaemic coma
 uraemia
 hepatic coma
 respiratory failure (hypercapnia)
 severe dilutional hyponatraemia

In arriving at a diagnosis it is often of value to know the rapidity with which the coma developed. The contrast between the rate of onset of cerebral thrombosis and cerebral haemorrhage is well known. Further, one should always ask exactly what the patient was doing at the time he was taken ill. The sudden occurrence of subarachnoid haemorrhage, from aneurysm or angioma, on vigorous physical exertion is well recognized. Any recent history of head injury will be of obvious importance. In the same way recent participation in such potentially traumatic activities as rugby football should be noted, even if there has been no obvious injury. Extradural haematoma is still misdiagnosed due to failure to recognize the lucid interval which may occur between the loss of consciousness of the initial injury and the later development of coma. In the elderly patient even trivial trauma may cause subdural haematoma, with a variable period of fluctuating impairment of consciousness and finally coma. This very variable interval of days or weeks makes it difficult to evaluate the significance of recent minor injury (Table 20.2).

It is important, if possible, to establish when the patient was last known to be well. With elderly patients living under circumstances of social isolation this may be very difficult to determine. Even the duration of actual coma before admission will often be uncertain. If the patient is known to have been unwell before coma developed the nature of his symptoms may indicate the present diagnosis. A variety of previous symptoms may be relevant. Previous depression and agitation may point to a present suicidal attempt. Headache, vomiting, and visual failure suggest a space-occupying lesion with raised intracranial pressure. Polyuria, polydipsia, and weight loss point to the hyperglycaemic coma of diabetes. A recent return from the tropics raises the possibility of cerebral malaria.

Before admission, signs may have occurred which will be of diagnostic value. Thus a relative may have noticed abnormal movements suggestive of epilepsy. If these have involved one side of the body it strongly suggests a focal lesion in the contralateral hemisphere. Frequently, little history can be obtained at the time

Table 20.2 Clinical features of extradural and subdural haematoma

	Extradural	Subdural	
		Acute	Chronic
Age:	Often young males	Often young males	Mostly over 50 y
Injury:	Often mild	Usually severe	Only in 50%; usually mild
Skull fracture:	80%	Common	Rare
Haematoma bilateral:	Very rare	15%	15%
Onset:	Less than 12 hours	Less than 3 days	Less than 3 months
Conscious level:	Progressive deterioration	Progressive deterioration	Fluctuant
Lucid interval:	50%	Uncommon	Indefinite
Focal signs:	Commonly moderate	50%, Moderate	Common, Mild
Fits:	Rare	4%	10%
Pupillary signs:	50%	50%	20%
CSF:	Usually clear	Usually bloody	Often xanthochromic

when it would be most valuable – immediately on admission. One source of information sometimes forgotten by the hospital doctor is the patient's general practitioner. Not infrequently he may have been bypassed, friends or perhaps the police having brought the patient directly to an accident and emergency department. The GP may be able to provide valuable information about past illnesses or present drug treatment.

PHYSICAL EXAMINATION

Many patients on regular therapy with potent drugs such as steroids, insulin, or anticoagulants, carry a card saying so. Similarly if they suffer from a rare disease such as porphyria or even a common condition like epilepsy there may well be a statement to this effect in their wallets or on a bracelet. This is a habit to be encouraged and can be of great value in helping one to arrive quickly at the correct diagnosis and treatment. In the future 'smart cards' (data storage cards), which can be read by computer, are likely to be available and will be able to contain unlimited information about an individual.

On occasion systematic clinical examination may have to be delayed to allow for urgent resuscitative measures, such as the establishment of a clear airway. A careful examination of all the body systems must be carried out scrupulously as soon as possible however, and this must include the back as well as the front of the patient! All findings should be carefully recorded with the date and time so that changes in the physical state and in particular in the level of consciousness can be easily assessed, if necessary by other observers. Such notes will also be of the greatest value if medicolegal complications arise.

General observation

One should observe the patient's colour, remembering that minor degrees of jaundice are easily missed in artificial light. Cyanosis will be of obvious importance, and one should also look for any abnormal pinkness suggestive of carbon monoxide poisoning. The pigmentation of Addison's disease must also be looked for. Any movements of face or limbs must be noted, paying especial attention to asymmetry. Focal epileptic discharge is of the greatest value in establishing the site of the lesion as well as narrowing down the list of possible causes of the coma. The rate, rhythm and depth of respiration are all of importance. Cheyne–Stokes respiration or other forms of periodic breathing usually indicate severe cortical or medullary damage and a less good prognosis. Respiration is often shallow, with marked reduction in tidal volume in barbiturate-induced coma. If there is the slightest doubt as to the adequacy of ventilation the question of urgent mechanical ventilation must be considered and blood gas estimations are of the greatest value in making the decision. Continuous non-invasive monitoring of oxygen saturation (oximetry) of the blood is now becoming widely available and again can be of great assistance. These tests frequently demonstrate the inadequacy of a purely clinical assessment of the effectiveness of respiration.

Respiratory failure due to lung disease, when severe, can be a cause of coma. There is disturbance of cerebral function, the high $p\mathrm{CO_2}$ causing increased cerebral blood flow, and this, together with the anoxia, leads to cerebral oedema. Brain swelling will cause a rise in intracranial pressure and dilated retinal veins and papilloedema may be seen. Although most patients with respiratory failure will present only with confusion, coma can develop rapidly at any time, particularly after ill-advised therapy with a high concentration of oxygen.

The typical sighing respiration of diabetic acidosis will usually be obvious and the breath should always be smelt for acetone. Hepatic or uraemic fetor are signs which may be of value but their detection is often difficult.

Examination of the skin can be helpful. The scars of the mainliner drug addict may be found, while diabetics on insulin may show areas of fat atrophy. Loss of body hair, pallor and thinning of the skin will suggest hypopituitarism. The various stigmata of liver disease must also be carefully sought, including spider naevi, clubbing, palmar erythema and Dupuytren's contractures. In the abdomen the discovery of polycystic kidneys or the enlarged bladder of chronic prostatic obstruction may point to uraemia as the underlying cause of the coma.

Temperature

One important measurement is usually left to the nurse: the patient's temperature. Although error is less likely in the detection of liver, hypothermia is easily missed. Hyperpyrexial coma is very rare in Britain but hypothermic coma has been increasingly recognized. If the temperature is low, even if the reading of the routine clinical thermometer is still above the minimum, it is worth checking using a low-reading thermometer inserted rectally. Hypothermia is mainly a disease of the newborn and the elderly, and the likelihood of it developing will obviously be related to the prevailing weather. At these extremes of age, the homeostatic mechanisms which maintain normal body temperature may be impaired. Drugs such as phenothiazines further impair the shivering response to cold. Intercurrent infection may lead to elderly people feeling too ill to keep themselves warm. Myxoedema is not a common cause of hypothermic coma, although hypothermia itself may produce a state resembling myxoedema.

The blood pressure

The blood pressure should be carefully checked, although it can on occasion be misleading. In the hypertensive patient, cerebral haemorrhage is more common, both from congenital anomalies and also from the intracerebral rupture of an arteriosclerotic vessel. A rise in blood pressure may, however, occur as a response to the cerebral catastrophe of haemorrhage, both subarachnoid and intracerebral, and can also occur with extensive cerebral infarction. Indeed anything which produces a rapid rise in intracranial tension seems capable of producing this response, the exact underlying mechanism remaining controversial. Usually the rise in pressure is modest but the blood pressure can occasionally be dramatically high. It will normally settle over the next few days and if continued for more than a week will usually turn out to be long-standing, and not due to the recent neurological damage. The finding of hypertensive fundal changes, together with the signs of left ventricular hypertrophy, will also support the latter interpretation. Hypertension is common in the older age groups and its presence must not weigh too heavily in the making of a diagnosis.

A rare condition to consider if the blood pressure is high and the fundi show Grade III or IV changes is hypertensive encephalopathy. This is sometimes loosely diagnosed whenever neurological signs occur in association with a raised blood pressure. It is however much more than this, being characterized by spasm of the cerebral vessels and widespread cerebral oedema. These changes fluctuate and the neurological signs may vary from hour to hour. Consciousness is impaired and convulsions are common. Sometimes, particularly in association with the renal failure of acute nephritis, the whole clinical picture may occur at levels of blood pressure which are not markedly raised. This probably reflects the widespread damage to small blood vessels seen in acute nephritis. Treatment in hypertensive encephalopathy is a matter of urgency, as disastrous cerebral haemorrhage or infarction can occur at any time. Lowering of the blood pressure in other situations of neurological deficit has aroused considerable controversy. In general all one can say is that firstly the higher the diastolic pressure, whatever the cause, the stronger the indication for treatment, and secondly that in the presence of neurological damage the pressure should be lowered slowly. Marked fluctuation in the pressure is to be avoided.

The pulse

A slow full-volume pulse may occur in raised intracranial tension from any cause. If this is due to respiratory failure then other features may be noted, such as the generalized vasolidation associated with hypercapnia. The presence of an arrhythmia should lead one to suspect a recent myocardial infarction, in which mural thrombosis may develop. This may cause cerebral embolism. However, consciousness is less often lost in embolism in comparison with cerebral thrombosis or haemorrhage. The presence of atrial fibrillation, with or without other evidence of heart disease, will also suggest this possibility. Cardiac arrhythmia of any origin, if it gives rise to profound tachycardia or bradycardia, may cause such a drop in cardiac output that, particularly in the elderly, cerebral perfusion is impaired and confusion results. Syncope may occur but coma is unlikely.

Trauma

Evidence of trauma must always be carefully sought. It may be the cause of the coma or have resulted from the abruptness of the patient's collapse. The temporal fossa should be felt for the boggy swelling due to a haematoma, which would suggest an underlying fracture and possible extradural collection of blood from a torn middle meningeal artery. Bruising about the head in an elderly person will raise the possibility of a chronic subdural haematoma. The skull itself should be carefully felt for depressed fracture and at the same time the nose and ears should be looked at for the bleeding or leakage of CSF which may indicate a fracture of the skull base. Usually with head injury the circumstances under which the patient has been found will indicate the diagnosis. The error is still made of regarding the confused and aggressive man smelling of alcohol as yet another drunk and his gradual lapse into coma as extradural blood collects is missed for want of careful neurological observation.

The nervous system

Examination of the nervous system is obviously limited in the comatose patient. Its main aims will be to establish the level of coma and to look for asymmetry or signs which may suggest the site of a lesion. The fundi may show papilloedema, hypertensive retinopathy, diabetic changes, or the subhyaloid haemorrhages of subarachnoid bleeding. Pupillary abnormalities must be noted and are often a sensitive index to change in the patient's level of consciousness. The constricted pupils of brain-stem haemorrhage or morphine poisoning are well known. Facial weakness can often be detected both by appearance and the way the face blows out on respiration. Neck stiffness should be looked for, but may be absent in deep coma, even in the presence of meningitis. In the limbs, posture, tone, spontaneous movement and reflex pattern should all be noted, together with any features suggestive of long-standing neurological disease. Sensory testing will usually be impossible but the response to deep and superficial pain should be assessed on each side.

INVESTIGATION

In the majority of cases initial investigations will not need to be extensive. Diabetic coma will usually be suggested by the clinical picture and easily confirmed by examination of the urine and blood. Measurement of blood sugar, even with modern techniques should not be left to the most inexperienced nurse! If hypoglycaemia is suspected an instant rough estimation of blood glucose can be done at the bedside, but because the test is inaccurate at low concentrations a therapeutic trial of intravenous glucose may be necessary. Blood should be taken first so that later a glucose estimation by the laboratory will confirm the diagnosis. If poisoning by drug or chemical is a possibility, blood and, if available, gastric contents should be taken and stored, even if immediate analysis of the sample is not possible locally. Later analysis may prove of value and occasionally in forensic problems the presence of such samples will prove of the greatest help. Rapid analysis, both qualitative and quantitative, for common causes of drug coma, such as salicylates and benzodiazepines can be of the greatest assistance. Not only can the precise diagnosis be established, but an assessment can be made of the vigour with which treatment must be pursued.

Suspected subarachnoid haemorrhage or meningitis must usually be confirmed by lumbar puncture. Provided there is nothing which suggests the presence of raised intracranial pressure the risk is negligible. Intracerebral haemorrhage commonly leads to blood in the subarachnoid space and lumbar puncture does not differentiate between the two types of haemorrhage. In subarachnoid haemorrhage, X-ray CT examination may be of great value, but if negative does not exclude the diagnosis.

In the patient where trauma has occurred or may reasonably be suspected, skull X-rays should be obtained. With the widespread availability of CT scanning of the brain, quick, reliable, non-invasive investigation can be undertaken, making other techniques such as angiography, ultrasound and isotope scanning obsolete. In selecting cases for investigation careful and repeated assessment of the level of coma is of the greatest importance in guiding management.

Commonly in cases of coma the cause is initially in doubt. Provided the patient is properly cared for so that deterioration does not pass unnoticed, he is unlikely to come to any harm, and with the passage of time the diagnosis will usually become clear. Deepening coma in an undiagnosed patient is an emergency requiring active investigation and the fullest possible consultation with other specialists, particularly neurosurgeons. The patient should be supported, if necessary by artificial respiration, while this is being done.

It remains true that many cases of coma are misdiagnosed or not diagnosed at all in the first few hours, because the patient has taken an overdose of one of the less obvious drugs under circumstances which do not suggest this diagnosis.

CLINICAL PROBLEM

T	P	BP	R
38·2	82	190/115	24

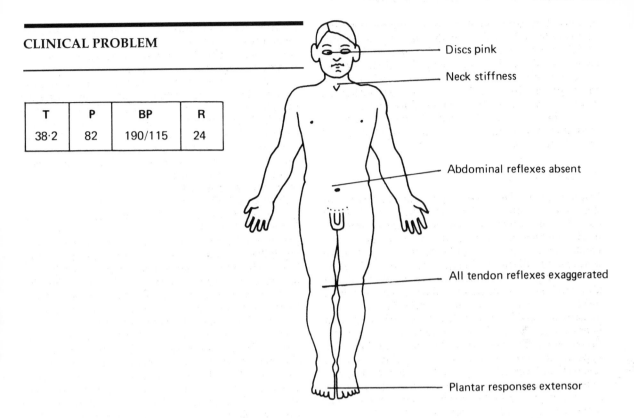

- Discs pink
- Neck stiffness
- Abdominal reflexes absent
- All tendon reflexes exaggerated
- Plantar responses extensor

A successful businessman, aged 55, was found unrousable in bed in the early morning by his wife. He was breathing stertorously. He had gone to bed early because he had felt unwell and tired, having woken the previous morning with symptoms of a mild head cold.

He was known to have been hypertensive for 5 years, a raised blood pressure having been found at a routine insurance examination. There were no symptoms referable to his blood pressure and his general practitioner had put him on a beta-blocker/thiazide combination which he had been taking ever since. His blood pressure, however, had not been checked for 6 months. He had been overweight for a number of years and 2 years previously had developed severe back pain after a long car journey. This settled on bed rest and was thought to have been due to a prolapsed intervertebral disc. He had smoked over 20 cigarettes daily for many years and was a moderately heavy social drinker. There had been no recent business or financial problems.

Examination by the GP showed him to be comatose, although he responded to painful stimuli. There were no signs of a hemiplegia and the plantar responses were flexor. He was admitted to hospital with a suspected cerebrovascular haemorrhage.

On admission he was found to have become more deeply comatose (see diagram). Pulse 82 regular. Blood pressure 190/115. Temperature 38.2°C. Respirations 24. The pupils reacted normally to light both directly and consensually. The discs were a little pink but otherwise the fundi were normal. No lateralizing features were present, the tendon reflexes being symmetrical, and muscle tone generally reduced. The abdominal reflexes could not be elicited, while both plantar responses were probably extensor. No abnormality was present on general examination.

Over the next few hours his condition deteriorated further, the tendon reflexes becoming exaggerated, with the development of some neck stiffness.

QUESTIONS

1. What are the most likely diagnoses?
2. What would be your initial management of this case?

DISCUSSION

The initial diagnosis of cerebral haemorrhage was reasonable, for the condition is common, particularly in hypertensive men of this age. Non-specific premonitory symptoms may occur, and once bleeding commences the development of coma is usually rapid. At the same time, onset during sleep is not typical and there will usually be some asymmetry of signs reflecting the site of the initial bleed. Bilateral signs will occur in brain-stem haemorrhage, but then there will often be pupillary changes, together with other features of medullary damage. The optic fundi in this patient were slightly pink, which raises the possibility of raised intracranial pressure. This is an unreliable sign and should not be taken as an absolute contraindication to lumbar puncture, but should indicate the need for caution.

Cases such as this strengthen the argument for initial lumbar puncture whenever there is the slightest doubt as to the diagnosis in a case of coma. Uniformly blood-stained CSF will strongly support the diagnosis of haemorrhage while the occasional unsuspected meningitis will be diagnosed early. In cases of cerebral haemorrhage, if focal signs develop and persist, further urgent investigation by CT scan may be needed to delineate the possible intracerebral haematoma. In the occasional patient this may cause a fluctuating clinical picture due to alterations in intracranial pressure, and some cases have been thought to have been helped by surgical evacuation of the clot. Carotid arteriography might also then be a reasonable investigation. It would not be part of the initial investigation of the patient.

Viral encephalitis is a less likely diagnosis because of the speed with which the coma developed. Lumbar puncture would aid in the diagnosis of the atypical case, but delay in arriving at the diagnosis is less important because of the lack of specific treatment in the majority of cases. Cerebral venous thrombosis also develops more slowly and often shows a fluctuant course. Coma is usually less profound and focal signs are commonly present. There will often be some other predisposing condition. Subarachnoid haemorrhage is a real possibility although neck stiffness would usually be an early rather than a late feature. It may be completely absent in some severe bleeds.

The possibility of drug overdose must be considered in any comatose patient. There is nothing to suggest this in the patient described here, but depression does become increasingly common with age.

Some 3 days after admission this man died and at postmortem a severe purulent meningitis was found, there being no other pathology. The diagnosis of pneumococcal meningitis had in fact been made by lumbar puncture on the second day of his illness. Examination of the CSF had been delayed because on admission a firm clinical diagnosis was made of intracerebral haemorrhage.

21. Visual failure

In most patients with impairment of visual acuity the cause is a simple error in refraction and correction is straightforward. There are, however, a wide variety of other possible reasons, which may be much less obvious, requiring careful examination and investigation before they can be diagnosed (Table 21.1). Many causes are due to disease elsewhere in the body.

The commonest causes of blindness in Britain are intrinsic diseases of the eye, such as senile cataract , macular degeneration, glaucoma, retinal detachment, and the retinopathy of diabetes mellitus. These will normally be obvious on direct examination of the eye. Patients often have difficulty in describing accurately the nature of their disability and it is important to establish whether there is a true impairment of acuity and not some other symptom such as diplopia.

HISTORY

It is essential to enquire whether the impairment has come on rapidly, in seconds, or over hours, days or months. Sometimes when the visual loss is unilateral the patient has only discovered it by chance, when for some reason he covered his sound eye. Alternatively, and particularly with field defects such as hemianopia or quadrantanopia where central vision is preserved and the loss is peripheral, the disability is only discovered on routine examination. Sometimes a patient may misinterpret a hemianopia, for example to the left, as being a failure of vision in the left eye. In other cases, the patient may be unaware that he has suffered visual loss and is thus unable to describe its development. The other information of the greatest help in diagnosis is whether the loss is unilateral or bilateral. Again this needs careful confirmation by examination. Another important symptom is of rainbow-coloured halos seen around lights which is a typical feature of the prodromal phase of acute congestive glaucoma. The main diagnostic difficulty tends to be with central nervous system disease presenting with visual failure.

Visual changes occur in a variety of systemic diseases, and even if they are of no direct importance, they will draw attention to the underlying disease. Symptoms must be sought therefore of conditions such as anaemia, vitamin B_1 or B_{12} deficiency, pituitary tumour, diabetes mellitus, cranial arteritis and carotid artery atheroma. Cardiac arrhythmias and infective endocarditis can give rise to emboli which may reach the retinal or cerebral vessels and impair vision.

When taking the history, it must be remembered that any alteration in vision, with its implied threat to sight, is alarming and distressing to the patient and this, allied to difficulties in description, makes it all too easy for the doctor to lose patience and consider a psychiatric diagnosis. While hysterical blindness does occur, it is uncommon. The visual loss is usually complete and frequently the patients appear little concerned by their disability. Other hysterical symptoms may be present, often related to the eyes.

The circumstances under which the visual impairment occurs may also be a clue to its nature. Thus defective vision in dim light will suggest night blindness. Although this is rare it is a feature not only of vitamin A deficiency but also of such diseases as

Table 21.1 Differential diagnosis of bilateral visual failure

1. Rapid bilateral blindness
Occiptal lobe ischaemia due to vascular disease
Cerebral oedema with or without hypertension
Occipital lobe trauma
Toxic damage to the optic nerves, e.g. methyl alcohol poisoning
Neuromyelitis optica
Hysteria
Cranial arteritis (usually affects one eye first)

2. Gradual bilateral blindness
Senile cataract
Senile macular degeneration
Chronic glaucoma
Retinal disease, e.g. diabetic
Optic atrophy:
a) optic nerve chiasmal compassion e.g. tumour/aneurysm
b) optic neuritis e.g. multiple sclerosis
c) toxic damage e.g. alcohol, tobacco
d) hereditary e.g. Leber's, amaurotic familial degeneration

retinitis pigmentosa and syphilitic retinitis. It may also be complained of in hysteria. A characteristic story is occasionally elicited from patients with hemianopic field defects: a temporal loss of vision leading the patient to repeatedly knock into both people and objects on that side, sometimes leading to traffic accidents if vehicles approaching on the hemianopic side are missed.

The past history must be carefully elicited with a record of all the drugs the patient is receiving, or has taken over the previous year. Earlier symptoms suggestive of multiple sclerosis will provide an explanation of a present attack of acute retrobulbar neuritis. Sarcoidosis can involve the optic nerve as well as the lungs, and polyarteritis nodosa the retinal vessels in addition to those of muscle and kidney. A wide variety of drugs and chemicals can damage the optic nerve. Quinine, lead and methyl alcohol are well known causes, as are various halogenated hydrocarbons and organic arsenicals. Visual failure may also occur with the potent antituberculous drug ethambutol. Retinal damage with serious and irreversible loss of vision is seen in long-term chloroquine therapy for rheumatoid arthritis, and can progress for some time after the drug has been stopped. Tobacco and alcohol consumption must also be checked. Excess in either of these habits, particularly when combined as they so often are, may lead to a chronic retrobulbar neuritis with defective vision.

The family history occasionally is of value. Rare conditions such as Leber's Hereditary Optic Atrophy, Amaurotic Familial Idiocy, and retinitis pigmentosa will usually be associated with a history of other affected members in the family. In young girls, basilar migraine can produce a confusing story, and a positive family history for migraine should be always sought because the patient herself may not have had previous typical headaches (see Ch. 20).

EXAMINATION OF THE EYE

It is as well to begin with the eyes, both to confirm and measure the patient's disability and also because the diagnosis may be immediately apparent and thus allow the remainder of the examination to be both more appropriate and rapid. Fortunately the diagnostic aids need only be very simple. The highest plus lens of the ophthalmoscope gives a good view of the front of the eye, of the anterior structures such as cornea, aqueous, iris and lens. The retina is examined in the usual way. Visual fields and blind spots can be usefully assessed by the traditional whiteheaded pin, even though the precise delineation of field defects and central scotomata will require formal perimetry and the use of a Bjerrum screen. These latter techniques, although simple, require some practice and are time-consuming. Undoubtedly in the future increasing use will be made of the newer methods of automatic screening.

A measurement which is commonly ignored by the general physician is a precise evaluation of visual acuity. Although the use of a Snellen chart is difficult unless the ward or clinic has been properly equipped, a reasonable idea of the acuity can be obtained by the use of a set of test types, such as Jaeger's Test Card. It can be surprising on occasion how poor is the correlation – in either direction – between the complaint by the patient and the degree of defect found. Measurement of acuity also allows the progress of the patient to be followed and for treatment to be initiated at an early stage. Although acuity is important it only reflects macular function and if normal does not exclude other defects. Gross reduction in visual field may occur with complete preservation of central vision.

As in the other areas of the body examination of the eye must be systematic. Proptosis is displacement of the eyeball forwards. It may be caused by primary or secondary tumour, granulomas such as histiocytosis X, and leukaemic infiltrations. It is also a characteristic feature of Graves' disease. Occasionally it may be combined with pulsation of the globe and a bruit, due to an aneurysm in the cavernous sinus or a vascular tumour. In all these situations there may be pressure on the optic nerve with visual failure. Apparent proptosis may occur when the large eyeball of high myopia is misinterpreted.

Ptosis can occur as a result of sympathetic or third nerve damage. It is a feature of neurosyphilis where there may also be optic atrophy. It may be a feature of myasthenia, and in younger patients as a congenital abnormality.

The ocular movements must be checked and the pupillary reflexes elicited both directly and consensually. In optic atrophy there may be a fixed dilated pupil which will only react to consensual stimulation. The pupil may also be fixed after previous iritis with adhesions. If visual impairment is due to damage to the optic radiation or occipital cortex the pupillary reflexes will be normal. Cortical blindness is not common and is often misdiagnosed, for there are no physical signs other than a failure to blink on menace. The pupillary reflexes are retained and the differential diagnosis is from hysterical blindness.

Cataract occurs commonly in diabetic patients. In juvenile diabetes a specific type of cataract may rapidly develop which has a characteristic snowflake appearance. In addition senile cataract occurs more frequently and at an earlier age but does not differ otherwise from that seen in the non-diabetic. Impairment of vision is also seen if the blood sugar is varying widely, probably due to osmotic changes altering the curvature of the lens. It responds quickly to control of the diabetes.

The cornea is examined for inflammation or ulceration or the presence of a foreign body. Cloudiness and oedema occur in acute glaucoma and the tension of the eyeball must always be carefully assessed, certainly by palpation and ideally by tonometry. The surrounding conjunctiva may show the generalized hyperaemia of conjunctivitis or the circumcorneal injection of iritis. Exudation of pus or blood may be seen in the anterior chamber, and keratic precipitates may be present on the back of the cornea due to an underlying iridocyclitis. The iris may be tremulous, due to lack of support by the lens because of dislocation, as seen in Marfan's syndrome or homocystinuria. Adhesions may be present from the iris to the back of the cornea or to the lens due to inflammation, with associated deformation of the pupil.

In the older age group, senile cataract becomes an increasingly important reason for visual impairment. Commonly, in the early stages, the opacification begins as streaks spreading in from the periphery of the lens like the spokes of a wheel. Later, without surgery, after a period of swelling the lens shrinks, losing fluid, and becomes generally opaque; this is the stage of hypermaturity when it is ripe for operation.

Ophthalmoscopic examination

When looking at the fundus, adequate illumination is essential and exhausted batteries and blackened bulbs remain the commonest reason for failure in diagnosis. Ideally the room should be darkened. If the pupil is small a suitable mydriatic should be used to allow adequate examination. Although mydriatics such as atropine have no effect on the tension of the normal eye they may precipitate an attack of glaucoma if the angle of the anterior chamber is narrow. For this reason the depth of the anterior chamber should be assessed before they are instilled. The usual diagnostic mydriatic is tropicamide, which is mild and short-acting and does not need to be reversed. An alternative is to use cocaine, which lowers the intraocular tension. The action of other mydriatics should be reversed after use. It is important not to be confused by normal variations such as opaque nerve fibres spreading out from the margins of the disc, or by choroidal pigments surrounding the disc. The nasal margin may be indistinct normally, and the disc generally may be less sharply seen in young long-sighted individuals. The physiological cup is usually a little paler than the rest of the disc and may occupy up to one-half of its area. It never occupies the whole disc.

Examination may reveal a wide variety of abnormal conditions, but the commoner changes are those of papilloedema, optic atrophy, retinopathy, retinal detachment, choroiditis and senile macular degeneration. Among the more important types of retinopathy are diabetic and hypertensive.

Papilloedema is an important finding and typically visual acuity is not greatly impaired early except for transient obscurations. Later on however, severe failure may occur very rapidly. When present bilat-

erally the commonest cause is cerebral tumour, particularly of the posterior fossa. It is unusual in cerebrovascular accidents, although it may occur transiently in subarachnoid haemorrhage. Viral encephalitis, toxic encephalopathy or trauma can also produce the necessary cerebral swelling and rise in intracranial pressure. Sometimes when there is marked CO_2 retention due to respiratory failure, papilloedema develops. An important although rare cause is benign intracranial hypertension, and sometimes surgical decompression is necessary in this condition to prevent visual loss. Its occurrence almost entirely in females, and the common relationship between the onset of the disorder and menstrual disturbances will help in the diagnosis (see Ch. 23). Unilateral papilloedema may occasionally occur on the side opposite to a frontal lobe neoplasm, but more often it reflects local disease of the eye or orbit. Central retinal vein thrombosis may give rise to blindness and is usually obvious on ophthalmoscopic examination. The optic disc is swollen and the retinal veins overfilled, with A-V nipping. Scattered large and small haemorrhages and exudates are seen. This condition may occur as a complication of hypertension, diabetes, atheroma, various clotting disorders and polycythaemia.

In contrast to papilloedema, optic neuritis usually produces marked impairment of visual acuity with little evidence of change in the optic discs and fundi. If inflammatory change occurs immediately behind the eye some swelling of the disc may occur but this is not usually marked, nor is it associated with other retinal changes. Demyelination is the most important cause and when unilateral is usually due to multiple sclerosis. Central vision is impaired with a central or paracentral scotoma. The eyeball is commonly tender, and there is retro-orbital or temporal pain. If bilateral it may be due to neuromyelitis optica where transverse myelitis occurs in association with bilateral optic neuritis. Nutritional deficiency, particularly of vitamin B_{12}, can cause an optic neuritis, as may drugs such as tobacco or methyl alcohol.

Optic atrophy can follow any of the above conditions and if it has been preceded by any degree of swelling of the disc there may be evidence of this. One may see sheathing of the disc with connective tissue, hiding the lamina cribrosa, while the veins will be turtuous and may be partially surrounded by fibrous tissue. Although optic atrophy can be diagnosed ophthalmoscopically little information will usually be gained as to its cause. Frequently it will be due to pressure on the optic nerve, chiasma or tract. Visual field and Bjerrum screen examination can provide most valuable data as to the site of the lesion in the optic nerve.

GENERAL EXAMINATION

Severe anaemia from any cause can occasionally lead to visual failure, with retinal haemorrhages and exudates. Impairment of vision may occur rapidly if there has been severe blood loss, probably due to a failure of perfusion of the retina and occipital cortex. Impairment is especially likely in severe pernicious anaemia, as in this case deficiency of B_{12} may lead directly to damage to the optic nerves. A plethoric colour suggests the possibility of polycythaemia with its tendency to both arterial and venous thromboses. The skin should also be examined for evidence of any bleeding tendency such as petechiae or ecchymoses, and for the septic emboli that may occur, especially in the finger pulps, from infective endocarditis. The peripheral pulses, if absent, will suggest vascular disease or perhaps embolization from endocarditis.

The blood pressure must always be measured. If the patient is on hypotensive drugs any postural drop must be noted, and always the effect of exercise on the blood pressure. When examining the head and neck the temporal arteries should be felt, as sudden blindness and also diplopia and field defects may occur abruptly, without warning, in the presence of cranial arteritis. Cortical blindness may also occur from this condition. In association with arteritis the muscles of the neck may be tender and some degree of cervical lymphadenopathy can occur.

The carotid and vertebral arteries should be felt and auscultated. Recurrent microembolization of the retina producing transient episodes of blindness may be caused by atheromatous ulceration of a carotid artery and effective treatment by surgical disobliteration or anticoagulation is effective in some patients.

Examination of the heart may reveal rheumatic or congenital disease which predispose to endocarditis. Cortical blindness can occur in acute nephritis, probably due to cerebral oedema resulting from vasoconstriction and damage to small vessels. There may be few signs pointing towards renal disease, so the urine should always be examined and the blood urea measured in any such case. Visual loss in the end stages of chronic renal disease may also occur but is unlikely to cause diagnostic difficulty.

Pituitary tumours producing compression of the visual pathways can lead to marked visual field defects which are often diagnosed late. They can also lead to endocrine failure and this may be clinically obvious. Skin texture and hair distribution should be noted particularly.

The examination of the nervous system is most important. A wide variety of diseases can affect any part of the visual pathway from the back of the eyeball to the occipital cortex. As well as the visual changes they will often produce symptoms and signs resulting from damage to other parts of the brain and spinal cord, which will commonly lead more easily to the diagnosis. An obvious example of this is multiple sclerosis, but it is also true for arterial aneurysm compressing the visual pathway in the region of the chiasma, and for tumours and areas of infarction within the cerebral hemisphere. The localization of the visual cortical areas posteriorly at the occipital poles means that they may be specifically damaged by localized trauma in this region, and also, since they are supplied by the posterior cerebral arteries, that they may be affected by ischaemic disturbances of the vertebrobasilar system.

The underlying diagnosis will usually be obvious in such conditions as meningitis, encephalitis and neurosyphilis. It is often obscure in chronic granulomatous disorders like sarcoidosis, and may only become established when lesions develop elsewhere, more accessible to biopsy.

SPECIAL INVESTIGATIONS

In the majority of the above diseases the diagnosis is reached on clinical grounds alone. Biochemical tests will be needed to establish the presence of diabetes and renal disease, and may be of value in identifying chemical toxins. Assay of vitamin B_{12} may show a deficiency despite a normal haemoglobin and the absence of the classical signs of subacute combined degeneration. Neuroradiology is essential to exclude neoplasm, if this is suspected, for example: glioma of the optic nerve, chromophobe adenoma of the pituitary, or meningioma of the base of the skull. While the diagnosis can sometimes be obvious from straight skull films, special views of the optic foramina, CT scan and angiography may all be needed. In diseases of the carotid arteries Doppler ultrasound imaging will be required.

CLINICAL PROBLEM

T	P	BP	R
37·2	92	180/115	26

Normal pupillary reflexes

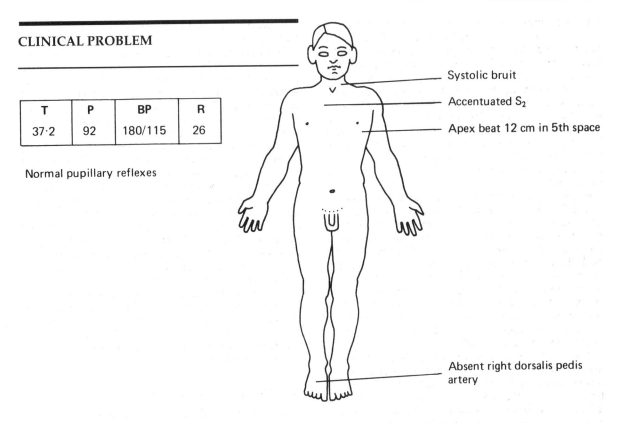

Systolic bruit

Accentuated S₂

Apex beat 12 cm in 5th space

Absent right dorsalis pedis artery

A man of 72 years, a retired publisher, was admitted to hospital because of the abrupt onset of total blindness. His vision had been completely normal and he had felt quite well until the morning of admission, when on standing up after cleaning the bath he became blind. He had rested for several hours but his vision did not improve.

In the previous few months he had been under some stress at home because of the illness of his wife with an inoperable carcinoma of the breast. Five years previously he had been found to have a raised blood pressure when he had consulted his GP because of recurrent episodes of dizziness. He had been treated since that time with a thiazide diuretic. He had smoked 20 cigarettes daily for many years, and had taken only moderate quantities of alcohol. There was nothing of relevance in his family history.

On examination he was distressed and agitated and said he could see nothing. The pupillary reflexes were normal, the pupils responding to both direct and consensual stimulation. His pupils constricted when he was asked to look towards the end of his nose. There was, however, a failure to blink on menace, in both eyes. The fundi showed minimal arteriosclerotic changes only. Pulse 92 regular. Blood pressure 180/115. Neck movements were full and pain-free. There was cardiac enlargement with a forceful cardiac impulse. The second sound was accentuated, but no murmurs were present in the heart. A systolic bruit however could be heard over the left carotid artery. The right dorsalis pedis artery could not be felt. There were no signs of heart failure and the lungs were clear.

No abnormality was otherwise present in the cranial nerves. Examination of the limbs was quite normal, there being no long tract signs. He appeared to be appropriately concerned about his sudden disability and there was no evidence of any gross psychiatric disturbance.

Initial investigations included chest and skull X-rays which were normal. There was no anaemia and no abnormality was seen in the peripheral blood film. The urine contained no sugar, but there was a trace of protein.

QUESTIONS

1. What is the most likely cause of this patient's blindness?
2. What further investigation would be of value?
3. What do you imagine will be the eventual outcome?

DISCUSSION

This patient's presenting complaint is straightforward: he has suddenly become blind. It is always important in such a case to analyse carefully the degree of visual loss, the speed with which it came on, and the circumstances under which it developed. Any past history of visual disturbance however transitory should also be sought. The rapidity of onset of symptoms in this case suggests a vascular cause, although a similar story is also commonly given by patients with hysterical blindness. The continuation of the blindness for at least several hours would indicate that there is probably some degree of structural damage and not simply a reversible functional impairment.

The patient's past history of hypertension and of heavy cigarette smoking also increase the likelihood of cerebrovascular disease. Furthermore when his hypertension was first diagnosed he was complaining of recurrent episodes of dizziness, presumably occurring on a basis of impaired cerebral perfusion, and suggesting that there was some degree of cerebrovascular disease already present. The drug treatment he is receiving for his blood pressure is unlikely to be relevant in this respect as it does not produce postural hypotension.

The recent illness of his wife with carcinoma of the breast can reasonably be supposed to be a cause of considerable stress and the possibility of a psychogenic reaction must be seriously considered. Gross hysterical symptoms such as blindness or paralysis are much less common now than in the past. They were particularly well described in battle casualties during the last war. They still occur occasionally, and are usually a response to some situation which the patient finds intolerable. Such a reaction is more common in those of low intelligence or poor education, and is undoubtedly predisposed to by previous head injury. The likelihood of the diagnosis of an hysterical illness being correct would be greatly increased if there had been previous reactions of an hysterical nature or some other evidence of a neurotic personality structure in the past. It is rare for an hysterical reaction to occur for the first time at the age of 72 years and the absence of any previous psychiatric history must therefore throw doubt on this diagnosis. However any form of organic cerebral disease may lead to the appearance of hysterical or affective symptoms for the first time at any age. It could therefore be argued that a background of developing cerebrovascular disease has predisposed this man to an hysterical response to his wife's illness. It is important in this type of case, both when taking the history and when examining the patient, to evaluate the mental state and to try and assess whether the patient's reaction to his symptom is appropriate. A lack of emotional response may be claimed as the 'belle indifférence' of Janet, but could just as easily be his habitual stoicism.

Examination of this patient revealed clear evidence of widespread vascular disease. His blood pressure is raised, a bruit is present over one carotid and a peripheral pulse in a foot is missing. The findings on examination of the eyes indicate that there is no damage to the peripheral visual mechanism, or to the visual connections with the brain stem, for the pupillary responses are all intact. The loss of the menace response supports his claim to be blind. His emotional response also suggests that his blindness is organic in nature. The likely diagnosis, therefore, is blindness due to ischaemia of the occipital poles of the cerebral hemispheres due to vascular disease. Such a syndrome can occur temporarily as a result of the vascular spasm of migraine, but this is not a relevant diagnosis here. Blindness due to vascular spasm associated with cerebral oedema may occur in hypertensive encephalopathy, and this syndrome can develop at relatively low levels of blood pressure if there is renal failure. The absence of significant retinopathy excludes this diagnosis, although it would be reasonable to check the blood urea.

Sudden blindness although not common, is a well recognized complication of vertebrobasilar disease. Although it may be complete as in this case, commonly as recovery occurs the visual loss takes the form of an homonymous hemianopia, and at this stage macular vision may be better preserved than peripheral. The final recovery of vision is often surprisingly good, although the overall prognosis is poor as there is usually generalized vascular disease. If there is doubt as to whether sudden bilateral blindness is hysterical or due to occipital cortical damage, an EEG may help by showing abnormalities posteriorly and failure to respond to photic stimulation. A CT scan may confirm bilateral occipital lobe infarcts. Using the radiopharmaceutical HMPAO (Ceretec), SPECT scanning of the brain will show areas of reduced or absent blood flow in the occipital lobes.

> This patient's cortical blindness slowly improved over 3 weeks. A presumptive diagnosis of basilar artery thrombosis was made.

22.   Dizziness

This is a common symptom, and often causes much difficulty in communication between doctor and patient. The word is frequently used loosely to cover many different sensations, ranging from the panic attacks of the housebound housewife when she ventures out of doors, to the rotary vertigo of Ménière's disease. The essential element which must be sought is a disturbance of the patient's subjective orientation in space, with an associated sense of movement, of the patient, of his surroundings, or of both. The term vertigo is sometimes used as an equivalent to dizziness, but it is better reserved for the sense of rotation most typically complained of in labyrinthine disease. In the majority of patients where a definite diagnosis is eventually arrived at, the complaint will have been of vertigo. Where the patient complains of non-rotatory dizziness it is common never to achieve a clear-cut explanation of his symptoms even though they are probably occurring on an organic basis.

It is convenient to classify the various causes of dizziness into those which give rise to a single attack which then improves, and where the diagnosis is more likely to be obvious from other associated features, and those where recurrent attacks occur, often over a long period. A second useful division is between those patients who have rotatory vertigo and those where the dizziness reflects a much less clearly defined sense of movement.

Unusual presentations of common disease may be much more frequent than typical cases of rare diseases. Thus the onset of acute vertigo can be the result of multiple sclerosis with demyelination involving the brain stem. This is not the most usual presentation of multiple sclerosis but undoubtedly is far commoner than, for example, syphilitic labyrinthitis.

Another feature which occasionally causes confusion is that vertigo, if severe, will almost invariably be associated with nausea, vomiting, sweating, ataxia and pallor. The presence of these symptoms does not, therefore, require some additional explanation. Severe vertigo even when due to some quite trivial cause is a very unpleasant and incapacitating symptom and the patient may both feel and appear to be quite disproportionately ill.

CLINICAL ASSESSMENT

History

As will already be obvious a careful history is needed and this may require considerable time and patience. As far as possible the precise experience of the patient must be determined, together with its time course. The patient should always be asked whether the occurrence of symptoms can be related to any particular position of the head or to any especial movement of the neck. Benign positional vertigo is a common condition and attacks follow movements of the head, such as occur on lying down at night or on getting up in the morning. It can be contrasted with the less clear-cut dizziness that may occur in patients with cervical spondylosis where the movement of the neck leads to compression of the often atherosclerotic vertebral artery and thus to brain-stem ischaemia. A sudden onset of vertigo without deafness in a young person, who may recently have had an upper respiratory infection, will suggest the diagnosis of vestibular neuronitis.

All associated symptoms must be noted and certain important ones such as deafness, tinnitus and aural discharge carefully looked for. If these symptoms are present their pattern must be analysed and their relationship to the primary symptom of dizziness established. Thus in Meniere's disease, some patients may not complain of the deafness or tinnitus that typically make up the clinical picture, because they are so minor that they do not concern them. If present, however mild, they add considerable support to this diagnosis.

Recent physical illness is unlikely to be missed but it is also important to note any head injury, however trivial. Non-specific dizziness, which may be positional in type, is common after head injury and its occurrence is not closely related to the severity of the injury. It usually settles within a few weeks or months, although sometimes it may continue much longer, particularly when the question of financial compensation remains unsettled. Assessment of the extent to which a functional element is present in such cases is very difficult.

Dizziness is a common symptom in menopausal women, and is often associated with other features due to vasomotor instability.

As always, any drug therapy that the patient is receiving must be noted. Streptomycin toxicity is unlikely to cause any diagnostic difficulty. It is related to the dose of drug given and is most likely to occur in the elderly and those with renal failure. Patients are still referred to hospital because of the side-effects of phenytoin, and some of these patients have signs of a cerebellar disturbance. Many patients, especially in the older age groups, are receiving hypotensive therapy. In the past, postural and exercise hypotension were common and troublesome side-effects which resulted in dizziness and syncope. Although now much less common, they still occur, particularly in the more arteriosclerotic patients.

Severe vertigo, ataxia and nystagmus may develop in alcoholics as part of the picture of Wernicke's encephalopathy. A history of excess alcohol intake must always be sought, and the rapid therapeutic response to thiamine which is usually obtained is of value as a diagnostic test.

The family history is not usually helpful, although sometimes a strong background of migraine may alert the physician to this possibility as the explanation of a series of vertiginous attacks. Brain-stem migraine is now a well-recognized condition, but because it is much less common than the classical form, mistakes in diagnosis continue to be made. It seems to be more frequent in young women, and may cause particular confusion in diagnosis when the presentation is recurrent disturbances of consciousness (see Chs. 19 and 21).

Physical examination

A full general examination is required, but particularly attention must be paid to the central nervous and cardiovascular systems, and also to the function of the auditory and vestibular mechanisms. Anaemia and polycythaemia must be looked for, and the blood pressure must be checked both lying and standing and, if indicated, after exercise. If the vertigo is related to exercise of the arms, the pressure should also be measured in each arm, as there may be a subclavian steal syndrome. All the pulses must be felt. A reduction of the carotid pulse or bruits heard over either the carotid or vertebral arteries will indicate extracranial cerebrovascular disease. One may also find an arrhythmia, which if intermittent can give rise to syncope or dizziness (see Ch. 19). Rarely, increased carotid sinus sensitivity can also give rise to such symptoms. In the heart there may be evidence of anaemia in the form of a tachycardia and apical systolic murmur. Movements of the cervical spine should be examined and the patient asked whether any position of the neck produces his symptoms.

In the general examination it is important to look for evidence of thiamine deficiency, as this will aid a diagnosis of Wernicke's encephalopathy. Most attention, however, must be to the central nervous system. In the majority of patients complaining of dizziness no abnormal signs are found that would suggest disease of temporal lobe, cerebellum, or brain stem. If present, however, the list of probable diagnoses changes considerably. Thus infarction in the territory of the posterior inferior cerebellar artery, tumours of the cerebellar vermis, multiple sclerosis involving the medulla, brain stem encephalitis, and basilar artery aneurysm can all give rise to recurrent vertigo, usually associated with other distinctive symptoms.

An important, although rare, cause of vertigo is a tumour of the cerebellopontine angle, the commonest being the acoustic neuroma. Although later on these will give signs of central damage from compression of the brain stem and hydrocephalus, every effort should be made to establish the diagnosis at an earlier stage while the tumour is still small. An important physical sign, absent in most of the other commoner causes of vertigo, is diminished corneal sensation and this must be always looked for with considerable care in all cases of dizziness.

Other important central nervous system signs in the diagnosis of dizziness are nystagmus and 8th cranial nerve involvement.

Nystagmus

This remains a physical sign that is often poorly elicited and analysed and its interpretation is perhaps the source of even more confusion. When testing for its presence the patient must not be asked to look to the extreme limits of his gaze, for then anyone may show spurious nystagmus. Furthermore at least 5 seconds should be allowed in each direction for it to develop. The presence of a few nystagmoid jerks, such as occur commonly in normal people when tired, should be ignored. If present, the position of the eyes when the nystagmus occurs, the deviation which produces the greatest amplitude, and the direction of the fast movement, should all be noted. Nystagmus is usually described by the direction of the fast component if present.

A number of types of nystagmus can be distinguished clinically. One is pendular nystagmus, where there is a rapid symmetrical horizontal oscillation on either side of the midline. This form of nystagmus is due to local ocular disease and is not important in the differential diagnosis of dizziness. The more common and significant form of nystagmus is jerk nystagmus, where there is a fast movement in one direction followed by a slow movement in the other. Jerk nystagmus can be present at rest or on deviation of the eyes, and can be horizontal, vertical, or rotary. Nystagmus of this kind always indicates disease of the labyrinth or its higher connections.

Dissociated or ataxic nystagmus is present when the abducting eye shows coarse and irregular nystagmus, while the adducting eye shows only a fine nystagmus associated with some degree of paresis of the medial rectus of that eye. It most commonly occurs in multiple sclerosis.

The eighth nerve

It is important to test both divisions of this nerve, whether or not the patient actually complains of deafness. Simple clinical tests can be surprisingly effective. Care must be taken to mask the other ear and also to exclude the presence of wax by inspection with an auroscope. At the same time obvious disease of the drum and middle ear can be excluded. If any impairment of hearing is found, Rinne's and Weber's tests should be done to differentiate between conductive middle-ear deafness and perceptive nerve deafness. Normally in the Rinne test the tuning fork can be heard twice as long by air conduction as by bone conduction from the mastoid. In Weber's test the tuning fork at the vertex of the skull will normally not be lateralized.

Investigation of labyrinthine function is rather more complex, and the caloric and rotational tests used are not normally performed as part of routine examination. The delineation in recent years of the condition of benign positional vertigo does, however, justify testing for positional vertigo and nystagmus as it can be done quickly and simply. Starting with the patient sitting on a couch, the head is turned to one side and then the patient is laid back with his head hyperextended over the end of the couch. Each side is tested in turn several times. The positive result obtained in benign positional vertigo develops after a latent interval of some seconds and disappears if the test is repeated several times (adaptation). The nystagmus is chiefly rotatory and is directed to the underlying ear. If, as in some less common cases, the positional vertigo is due to a central lesion of the posterior fossa the nystagmus appears immediately and does not show adaptation.

Simplified tests of caloric function can be used. One is to irrigate each auditory meatus in turn with 5 ml of 5°C water, the patient sitting upright with his head tilted 60° backwards. The time is noted to the onset of the typical symptoms of nausea and dizziness. There is horizontal nystagmus away from the side irrigated. Vestibular damage is indicated by a delay and reduction in the response.

SPECIAL INVESTIGATIONS

In the majority of patients these will not be needed. If any impairment of hearing is detected or suspected, this should be delineated accurately using the audiometer to measure the threshold at different frequencies. A valuable test is for loudness recruit-ment. Here the relative loudness of two sounds, one presented to the normal ear and one to the deaf ear, is assessed at differing overall levels of intensity. In some patients as the overall loudness is increased the difference between the two sounds decreases – the phenomenon of loudness recruitment. It appears to be due to a lesion producing selective destruction of the low intensity elements of the cochlea itself. Lesions of the cochlear nerve and central nervous system usually affect fibres from the low and high elements equally and then loudness recruitment is less likely to occur. The test is positive in all cases of Ménière's disease where the low intensity elements are especially affected. Loudness recruitment does not occur in cases of vestibular neuronitis, where the cochlea is unaffected and the hearing usually normal. It is positive only to a minor extent in a few cases of acoustic neuroma.

Caloric testing (Fig. 22.1) is based on the warming and cooling of the lateral semicircular canals by water, usually at 44° and 30°C. Convection currents are set up resulting in movement of the cupolas: the normal finding with cold water will be nausea, horizontal nystagmus to the opposite side, and falling to the stimulated side. With warm water, the opposite results are obtained. The exact onset and duration of the nystagmus can be assessed clinically or more exactly be recording electrodes around the eye – electronystagmography. The simplest and commonest abnormality which is detected is canal paresis, where the duration of the nystagmus is reduced when the affected side is irrigated by both hot and cold water. Canal paresis results from damage to the vestibular system, particularly to the cupolar sense organs or their connections. A second type of abnormality that may be seen is directional preponderance, Here nystagmus in a particular direction is reduced, while in the other direction it is increased. Such a pattern occurs particularly with lesions of the central connections of the labyrinth, the nystagmus being towards the side of the lesion. This pattern (rather more than the canal paresis pattern) may also occur with lesions of the cerebellum or the posterior temporal lobe if these involve vestibular connections.

Examination of the CSF will be of value in encephalitis and occasionally can help in the diagnosis of multiple sclerosis. In acoustic neuroma the protein content is usually markedly increased and the extent of the rise correlates roughly with the size of the tumour. In one series, however, 25% showed a normal protein.

Neuroradiology will be of little value in the majority of cases. X-ray of the cervical spine may show the changes of cervical spondylosis, or the calcified arteries of extracranial cerebrovascular disease. Skull views are important in the diagnosis of acoustic neuroma, particular attention being paid

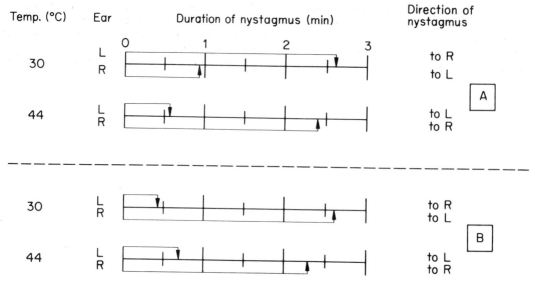

Fig. 22.1 Patterns of caloric response

Normally nystagmus continues for 2–3 minutes and is equal on each side. Cold water induces nystagmus to the opposite side, hot water the reverse. In canal paresis the duration of nystagmus is reduced in the affected ear for both hot and cold water. In directional preponderance the duration of nystagmus is reduced when the nystagmus is provoked towards the side of the lesion.

A. Nystagmus is reduced in duration to the left, when either ear is irrigated. There is therefore directional preponderance to the right. This was due to a L temporal glioma

B. Nystagmus is reduced when the left ear is irrigated by hot or cold water. This is left canal paresis, due to Ménière's disease

to the internal auditory meatus. The slightest difference in diameter of the two canals is suspicious, as is any erosion or alteration in shape. Congenital or acquired lesions of the base of the skull may also be seen. If a space-occupying lesion of the posterior fossa is suspected then a CT scan should be obtained. Contrast studies either by air encephalography or myodil ventriculography are now only rarely required.

In those cases where episodes of cardiac arrhythmia are a possible cause of dizziness, ambulatory monitoring of the ECG will often allow a precise diagnosis to be made.

DIFFERENTIAL DIAGNOSIS

In the majority of patients who give a history of clear-cut recurrent attacks of vertigo the diagnosis will usually lie between Ménière's disease, acute labyrinthitis secondary to middle ear disease, vestibular neuronitis, and benign positional vertigo. Ménière's disease is uncommon before middle age, and the presence of deafness and tinnitus is of the greatest help in diagnosis. As the deafness increases, the vertigo settles.

Chronic ear infection is usually obvious both from the history and on clinical examination. Vestibular neuronitis is more a disease of younger patients and

the pattern of the illness often suggests an infective process. Indeed sometimes it may occur in minor epidemics. There is never evidence of any cochlear damage and symptoms will usually gradually settle, although for a long time they may be precipitated by sudden movements of the head.

Vertigo may occur as part of an epileptic seizure, usually due to a temporal lobe focus. There will commonly be a loss, or at least disturbance, of consciousness and the EEG may help in the diagnosis (see Ch. 19).

Vertebrobasilar migraine can be a difficult diagnosis as here also there may be vertigo and loss of consciousness. In migraine other details of the history and family background will help. The EEG is normal between attacks but during an attack may show gross abnormalities. Similar symptoms due to ishcaemia can occur in the elderly due to atherosclerosis. A precise diagnosis can be difficult unless other features are present. To what extent such cases should be treated by anticoagulants and antiplatelet agents remains uncertain.

Although posterior fossa tumours are rare compared to these other conditions, it is obviously important to make such a diagnosis, especially with regard to acoustic neuroma. The removal of the tumour at the 'otological' rather than the 'neurological' stage has greatly improved the prognosis. The proximity of the tumour to the facial nerve can result in minimal degrees of facial nerve damage that may be present early, and be detected provided they are carefully looked for. Thus taste may be impaired, the blink reflex delayed, and the secretion of tears reduced on the affected side.

In any series of cases of dizziness, a significant number of patients will never have any diagnosis established. In some of these cases psychological factors are probably important, although it is uncommon for any specific psychiatric diagnosis to be made.

CLINICAL PROBLEM

T	P	BP	R
37	72	125/80	22

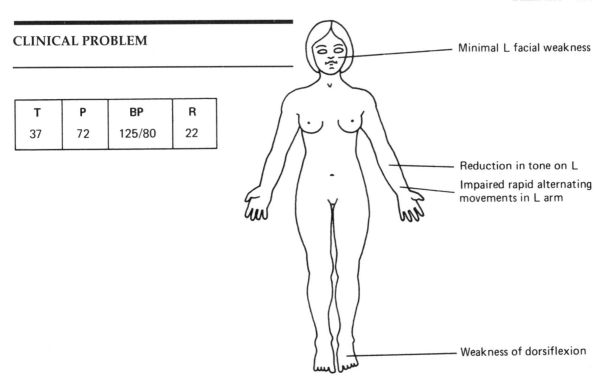

Minimal L facial weakness

Reduction in tone on L

Impaired rapid alternating movements in L arm

Weakness of dorsiflexion

A 26-year-old housewife developed recurrent attacks of dizziness, which initially lasted for about one minute. During these attacks her surroundings appeared to move, but there was no actual rotation. She felt unsteady and had to sit down. The attacks began and stopped suddenly and occurred for no obvious reason. She had not noticed that any particular activity appeared to precipitate her attacks, which had occurred at all hours of the day. Over about 3 weeks they increased in frequency, until finally they were occurring hourly. With some of the attacks she had felt a little nauseated, but at no time had she vomited. There had never been any tinnitus or impairment of hearing. Over the same few weeks she also had the feeling that her walking was disturbed, and she had the sensation that she was being pulled to the left. She felt that her left leg was tiring more easily than normal, and she had noticed occasional cramps in the calf of that leg at night.

She was given symptomatic treatment with prochlorperazine and over the next week her symptoms improved considerably. The attacks of dizziness settled completely, although she continued to feel that her walking was not quite normal. However, a month later the attacks recurred and in addition she also noticed double vision. The images were only slightly separated and the symptom was more marked towards the end of the day when she was tired.

In the past she had always been well and had had no previous illnesses except appendicitis 4 years earlier. Her mother had suffered from 'sick headaches' for many years, thought to be due to migraine.

Because of the further development of her illness she was admitted to hospital for investigation. No abnormality was present on general examination, abnormal signs being confined to the nervous system. The fundi were normal, and examination of the cranial nerves revealed nothing except some degree of facial asymmetry which suggested the presence of minimal weakness of the lower half of the face on the left. Rapid alternate movements were a little impaired in the left hand, but she was a right-handed person. Tone appeared reduced in both the left arm and leg. There was some weakness of dorsiflexion of the foot on the left, and the left plantar response was equivocal.

QUESTIONS

1. What are the most likely causes of this woman's illness?
2. What further investigations may be of value in arriving at the diagnosis?

DISCUSSION

This woman's major complaint is of dizziness which is non-vertiginous in nature. Her attacks have no obvious precipitating cause and in particular there are no associated symptoms that might suggest disease of the middle or inner ear. If dizziness or vertigo occur for any reason there is commonly some nausea or vomiting and her feeling of nausea has therefore no extra significance. The disturbance of her gait is an important symptom. The feeling that her left leg tires more easily and the occurrence of occasional cramps raise the possibility of an upper motor neurone lesion involving that limb, although the sensation of being pulled to the one side while walking could also occur with a lesion of the cerebellum or its connections. The fact that her symptoms improved with prochlorperazine is of no value in establishing the diagnosis as this is a non-specific effect. Her walking would be unlikely to improve on such treatment and the fact that this also improved suggests that the natural course of her illness is fluctuant, and that a spontaneous improvement may be occurring. Her final complaint of diplopia also suggests, in this context, that there may be disease involving the cerebellum or its connections.

This overall pattern of symptoms is strongly suggestive of organic disease. Dizziness, ataxia and diplopia may occur in drug intoxication, for example with barbiturates, but would usually give rise to more symmetrical symptoms and not involve particularly one side of the body. It is likely therefore that some more localized pathology is present involving particularly the brain stem.

The findings on examination support this interpretation. The signs are minimal and their exact significance must initially be in doubt, but the asymmetry disclosed in the face, the arms and the legs all suggest organic pathology. The weakness and equivocal plantar response support the possibility of a left-sided pyramidal disturbance, while the impairment of rapid alternate movements and the reduction in tone may indicate an additional cerebellar lesion. The fact that both sets of sign involve the same side of the body suggests that they may be due to separate lesions, for unlike pyramidal signs resulting from a brain-stem lesion, cerebellar signs are homolateral.

A number of possible diagnoses must be considered.

Brain stem encephalitis is uncommon, most viruses showing more widespread neurotropism. There is usually some disturbance of consciousness and also symptoms such as headache due to raised CSF pressure. Ménière's disease is uncommon at this age and is usually associated with deafness and tinnitus and also would not explain the symptoms in the left arm suggestive of a cerebellar lesion.

The story is fully compatible with a diagnosis of multiple sclerosis and the time course of the first episode is quite typical. Vertigo is a well-recognised early symptom occurring in between 5% and 15% of cases. Less clearly defined dizziness is as common as true vertigo. A feeling of being pulled to one side is also described in association with vertigo. During an attack there will usually be nystagmus, and some cases may show a continuous dissociated (or ataxic) nystagmus. Such a finding is always highly suggestive of the disease but is not completely pathognomonic.

The diagnosis of acute vestibular neuronitis is rendered untenable by the presence of symptoms and signs elsewhere in the central nervous system. Acoustic neuroma must be considered in a case such as this, although the age of the patient and the time course of the symptoms would not support the diagnosis of a progressive space-occupying lesion. Furthermore the presence of cerebellar and possible pyramidal signs would be very unlikely in the absence of any evidence of damage to the trigeminal nerve.

In the investigation of this case, audiometry and caloric testing would be reasonable although not essential. They showed in fact no impairment of hearing, but bilateral reduction in caloric responses compatible with a bilateral brain stem lesion. EEG and isotope scan would be very unlikely to give information of value, both techniques giving little information about lesions in the posterior fossa. Vertebral angiogram is rarely required in this type of case. Occasionally these symptoms may arise from a basilar aneurysm, or vertebrobasilar angioma, but delay in establishing such a diagnosis is not usually of importance. These investigations were not therefore performed. Skull X-rays were done and were normal, and views of the internal auditory meati showed no evidence of expansion. An X-ray CT scan was also completely normal. A lumbar puncture revealed clear fluid at a normal pressure, with a free rise and fall on jugular compression. The number of white cells was slightly raised at $10/mm^3$. The protein was also a little increased at 50 mg/dl and immune electrophoresis showed a rise in IgG with discrete oligoclonal bands. There was impairment of visually evoked responses on the EEG compatible with retrobulbar neuritis.

It was thought that the most likely diagnosis was multiple sclerosis, and this was confirmed by the later history of the patient.

23. Headache

This is one of the commonest symptoms which brings a patient to his doctor. That there is no serious underlying cause is usually realized by both, but the patient requires symptomatic relief and reassurance. The physician must decide how far investigation should be taken to be reasonably certain that no serious organic disease is present. A careful history is of the greatest importance for there will be no physical signs in the majority of patients, and a firm diagnosis must frequently be reached on the history alone. A knowledge of the psychological stresses to which the patient is exposed, together with knowledge of the family background is often of the greatest help in diagnosis and many patients can and should be fully dealt with by their general practitioner. Table 23.1 is a simple classification of the wide variety of possible causes.

Table 23.1 Causes of headache

Psychogenic
Migrainous
Vascular
Raised intracranial pressure
Post-traumatic
Local pathology of skull, spine, sinuses and orbits

The first two groups contain the large majority of patients and in neither of these groups will there usually be physical signs or abnormal findings on investigation.

Psychogenic

Tension headache is experienced by the majority of people at some time. If frequent or severe it may bring the sufferer to his doctor, usually after simple analgesics have been found ineffective. The pattern of the headache is often very typical. It is described as severe, continuous, and more a sense of pressure or tightness than an actual pain. The distribution is often over the vault, or less frequently occipitofrontal. It is usually bilateral. Other somatic pains suggestive of muscle tension may also be present. Many patients admit that the symptom is worse when they are under unusual stress at work or at home, and it may be possible to date the onset of the headache to some alteration in their circumstances. A rough but useful rule is to enquire in a man about his work and financial affairs, and in a woman about her marriage and children. Examination reveals little. Occasionally the increased tension in the frontal and occipital muscles is associated with some actual tenderness, but this is rarely so marked as to cause confusion with cranial arteritis. The longer a headache of this type has been present, the easier becomes the diagnosis and also, unfortunately, the more resistant it is to treatment. Further treatment with analgesics is of little value, and even though the headache is psychogenic, sedatives and tranquillizers are of less value than might be expected. Failure of this form of treatment does not mean the headache has an organic cause. Social manipulation, if feasible, can sometimes be very effective. In some patients where there is the specific worry that they may have a cerebral tumour or some other serious disease, strong reassurance supported perhaps by a few selected investigations designed to impress the patient, can be successful.

Tension headache due to anxiety may be a part of a mixed depressive illness. This is an important diagnosis to make, as effective treatment is now possible. Unfortunately the underlying primary mood change which is usually not severe, is often missed. Enquiry should be made for the somatic accompaniments of depression – loss of appetite, weight and libido, together with constipation and disturbance of sleep rhythm. The headache itself may show the same diurnal variation as the mood change, being worse on waking and improving gradually throughout the day. This variation is not so marked as with the headache of raised intracranial pressure and improvement takes place more slowly during the course of the day. Some response will occur in the majority of these patients to drugs of the tricyclic group, the headache improving along with the depression.

Migraine

Migrainous headache is extremely common and a wide variety of partial and atypical patterns are seen.

Diagnosis here can be difficult, and the past history and family history must be carefully taken.

In the typical patient there is a history of recurrent episodes of headache starting in adolescence, lasting from 2 hours to 2 days. The pain is more often uni-lateral, in contrast to tension headaches. It is frequently accompanied by photophobia, nausea and vomiting. Many patients also experience an additional aura usually of visual disturbances, such as various forms of flashing lights (teichopsia), scotomata or even hemianopia. These last considerably longer than the aura seen in epileptic patients. Paraesthesiae may occur around the angle of the mouth or in the hand and rarely there may be the development of hemiparesis or hemiplegia. Fortunately, this is usually transient, clearing within hours, although the exceptional case has been recorded of fatal cerebral infarction due to intense and long-lasting vaso-constriction. If the major hemisphere is involved, there may be dysphasia.

An interesting variant is basilar migraine where the initial vasoconstrictor phase involves the vertebrobasilar arterial system and produces dysfunction of the brain stem. This unusual form is more often found in adolescent girls and may present with such symptoms as diplopia, vertigo, and loss of consciousness. When loss of consciousness has occurred, the differential diagnosis from epilepsy is of the greatest importance and may be difficult unless a very detailed history is taken (see also Ch. 19 and 22).

The phenomena of the aura are of great help in the diagnosis of the headache which follows, as the headache alone may be non-specific in its charac-teristics. The circumstances under which the attacks occur can also be of diagnostic value. Migraine has been said to be commoner in the intelligent, the hardworking and the conscientious. It often occurs not during the period of concentration, but later, when the patient is relaxing in the evening or over the weekend. Some experience attacks after a partic-ular food. In women attacks may occur in relation to their periods. The contraceptive pill can both initiate migraine and also aggravate existing attacks. The majority of patients give a positive family history, while a few have an earlier history in childhood of the cyclical abdominal disturbances thought to be aetiologically related to migraine.

Although it is widely and correctly taught that on occasion migraine can be secondary to some under-lying cerebral disease, particularly vascular mal-formations such as aneurysm or angioma, in practice this is rare, and full neurological investigation is not usually required. Definite and persisting physical signs, such as ocular palsy, are an indication for further investigation, initially by CT scan. One should always be suspicious of migraine developing for the first time in middle age, in the absence of a family history.

Vascular causes

Here one must consider hypertension, arteriosclerosis and arteritis. Headache is common in hypertension and may be the symptom which first brings the patient to medical attention. Headache is usually a symptom of moderately severe hypertension. Tension headache can also occur after the diagnosis of hypertension has been made, and reflects the anxiety of the patient concerning his illness. Nowadays headache is a less common presentation as hyper-tension is frequently diagnosed on routine exam-ination in asymptomatic patients.

In severe hypertension, particularly in the malig-nant phase, headache is commonly severe and will often show the pattern associated with raised intracranial pressure (see below). It will usually be associated with papilloedema, fundal haemorrhages and exudates, and evidence of progressive renal damage. Hypotensive treatment is a matter of considerable urgency and the headache will respond only to lowering of the blood pressure.

Inflammatory disease of cerebral and cranial vessels can be associated with pain and the best known syndrome is that of temporal arteritis. The involved vessels will be tender and may be occluded so that it no longer pulsates. The inflammation is often widespread and may also involve the occipital artery with a corresponding change in the pattern of the headache. Occasionally the distribution of the arteritis is even more atypical and symptoms are maximal in the neck or jaw. The diagnosis can then be easily missed. Whatever the pattern, the danger of retinal artery involvement with resulting blindness is always present, so that early diagnosis and urgent treatment is essential. Symptoms of a generalized illness are present, with fever, weight loss, arthralgia, myalgia and general malaise. There is often hyper-aesthesia of the scalp. The ESR is invariably high. If the diagnosis is in doubt a therapeutic trail of steroids can be of great value. Whenever possible the affected artery should be biopsied, and this should be done before the commencement of steroids as the histological changes can resolve very rapidly. In cases where the clinical diagnosis is reasonably secure, treatment must not be unduly delayed to allow for biopsy as the risk of blindness is great. Temporal arteritis is part of a spectrum of vasculitis which includes polymyalgia rheumatica. Both show a dramatic response to steriods. Treatment may have to be continued indefinitely, attempts to discontinue steroids being followed by a rise in ESR and relapse.

Raised intracranial pressure

Although this is one of the most serious causes of headache, it is one of the least common. Many different mechanisms can lead to a rise in pressure, but the usual cause is space occupation within the skull by tumour, abscess or haematoma. If these occur below the tentorium cerebelli they will tend to cause interruption of the circulation of CSF at an early stage so that the headache increases rapidly in severity. Space-occupying lesions above the tentorium will also eventually produce obstruction to CSF flow as a result of impaction of the medulla in the foramen magnum (medullary coning). The typical features of the headache of raised intracranial pressure are its severity, its occurrence particularly on waking with gradual improvement over the next few hours, its aggravation by coughing, sneezing, and straining, and its common association with nausea and vomiting. The headache is often throbbing or bursting in character, it may be worse on lying down and is relieved by sitting or standing. As it becomes more severe it becomes continuous, and paroxysms of even more severe pain may be superimposed. The distribution of the pain is usually ill-defined, and of little value in localizing any intracranial lesion. There is some tendency for the headache of subtentorial lesions to be felt posteriorly, and to radiate down the back of the neck. Although physical examination will often reveal papilloedema, visual impairment is usually a late feature. This contrasts sharply with optic neuritis where the visual loss is usually marked although the papilloedema is only modest.

Headache is the main feature of the rare but interesting condition of benign intracranial hypertension. Here there is papilloedema, which may lead to visual failure, and the CSF pressure is markedly elevated. It is necessary to undertake full neuroradiological investigation to exclude a space-occupying lesion or a venous sinus thrombosis. The condition occurs mainly in women, particularly at the time of the menarche or the menopause, during pregnancy, or in association with menstrual disorders and the use of the contraceptive pill. This is of help in arriving at the diagnosis. Initially the visual impairment can consist of brief recurrent obscurations of vision which can be of any degree of severity. These, together with the severity of the headache, will indicate the need for treatment, which is usually by repeated lumbar punctures. Diuretics and steroids are sometimes used but their effect is uncertain. Even without treatment the condition appears to be self-limiting, but permanent visual impairment may occur as a result of the papilloedema.

In the headache of some pituitary tumours the pain can arise from pressure within the sella turcica pressing upon the diaphragma sellae. With progression of the tumour and destruction of the fibrous diaphragm the symptom may paradoxically remit only to return later, when there is a general rise in intracranial pressure.

It is unusual with intracranial space-occupying lesions for there to be a prolonged period when there are no symptoms or signs, other than those of raised intracranial pressure (ICP). This may appear to be the case with some infiltrating gliomas but usually there will be evidence of personality change and some degree of intellectual deterioration. If there are no signs on detailed examination of the patient with long-standing headache, raised ICP is unlikely to be present.

There are many other causes of raised intracranial pressure. Cerebral oedema may be caused by inflammation as in virus encephalitis, from toxic damage, as in lead encephalopathy and in porphyria, and from ischaemic damage as in malignant hypertension. In most of these cases the diagnosis will be obvious from the history and examination, but the toxic causes in particular can easily be missed. Severe headache occurs in any form of meningeal irritation as in meningitis or in subarachnoid haemorrhage, where in addition there is usually some rise in intracranial pressure. The onset is typically rapid and there are associated typical signs of meningeal irritation such as neck stiffness and a positive Kernig's sign. Diagnosis is usually straight-forward and is confirmed by the findings at lumbar puncture.

A common iatrogenic headache is that following lumbar puncture. Here the cause is a low rather than high intracranial pressure, resulting however in a similar distortion of the pain-sensitive intracranial structures. Although usually short-lived it may continue for a number of days without being of any significance.

Trauma

Headaches are common after most head injuries. They normally do not persist, but on occasion do continue, usually as part of the post-concussional syndrome. The headache is typically described as severe, continuous and poorly localized. It is made worse by any exertion, by noise or any form of emotional excitement, and resembles in most respects the pattern seen in psychogenic headache. The commonest associated symptoms are of giddiness and inability to concentrate. Although in many of these patients psychoneurotic and medicolegal factors are operating to perpetuate their complaints, nevertheless the syndrome may occur even in those of previously good personality without any question of financial compensation. It is especially likely to occur if the patient has been mobilized and returned to work too soon after a head injury. Rest and adequate sedation is essential after head injury and convalescence must be gradual. If headaches return as activities are increased then a further period of rest is called for. In those patients for whom litigation is still proceeding, it is unusual for medical treatment to have any effect on the symptoms.

Extracranial disease

A variety of other diseases may cause or even present with headache. Both acute and chronic sinusitis are painful but only in chronic inflammation of the frontal sinuses is it likely that any diagnostic problem will arise. Supraorbital or retroorbital pain can occur with eye disease, particularly glaucoma, iridocyclitis, and errors of refraction.

Headache may occur with disease of the skull bones, although it is uncommon. Paget's disease of the skull, as in other bones, can give rise to pain, and is easily diagnosed on X-ray or isotope bone scan. Deposits of tumour, both primary and secondary, in the skull, can also give rise to local headache.

A common cause of occipital headache is cervical spondylosis. This is a common radiological finding in the ageing population and is often asymptomatic. Support for the clinical diagnosis can be obtained by reproducing or exacerbating the pain by testing the full range of neck movement.

EXAMINATION AND INVESTIGATION

In the majority of patients the diagnosis can be made on the history alone. Important points on examination are the presence of papilloedema, the blood pressure, evidence of meningeal irritation and any signs of focal neurological damage. If there is any doubt as to the diagnosis then further investigation is required.

Chest X-ray may show primary bronchogenic carcinoma which has given rise to cerebral secondaries. Straight X-ray of the skull will reveal most diseases of the skull bones, and may also show evidence of raised intracranial pressure or cerebral neoplasm. In raised intracranial pressure there may be erosion of the posterior clinoid processes, and porosis of the dorsum sellae. If the pineal is calcified, its displacement by a space-occupying lesion may be obvious. Rarely abnormal calcifications may occur with a cerebral tumour, especialy craniopharyngiomas. If there is any suspicion of encephalitis, meningitis, subarachnoid haemorrhage or syphilis then lumbar puncture is mandatory. It is not of great value in the diagnosis of intracranial tumour and may be dangerous if there is a significant rise in intracranial pressure due to a space-occupying lesion, as it may precipitate coning.

Difficulty may arise as to the safety of lumbar puncture in some cases of possible subarachnoid haemorrhage or encephalitis, where the diagnosis is not certain and blurring of the discs or even definite papilloedema is present. A CT scan should be obtained first, and if there is still doubt, referral to a neurological centre considered.

There remains the occasional patient where the diagnosis is still unclear and in the past it was often a difficult decision whether to proceed to angiography or air encephalography. The development first of isotope and then CT scanning has made this decision much easier. Although these techniques are expensive, they are non-invasive and of the greatest value in the diagnosis of space-occupying lesions.

In cases of headache it is important not to miss the occasional case with serious but treatable organic disease, but one must try and do this without over-investigating the rest of one's patients.

CLINICAL PROBLEM

T	P	BP	R
37·2	68	110/70	22

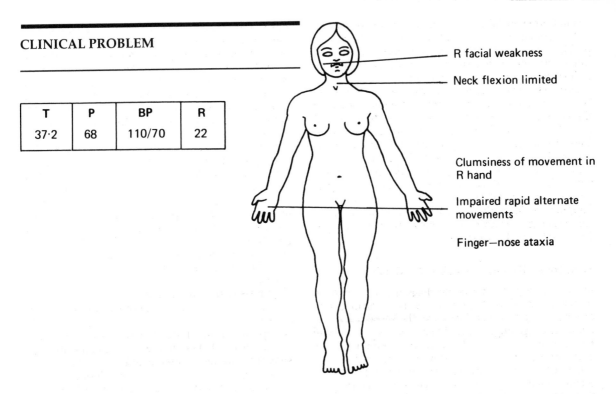

R facial weakness

Neck flexion limited

Clumsiness of movement in R hand

Impaired rapid alternate movements

Finger—nose ataxia

A 17-year-old student had been well until 2 months previously when she had crossed by boat from France to England. During the voyage she had suffered from severe sea-sickness, which was unusual for her, and her symptoms continued to some extent for several days after the end of the voyage. Furthermore, when she first left the boat she found her legs seemed a little unsteady, and this continued for about 10 days before settling. There was then an interval of a week during which she felt her normal self. She had consulted a doctor because of these initial symptoms and had received tablets which improved the vomiting but had not helped the unsteadiness.

The next symptom was of recurrent headaches. These began gradually and over the next 6 weeks became steadily more severe. They had been particularly bad at the time of her recent period. The headaches were dull and throbbing in character, and tended to be most severe over the back of the head, spreading a little way down the back of the neck. For two weeks she had noticed some stiffness of the neck, particularly when the headache was severe. There had been no further vomiting, although she had felt a little nauseated occasionally, and her appetite was poor.

She had broken her right humerus 18 months previously when riding and had suffered most of the common childhood fevers. She had had no infections of any sort in the previous year, and had been quite well during her recent holiday in southern Italy. There was nothing of note in her family history except that her father suffered from diabetes.

On admission she looked a very fit girl, who was in no way distressed by her illness. She was afebrile, and the pulse and blood pressure were normal. No abnormality was present on general examination. The fundi were normal, but there was some weakness of the face on the right, which appeared to involve both the upper and lower halves of the face equally. There was marked limitation of neck flexion and attempting this produced pain. Rapid alternate movements were impaired in the right hand (she was right-handed) and there was some ataxia on the right on finger–nose testing. When walking she appeared slightly unsteady and tended to veer to the right.

QUESTIONS

1. What investigations should be carried out on this girl?
2. What do you consider to be the more likely diagnoses?

DISCUSSION

Even though sea-sickness is a common experience, and symptoms may be of any degree of severity, it would be very unusual for them to continue for as long as 10 days, particularly after only a very short voyage. It suggests therefore that the channel crossing only unmasked an illness which was already developing, but until then subclinical. Vomiting and unsteadiness suggest a disturbance of the brain stem, involving in particular the labyrinthine system or any of its higher connections. Her next symptom was of headaches, and their pattern should lead one to consider the possibility of a rise in intracranial pressure. They are severe, progressive, dull and throbbing, associated with nausea and worse at the time of her period. Other features not complained of which would also suggest such an interpretation would be if they were more marked on waking in the morning, and if they were exacerbated by such manoeuvres as coughing, straining, and sneezing. Their localization posteriorly is more difficult to evaluate. The headache of raised intracranial pressure is commonly frontal or occipital whatever the site of the tumour. Increasing occipital headache also suggests the possibility of medullary coning, with impaction of the brain stem in the foramen magnum. Occipital headache spreading down the back of the neck is also common in meningeal irritation, as may occur from blood, as in subarachnoid haemorrhage or as a result of meningitis. Headache of this type is also often complained of by elderly patients suffering from cervical spondylosis.

The findings on examination in this patient are few. The most important is marked neck stiffness, which suggests meningeal irritation or early coning. The absence of papilloedema is against the latter interpretation. Her facial weakness indicates a lower motor neurone lesion, while the impaired rapid alternate movements with ataxia on finger–nose testing and on walking suggests a lesion of the cerebellum or its connections on the right.

The illness has been short and progressive. The focal neurological signs are against a diagnosis of migraine as is the pattern of the headache, although this diagnosis should always be considered in patients of this age. Some form of meningitis is possible and this diagnosis could be excluded by lumbar puncture. The duration of the illness would be long for a pyogenic infection, but is quite compatible with a tuberculous meningitis. Viral meningoencephalitis should also be considered, but again the time course would usually be more rapid and one would expect some clouding of consciousness. Although uncommon a posterior fossa tumour must also be excluded, as this may cause cranial nerve palsies and cerebellar signs, and commonly produces a rise in intracranial pressure with medullary compression at an early stage.

Initial investigation of such a patient would be by CT scan, with particular attention to the posterior fossa to exclude a space-occupying lesion. If this were normal it would be reasonable to exclude meningitis by examination of the CSF. Straight X-rays of the skull and of the cervical spine should be done, but are unlikely to be of value. If a cerebellopontine angle tumour is possible, as is the case here, views of the internal auditory meatus should be obtained. Audiometry and caloric testing should be carried out. They would help to exclude any congenital lesion at the level of the foramen magnum. EEG and isotope scan are also of limited value in the investigation of posterior fossa lesions. Isotope scan will be normal in the majority of cases of encephalitis, although there may be focal concentration of isotope in herpes simplex encephalitis. If a tumour is demonstrated then exploratory craniotomy will usually be required.

Investigation, culminating in craniotomy, established a diagnosis of medulloblastoma. A course of radiotherapy initially produced a marked improvement but 15 months later she relapsed and died 20 months after her first symptoms.

24.   Pain in the face

Although this is not a common symptom, it must be analysed with care, for the diagnosis has frequently to be made on clinical grounds alone – even the most sophisticated investigations may provide no additional information. Often a conclusion must be reached on the history alone, physical examination being important only to exclude certain of the diagnostic possibilities. The causes of pain in this area vary from the trivial, such as dental caries or malocclusion, to the most serious, for example carcinoma of the nasopharynx. In some patients a firm diagnosis will unfortunately never be arrived at and in these treatment will usually prove ineffective. To minimize the size of this group every effort should be made to establish a precise diagnosis early on before the patient's story has become contaminated by discussion with too many doctors. Specific treatment can then be given if appropriate, and, of equal importance, avoided in those cases where it is not indicated. One still meets the occasional patient who has passed through the hands of so many physicians and surgeons and received such a variety of therapies, often including some at least of the various surgical attacks possible on trigeminal neuralgia, that the original diagnosis must forever remain in doubt. Indeed, one is often at a loss to know what are the primary symptoms and what are the result of treatment.

A. FACIAL PAIN WITHOUT ABNORMAL SIGNS

Trigeminal neuralgia (tic douloureux)

This is an important diagnosis. The story is usually very typical of short, sharp and severe pains coming in bursts, always unilateral, and confined to the trigeminal distribution. Usually the patient is elderly, and initially at least the pain only occurs in the territory of the second or third divisions of the nerve. Often quite trivial sensory stimulation of the face will precipitate a paroxysm of pain, and perhaps because of this characteristic, the pain rarely occurs during sleep. The cause of this syndrome is completely unknown except in the unusual case where similar symptoms occur in a patient with established multi-

ple sclerosis or neurosyphilis. The diagnosis is rarely in doubt in such cases as there are almost always the physical signs of widespread disease of the central nervous system. A further help in diagnosis is the excellent response to carbamazepine in the majority of patients. The dosage should be built up gradually until adequate relief is obtained, and in this way the troublesome side-effects of drowsiness and unsteadiness can be minimized. As the attacks of pain tend to occur in groups with periods of temporary remission, many patients need only take the drug intermittently, and thus the risk of toxic complications is further reduced.

Glossopharyngeal neuralgia

The quality and characteristics of the pain in this rare condition are similar to that in trigeminal neuralgia. The difference lies in its distribution, the pain being felt in the throat in the region of the tonsillar fossa, and deep in the ear. Sometimes the pain is felt in the back of the tongue. Again, carbamazepine should be tried, before considering surgery such as glossopharyngeal nerve section.

Migrainous neuralgia

This is a condition to be aware of as again there is a specific remedy – ergotamine – which is effective in the majority of patients. It is often misdiagnosed, perhaps due to confusion from the variety of names which have been given to the syndrome in the past. The age of onset is earlier than with trigeminal neuralgia and the patient is more often male. Attacks of severe pain occur in clusters, each episode lasting for up to half an hour. The pain is unilateral, centres around the eye, and may be associated with lacrimation or stuffiness of the nose on that side. Attacks typically occur only once or twice in 24 hours, and unlike trigeminal neuralgia the pain usually occurs at night and wakes the patient 2 or 3 hours after going to sleep. Despite the name the majority of these patients do not usually experience the typical symptoms of migraine such as headache, nausea, and visual disturbances. They do, however, give a past history or family history of migraine more frequently than might be expected on chance alone. Perhaps the main reason for believing the condition to be related to migraine is the excellent response to subcutaneous ergotamine. Migrainous neuralgia responds rapidly and the attack will remit even though the pain will probably return in a few months' time. In those occasional cases resistant to treatment, it has been claimed that stellate ganglion block is effective, either temporarily by local anaesthetic or permanently by surgery. A good response occurs in perhaps a half of the cases so treated, the reason for this being as obscure as the cause of the condition itself.

Facial pain associated with depression

Many psychiatric patients complain of symptoms more suggestive of organic rather than mental disease. These often enable the patient to gain the sympathy, interest and help that he feels he needs. Similarly, physical complaints may be part of a hysterical illness, the symptoms being used by the patient in his manipulation of the world around him. Facial pain can be the somatic complaint in either of these mechanisms. The pain has no specific localization but is commonly described as continuous and unrelieved by any treatment. Diagnostic problems occur frequently when facial pain is one of the somatic symptoms in the agitated endogenous depression that occurs commonly in the middle and older age groups. It is all too easy to concentrate attention on what seems a clear-cut organic symptom, the investigation of which is straightforward, and to neglect even to enquire for the symptoms of endogenous depression. It is important to recognize that depression may present in this way, for it is in this type that drug therapy with the tricyclic antidepressants is so often successful. Usually the facial pain fades as the depression lifts.

Atypical facial pain

It is important to separate another unfortunate group where such depression as is present is not primary, but secondary to the facial pain and as a consequence of varied advice, diagnoses and failed treatments to which the pain has exposed the patient. The majority are middle-aged women, but having said this, there is little else that is generally agreed. The clinical picture is highly variable and the description of the pain does not consistently fit any of the previously described categories. The pain is commonly diffuse, often bilateral and the duration of each attack can be much less clearly delineated. These cases can reasonably be labelled atypical facial pain. Most forms of therapy prove unsuccessful or only of very temporary value, and in the few patients investigated, psychiatric assessment reveals little of convincing aetiological significance. All lesser treatments having failed, many of these patients in the past had surgical division of the trigeminal sensory root and were left with the painful paraesthesiae of anaesthesia dolorosa in addition to their original symptoms. Addiction to one of the major analgesics is also a very real danger. The ultimate clinical picture is so complex and confusing that no one is able to reach a diagnosis.

B. FACIAL PAIN WITH PHYSICAL SIGNS

Dental causes

Many patients with facial pain of obscure origin eventually have a dental clearance, usually with little effect. Pain arising from the teeth can usually be diagnosed by the typical history of a relationship to chewing and to temperature changes, and the site of the trouble found by thorough dental and radiological examination. Pain may originate from the temporomandibular joint in some edentulous patients. This arises as a result of overclosure of the jaws leading to the mandibular condyle sliding forwards and so in time causing arthritis. A similar syndrome can occur in the non-edentulous as a result of rheumatoid arthritis. Symptoms are more likely to occur in nervous and tense individuals, and perhaps as a result of this, correction of the bite is not always successful in removing the symptom.

Other extracranial sources of pain

Many diseases involving a variety of structures in the region of the mouth, throat and neck can give rise to facial pain. Usually the diagnosis will be obvious from the nature of the accompanying symptoms and signs, even if the pattern of referred pain is unusual. Examples are the pain of the acute parotitis of mumps, of acute inflammation of any of the nasal sinuses, of salivary duct obstruction by stone, and the pain arising from local lesions, whether inflammatory ulcer or carcinoma, of the tongue, mouth and pharynx. Although chronic sinusitis is commonly diagnosed as a cause of pain and treated with vigour, success is less often achieved as judged by improvement in the original symptom. The nasopharynx is not easily accessible to clinical examination and lesions here can all too easily be missed. Nasopharyngeal carcinoma spreads upwards to the base of the skull early and many patients present with multiple cranial nerve palsies before either pain or bloody discharge from the nose.

Similarly tumours may arise in the bones of the orbit. These are usually lymphoma or secondary carcinomas and may cause facial pain and proptosis.

Post-herpetic neuralgia

This remains a source of great suffering for many elderly patients, particularly when it affects the first division of the trigeminal. Diagnosis should not be in doubt if a careful history is taken, and examination, even some considerable time later, will often reveal thin scars and areas of hyperaesthetic or even anaesthetic skin. Sometimes the patient presents with severe pain before the eruption appears and then diagnosis can be difficult, although within a few days the development of the typical vesicles will resolve the problem. Usually the pain of herpes zoster is most severe early on, and its natural history is for steady improvement to occur over the next 18 months. The pain is severe and may last continuously for up to 30 minutes. It does not occur only in response to reflex stimulation and may therefore disturb the patient's sleep. When the rash is marked the pain is usually severe, but this correlation is not close. A more important factor in determining how severe and how long-lasting is the pain of ophthalmic herpes is the age of the patient. In those over 60 the great severity of the pain commonly produces marked depression, which on occasion has led to suicide. Treatment is therefore of the greatest importance and analgesia must be adequate, particularly in the early stages. In view of the natural tendency of the condition to remit, particularly if the early pain has been adequately controlled, there is every reason to use opiates. If the diagnosis is made within the first 72 hours, some would advocate the use of steroids. Later on they have no effect, but if used at the stage of acute inflammation of the nervous tissue and continued for several weeks, the incidence and severity of the neuralgia is considerably reduced. The specific antiviral agents active against herpes provide effective treatment if used early in the attack. Corneal ulcers must be treated with topical idoxuridine.

Tumours of the skull and intracranial region

Any space-occupying or malignant process arising from or spreading to the region of the orbit or base of the brain can give rise to facial pain. This is due to pressure upon, and destruction of, the trigeminal sensory fibres. Commonly in such cases there will be objective evidence of a sensory deficit with depression of the corneal reflex on that side, and other cranial nerves will soon be involved. The exact clinical pattern will vary with the site of the lesion.

Aneurysms of the internal carotid may give rise to symptoms as a result of distortion and pressure upon local structures. Aneurysm may develop within the cavernous sinus, particularly in middle-aged women, and give rise to pain felt in any of the divisions of the trigeminal nerve (see Fig. 24.1). Classically, symptoms both begin and progress abruptly, but the onset can be insidious and the progression gradual. As with a tumour arising within the pituitary fossa, erosion of the clinoid processes can occur. The other types of internal

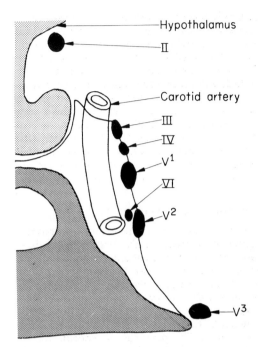

Fig. 24.1 Anatomy of carvernous sinus

carotid aneurysm that can give rise to pain in the face are those arising from the point of origin of the posterior communicating artery. These may give supraorbital pain, and because they are commonly diverted backwards and press on the oculomotor nerve, this can be associated with a dilated pupil, external strabismus and ptosis. An important and difficult differential diagnosis is ophthalmoplegic migraine (see Ch. 23).

Facial pain is a recognized, although not a common symptom of tumours arising in the cerebellopontine angle (see Ch. 22). The commonest cause is an acoustic neuroma arising on the vestibular division of the eighth cranial nerve, just inside the internal auditory meatus. Such tumours are very slow-growing and symptoms and signs typically develop gradually over a number of years. The main symptoms will be of deafness, tinnitus and vertigo, while the most important early sign is of diminished corneal sensation. Later there will be cerebellar ataxia, nystagmus and perhaps other cranial nerve palsies. In both neuroma and the less common meningioma, examination of the CSF will usually show a great increase in the protein, but if this is normal it does not exclude a tumour of the cerebellopontine angle. Cholesteatoma, although less common, can give rise to a similar clinical picture.

Cerebrovascular disease

Ischaemia of the brain stem is common, but fortunately infarction is rare. Although diagnosis is not usually difficult it is worth noting that following such episodes, particularly when they occur in the territory of the posterior inferior cerebellar artery, giving rise to some variant of lateral medullary syndrome, facial pain can occur. This can be of any degree of severity. It can posses features suggestive of trigeminal neuralgia but the story is never completely typical and physical signs will be present on examination. Some improvement may occur with carbamazepine, which is worthy of trial even though the majority will not respond. In some patients the pain has many of the qualities commonly called 'thalamic'. Thus it is described as agonizing, burning, diffuse, persistent and at the same time may be subject to sudden exacerbations, either spontaneously or as a result of external stimulation. Such a pain is usually most resistant to any form of treatment.

CONCLUSION

A careful history and examination will allow a diagnosis to be made in the majority of cases where any clear-cut and treatable diagnosis is possible. If signs are present of neurological deficit, more detailed neuroradiological examination will be needed. It is important to recognize such conditions as trigeminal and migrainous neuralgia, as effective and specific treatment is available. Similarly aneurysms of the internal carotid may be successfully treated by carotid ligation and it is obviously better that this should be done before subarachnoid haemorrhage has occurred. Acoustic neuroma has a significant morbidity and mortality when treatment is attempted late, and every effort must be made to establish the diagnosis while the tumour is still small.

Finally, in those cases where depression is an important factor, drug treatment can be effective.

CLINICAL PROBLEM

T	P	BP	R
37·2	110	150/90	24

Anaemic

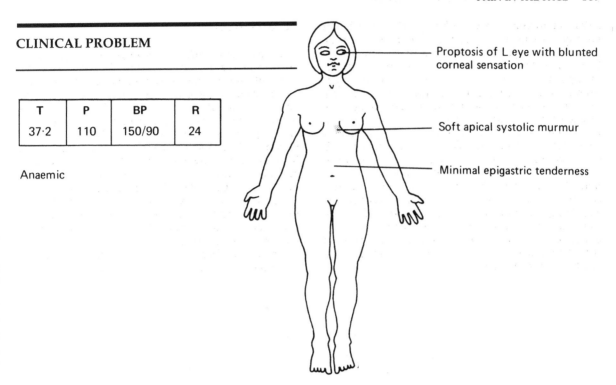

Proptosis of L eye with blunted corneal sensation

Soft apical systolic murmur

Minimal epigastric tenderness

A 50-year-old woman was referred to the outpatients' department because of pain in the face for 6 months. The pain was centred around the left eye, and when it was most severe, spread downwards into the left cheek. At first for several months the pain had been intermittent, lasting for up to half an hour at a time, but more recently it had been present to some extent continuously with occasional exacerbations. The severity of the pain had also slowly increased so that it now sometimes reduced her to tears. For the last month the pain had been particularly troublesome at night. She described the pain as dull and boring. It came and went slowly rather than abruptly, and occurred for no obvious reason. It did not seem to be provoked by going out into the cold, or by washing the face, and she had noticed nothing herself which either produced or relieved it.

Over the last year she had felt generally less well. She had felt anxious and depressed on occasion for no obvious reason and her appetite had been poor. She thought she had lost about a stone in weight, but was pleased by this as she was still a little obese.

She had also noticed a little epigastric discomfort after meals, but since avoiding fatty food this had seemed better. For the last few months she had also been troubled by occasional dull aching pains in her limbs, unrelated to exercise, which were most notice-able when she went to bed at night.

On examination she was pale and obviously anxious. The pulse was 110/min regular. The left eye seemed a little prominent and congested but there was no pulsation and no bruit could be heard. The sclera was visible above and below the cornea on the left, but not on the right. Neurological examination was normal except that corneal sensation on the left was blunted subjectively. General examination was normal except for the presence of a soft systolic murmur, heard best a little internal to the apex, and minimal epigastric tenderness.

QUESTIONS

1. What do you consider to be the most likely cause of the facial pain?
2. What investigations would be appropriate in this patient?

DISCUSSION

The history strongly suggests that this patient's pain is organic in origin, and there are in addition features which indicate that there is probably systemic as well as local disease. The nature of the pain is not that of trigeminal or migrainous neuralgia. When considered in association with the physical sign of unilateral proptosis it must suggest a local destructive lesion of the orbit. The subjective blunting of corneal sensation is a sensitive indication that there is beginning to be loss of trigeminal sensation, which will later lead to an objective impairment of the corneal reflex.

There are elements in her story which could be taken as indicating a psychiatric disturbance. Thus she has sometimes been tearful and sometimes has felt anxious and depressed for no obvious reason. Furthermore her appetite has been poor and she has lost weight – two frequent accompaniments of an effective disorder. However these symptoms are also very commonly associated with organic disease and this is strongly suggested by the findings on physical examination.

The presence of pallor, tachycardia and an apical systolic murmur are all typical of anaemia. This association of significant anaemia with pain, which might be coming from bone, must suggest the possibility of diffuse infiltration of the marrow. Widespread infiltration of the marrow by malignant cells will usually give rise to anaemia and may also be sufficient to cause bone pain and tenderness. Bone pain

for any reason is also often worse at night, and this patient has found the aching that she complains of in her limbs to be particularly troublesome at night. The history of weight loss, epigastric pain and tenderness suggests an intra-abdominal malignancy. Further investigation of this possibility will include gastroscopy, liver function tests and liver ultrasound. Marrow infiltration commonly causes a leucoerythroblastic picture in the peripheral blood, with nucleated red cells and immature white cells. Severe anaemia is not uncommon. In both the lymphomas and some carcinomas deposits of malignant cells in the bones may be large enough to give rise to local tumours, and the orbits are not an uncommon site for this. It is a particularly common occurrence in the Burkitt lymphoma, seen mainly in children in equatorial Africa.

Skull X-rays in this patient showed evidence of bone destruction in the left orbit. Examination of the peripheral blood revealed a severe degree of anaemia, the haemoglobin being only 6.0 g/dl. The blood film showed a leucoerythroblastic pattern, but did not contain any malignant cells. Bone-marrow aspiration produced only scanty amounts of marrow, but in the smears several clumps of highly abnormal cells were seen, resembling adenocarcinoma. Gastroscopy showed a lesion typical of carcinoma of the stomach. Biopsy confirmed this. Liver function tests were normal except for a moderate rise in the alkaline phosphatase. Liver biopsy also revealed adenocarcinoma. Her condition rapidly deteriorated and she died only 6 weeks after her admission to hospital.

25.   Weakness of the legs

A patient may complain that his legs have become weak for a wide variety of reasons. These range from the trivial such as the common weakness that occurs after a period confined to bed, to the most serious. The weakness may result from the general effects of some systemic disease such as severe anaemia, or be the inevitable consequence of the profound tissue wasting that is seen in disseminated malignancy, severe malabsorption state or occasionally in cardiac cachexia. Usually however the underlying diagnosis is then obvious and there is no difficulty in understanding the patient's complaint.

Weakness of the legs may also occur as the major symptom in many of the diseases which primarily affect the peripheral and central nervous systems, the muscles or the joints. The diagnosis here may be more difficult to arrive at, particularly in the early stages of the condition. Weakness can result from interference with the motor pathway at any point from the precentral cortex down to the muscle. Furthermore a patient will often complain of weakness of his limbs when perhaps more accurately he should have spoken of difficulty in the control of his limbs. The end result however may be the same – difficulty in walking, and this he describes as weakness. One must therefore also consider disturbances that result from diseases of the basal ganglia, cerebellum and of the sensory pathways from the limbs.

MODE OF PRESENTATION

Details of history

As with any symptom, what the patient is actually experiencing must be analysed with great care. One should enquire as to what activities are interfered with by his weakness and under what circumstances it is most noticeable. An example of the value of this is the difficulty which a patient with weakness of the muscles of the pelvic girdle typically experiences in getting up from a chair, or the tendency of the patient with a pyramidal lesion of one leg to trip easily on minor projections because of his weakness of dorsiflexion. Any weakness is usually more noticeable when the patient is tired, but if this feature is pronounced in that weakness only occurs after repeated

use of the involved muscles, then the diagnosis of myasthenia gravis must be considered. Weakness of the legs after physical activity may be due to the rare syndrome of 'claudication of the cord'. The development of weakness after a hot bath or any other manoeuvre which raises body temperature has been described in multiple sclerosis. If the weakness is more marked in cold weather, and prolonged contraction of the muscles occurs with very sudden exertion, the possibility of dystrophia myotonica is suggested. In the sensory ataxias symptoms will commonly be worse or, at first, only present when the lighting is poor or if the eyes are closed, and visual sensory information is no longer available.

Patients often complain of weakness in one leg only. This can be misleading as abnormal signs may be found in both legs. It remains true however that certain diseases, such as peripheral neuropathy typically, give rise to symmetrical weakness of the limbs, while in others such as poliomyelitis and prolapsed intervertebral disc, the weakness is usually asymmetrical.

Children and adolescents

The age of the patient is obviously important. In young patients a history should be obtained, if possible, from the mother and details sought of the pregnancy and labour. Any form of respiratory distress after birth may also be of significance, anoxia being a potent cause of cerebral damage. Convulsions in early life may be an indication that brain damage occurred at birth. Congenital disease will usually be apparent at an early age, with spastic weakness of the limbs and may be of any degree of severity. There are often associated involuntary movements and there may, in addition, be evidence of intellectual defect, with impairment of emotional control.

Another important group of diseases in children and young adults are the muscular dystrophies. The common form which presents early on is the pseudohypertrophic type due to a sex-linked recessive defect. The weakness is most marked in the proximal musculature especially of the hip girdle, and leads to the typical waddling gait. The other dystrophies are also genetically determined but the pattern of inheritance

Table 25.1   Important causes of a bilateral pyramidal lesion affecting the lower limbs

Cord compression
Trauma
Multiple sclerosis
Transverse myelitis
Cervical spondylosis
Motor neurone disease
Vitamin B_{12} deficiency
Cerebrovascular disease
Spinal vascular disease
Falx meningioma

Table 25.2   Important causes of cerebellar ataxia

Multiple sclerosis
Alcoholism
Drug intoxication, e.g. phenytoin
Posterior fossa tumours
Carcinoma (non-metastatic)
Hereditary degenerations (e.g. Friedreich's)
Congenital malformations at the level of the foramen
  magnum
Myxoedema

and the degree of clinical expression often vary considerably. As a result, although a family history must always be taken carefully, it may be of little value in an individual patient. If relatives of the patient have suffered from a dystrophy its pattern should be defined because the facioscapulohumeral form has a much better prognosis than the pseudohypertrophic. In general the later the onset of symptoms the better the prognosis.

In the young adult the muscular dystrophies become progressively less common, but other diseases appear. Trauma to the spinal cord may cause any degree of paraplegia, and this is a common consequence of both road and industrial accidents. While the long-term management of these young and otherwise fit patients may pose great problems, the diagnosis will not be in doubt. Multiple sclerosis commonly presents in early adult life and must be considered in the differential diagnosis of most neurological syndromes at this age. Poliomyelitis was also a common infection in this age group in more advanced societies, but has now been eradicated by immunization. Congenital vascular anomalies, although uncommon, often present in young adult life. Cerebral angioma may present as a progressive hemiplegia in addition to the usual presentation as convulsions or subarachnoid bleeds, while the rarer spinal angioma may cause either a progressive or intermittent paraplegia (Table 25.1).

Neoplastic causes

Neoplasms can develop at any age. In children and young people cerebral tumours are usually primary, while, with increasing age, secondary deposits from extracranial neoplasms, such as carcinoma of the bronchus, are common. In children, primary tumours are particularly likely to occur below the tentorium cerebelli, in the posterior fossa. In adults the situation is reversed, supratentorial tumours being more common. Posterior fossa tumours will usually cause a rise in intracranial pressure at an early stage and this will determine the nature of the initial symptoms. They commonly cause ataxia from interference with the cerebellum and its connections, and sometimes an ataxic difficulty in walking is the first sign of the disease (Table 25.2).

Tumours of the cerebral hemispheres and the meninges will not usually present solely as difficulty in walking. A well-recognized exception is a falx meningioma, which by pressing on the underlying leg areas of each precentral motor cortex may initially give rise to the symptoms and signs of a spastic paraplegia, mimicking a spinal cord lesion. Usually, cerebral tumours cause fits, symptoms resulting from a general rise in intracranial pressure, personality change, and focal symptoms and signs arising from damage and irritation at the site of the tumour. Hemiplegia is a common occurrence and its association with some of the other features mentioned will usually point to the underlying diagnosis.

Difficulty in walking is one of the main features of spinal tumour and frequently this is the initial presentation. The neoplasm may be primary, and arise from the nerve roots, meninges, or from the cord itself. The spinal cord can also be involved in lymphoma and leukaemia, commonly as a result of compression by extradural or subarachnoid deposits. Commonly there will be evidence of these diseases elsewhere with lymphadenopathy, hepatosplenomegaly, anaemia and bleeding, but a rapidly developing paraplegia may be the first sign of the disease. Neurological evidence of cord damage may also occur in leukaemia and lymphoma which has apparently been successfully treated, with full remission of the peripheral blood and bone marrow abnormalities. This results from the failure of many of the drugs used in these disorders to cross the blood–brain barrier and so deal with malignant cells in the subarachnoid space. These syndromes are less common now with the use of prophylactic intrathecal therapy in leukaemia. Cord compression can also occur as a result of secondary carcinoma or multiple myeloma and this is seen more frequently in the older age groups. Bloodborne metastases may develop directly in the cord or meninges, or secondary deposits may spread from the vertebral bodies. Local pain is usually a major feature and there is often a rapidly developing paraplegia with a sensory level. A history of heavy cigarette smoking

Table 25.3 Important causes of peripheral neuropathy

Diabetes mellitus
Acute infective polyneuritis
Vitamin B$_{12}$ deficiency
Chronic alcoholism
Polyarteritis nodosa
Carcinomatous neuropathy
Porphyria

will increase the likelihood of this diagnosis, as carcinoma of the bronchus is a common cause.

Non-metastatic complications of carcinoma may also cause difficulty in walking. A pure sensory neuropathy with sensory ataxia can occur, although a non-specific mixed peripheral neuropathy is more common (Table 25.3). Degeneration of the Purkinje cells of the cerebellar hemisphere is also described and can cause a rapidly progressive ataxia, but is rare. Another rare syndrome is a pure motor neurone disease resembling the idiopathic form.

Vascular causes

In the elderly population vascular disease, both cerebral and spinal, is widespread and walking may be impaired in many ways. Hemiplegia due to cerebral thrombosis is a very common problem, the story usually being typical, and the diagnosis not difficult. Arteriosclerotic disease of the basal ganglia is also common, producing the typical Parkinsonian picture.

Primary spinal vascular disease is an uncommon cause of spastic paraplegia of sudden or slow onset. Symptoms are usually predominantly motor, as a result of occlusion of the anterior spinal artery. Arteritis of the spinal arteries also occurs, most commonly resulting from involvement of the vessels by a chronic inflammatory process. In the past this was seen as a meningovascular manifestation of syphilis, and also as a result of vertebral osteomyelitis due to tuberculosis. The tuberculous granulation tissue spreads from a vertebral body, and particularly when associated with some degree of vertebral collapse, can cause mechanical compression of the cord, but the major cause of neurological damage was probably due to the associated arteritis.

Systemic diseases

Collagen diseases such as polyarteritis nodosa may be a cause of arteritis involving the brain and spinal cord, and a wide variety of neurological syndromes can result. The pattern of these may appear bizarre and diagnosis can be difficult unless there are other features present to suggest this type of multi-system disease. Dermatomyositis and polymyositis also cause muscle weakness which is usually proximal and may be profound. The diagnosis will usually be suggested by other features of the disease, particu-

larly the skin manifestations. In adults half of the patients with dermatomyositis will have an underlying carcinoma of which the myositis may be the first sign.

Polymyalgia rheumatica is a common disease of the elderly, characterized by muscle pain, stiffness, and weakness associated with malaise, weight loss, and a very high ESR. The leg symptoms may predominate.

In our ageing, obese population diabetes mellitus is seen with increasing frequency. Many neurological complications occur, peripheral neuropathy being common. This may be predominantly sensory, and a sensory ataxia can occur which mimics that seen with neurosyphilis, even with the occurrence of Charcot's neuropathic joints. Cerebrovascular syndromes are also common, due to the widespread atherosclerosis usually found in long-standing diabetics.

Another disease more often seen in the elderly is myxoedema. Normally walking is not affected (although sometimes it is the characteristically delayed relaxation of the ankle reflex which suggests the diagnosis). Occasionally however, cerebellar syndromes occur, and the patient presents with ataxia.

Pernicious anaemia can present with neurological symptoms. This has become a somewhat misleading name, for it is now realized that patients who become deficient in vitamin B$_{12}$ may, rarely, develop the neurological complications while the peripheral blood and even the bone marrow appear normal. The classical picture of subacute combined degeneration of the cord will normally present little diagnostic difficulty. Paraesthesiae are usually a prominent symptom, while examination will often reveal a combination of depressed tendon reflexes due to the neuropathy with extensor plantar responses as a result of the pyramidal lesion. Symptoms and signs may, however, be minimal and frequently the diagnosis is only made by estimating the serum B$_{12}$. This justifies the routine measurement of serum B$_{12}$ in all cases of neurological disease where the diagnosis is at all in doubt (Table 25.4).

Motor neurone disease

After the age of 50 motor neurone disease becomes increasingly common and the typical combination of upper and lower motor neurone signs in the absence

Table 25.4 Important causes of sensory ataxia

Chronic peripheral neuropathy (multiple causes)
Vitamin B$_{12}$ deficiency
Multiple sclerosis
Tabes dorsalis
Rare hereditary neuropathies

Table 25.5 Important causes of a bilateral lower motor neurone lesion affecting the lower limbs

Peripheral neuropathy
Motor neurone disease
Cauda equina lesions
Prolapsed intervertebral disc
Poliomyelitis
Diabetic amyotropy

of any sensory loss, will normally allow a confident clinical diagnosis to be made. Pure bulbar and predominantly lower motor neurone forms occur, and then diagnosis is less straightforward (Table 25.5). The various motor peripheral neuropathies must be considered before a pure lower motor neurone disease is diagnosed.

Metabolic causes

Occasionally other metabolic and endocrine disorders present with muscle weakness, and thus difficulty in walking. In the past, potent diuretics were often used without potassium supplements and patients were occasionally seen with profound weakness due to hypokalaemia. Fortunately this is now rare, but other causes of hypokalaemia such as chronic purgative addiction, carbenoxolone, and primary hyperaldosteronism can still be difficult to diagnose, usually because the possibility has not been considered. Muscle wasting is common in thyrotoxicosis and sometimes this may be so severe as to constitute a definite myopathy which is mainly proximal. Usually the other clinical features will indicate the diagnosis. In disorders of calcium metabolism myopathy has been increasingly recognized, and occurs in both rickets and osteomalacia. Muscle weakness, often most obvious in the limb girdles, may be profound, and constitute a major source of disability.

One of the commonest causes of proximal muscle weakness and wasting is corticosteroid treatment, particularly with the fluorinated preparations such as triamcinolone. Muscle weakness also occurs in Cushing's syndrome itself, whether primary or a non-metastatic manifestation of malignancy.

PHYSICAL EXAMINATION

A thorough general examination is essential to exclude many of the diseases already discussed. Diseases of the bones or joints will usually be obvious, but a common error is to misinterpret the pain, wasting and weakness in the leg that can result from osteoarthritis of the hip as being of neurological origin. The spine should be carefully examined, tenderness looked for, and the full range of movements elicited. Any local deformity is

particularly important. Straight leg raising should be measured on each side. Any slight asymmetry of the body should be noted, for congenital lesions of one hemisphere may lead to underdevelopment of the skull on that side, and the rest of the body on the other. A full neurological examination is mandatory but perhaps the single most important thing is to watch the patient walking over a reasonable distance. If the walking appears normal his performance should be stressed by asking him to walk heel to toe along a straight line. One should note whether there is any special difficulty in starting or stopping walking, and whether turning to left or right presents any particular problem. It is obviously important that the patient is properly observed and this is not possible if a long dressing gown or nightdress is being worn. Ill-fitting carpet slippers should also be removed and ideally the patient should walk barefoot. Careful attention should also be paid to the stance of the body generally, and to the presence, nature and symmetry of associated movements of the upper limbs. Any abnormal movements should be carefully noted.

Some patterns of disturbance are so characteristic that they are recognized at a glance.

The typical stooped and shuffling gait seen in Parkinsonism is usually obvious provided the patient has been properly observed. There will often be an expressionless face and a loss of swinging of the arms while walking. The patient frequently has difficulty in the initiation of walking, and once started commonly shows impairment in maintaining his balance. This is often particularly obvious when he attempts to turn. He may find it easier to walk backwards than forwards.

A spastic disturbance of gait is frequently seen, commonly as a result of cerebrovascular disease, and with severe disability so that the diagnosis is immediately apparent. Minor degrees of spastic weakness can be more difficult to detect, and if suspected the patient's shoes should always be inspected for the excessive wear of the toe which tends to occur.

The difficulty in walking may result from ataxia, due either to impairment of the proprioception or to disease of the cerebellum and its central connections (Table 25.2). If there is a loss of joint position sense patients may show the classical high-stepping gait, stamping their feet down, and Romberg's sign will be positive.

Cerebellar ataxia is uncommon and is usually associated with nystagmus. There may be some degree of dysarthria and the tendon reflexes may be decreased. If the vermis of the cerebellum is mainly affected, the limbs may show little ataxia on formal testing but there will be marked truncal ataxia. Bilateral hemisphere involvement typically leads to a broad-based 'drunken' gait, while involvement of one hemisphere causes the patient to stagger to that side.

INVESTIGATION

This will be guided by the history, the findings on examination and the diagnoses likely at any particular age. In the muscular dystrophies muscle enzyme estimations are of the greatest value. Family studies will allow the pattern of inheritance to be worked out even if there is no clinical disability. A wide variety of muscle enzymes can be measured, aldolase, lactic dehydrogenase, transaminase and creatine phosphokinase all being of value. The urinary excretion of creatine and of amino acids may also be increased. All these biochemical tests are of most use when there is active muscle wasting and are particularly likely to be positive in the Duchenne type of dystrophy. Muscle enzymes are also abnormal in the majority of patients with polymyositis, and here there may be elevation of the ESR and a rise in the serum gamma globulin.

The various metabolic myopathies are clinically similar and can only be distinguished by biochemical analysis. Potassium loss for any reason can cause profound muscle weakness, and although, in general, total body potassium only correlates poorly with serum potassium levels, if marked muscle weakness is present there will be hypokalaemia. Myopathy is also a feature of osteomalacia or rickets and again there is not necessarily a close correlation between the bone disease and the muscle weakness. The serum calcium and alkaline phosphatase should therefore always be estimated, taking particular care to avoid any haemoconcentration when the blood is being taken. Muscle weakness and wasting can be prominent in thyrotoxicosis and occasionally the other features of the condition may not be apparent. A myopathy may also rarely occur in myxoedema, and for both these reasons therefore the plasma thyroxine or TSH should be measured in any obscure myopathy.

Subacute combined degeneration of the cord may occur with little posterior column degeneration and the serum B_{12} level must be measured in any obscure peripheral neuropathy or pure pyramidal lesion. Rarely, neurological complications such as neuropathy and neuromyopathy may occur in malabsorption syndrome. Although folate deficiency may be present, it is by no means clear if this is the cause; other deficiencies are probably present.

Peripheral neuropathy is common in diabetes mellitus, and although the diagnosis is usually obvious, occasionally neuropathy is the initial presentation. The urine therefore must always be checked for sugar and in older patients who may have a high renal threshold for glucose, hyperglycaemia should also be excluded. Porphyria is a rare cause of peripheral neuropathy and should be excluded.

Alcoholism is often associated with neuropathy and may be suspected both clinically and from macrocytosis and abnormal liver function tests. Some patients after portocaval anastomoses may develp a slowly progressive spastic paraplegia due to pyramidal tract degeneration, while more rarely Parkinsonian or cerebellar syndromes may develop.

Serology on blood and CSF will usually confirm the presence of neurosyphilis and may also be of value in exotic disorders like rickettsial transverse myelitis. Lumbar puncture is of the greatest importance. The opening pressure and the rise and fall on jugular compression should be carefully assessed and may provide the first indication of spinal cord compression by tumour. Any abnormality should be followed up by myelography, which should include examination of the foramen magnum region for congenital abnormalities. The fluid itself may be xanthochromic and a large rise in the protein content will also usually be found in spinal compression. A rise in the protein content of any extent with minimal elevation in the cell count is a feature of acute infective polyneuropathy, which is a condition of widely varying severity and rapidity of onset. A more modest rise in the CSF protein occurs in about 30% of cases of multiple sclerosis and may be associated with a paretic Lange curve even though the WR is negative. In a large number of cases a rise will be found in the CSF gamma globulin content after concentration and electrophoresis. Serological tests for syphilis must always be done on the CSF even though sometimes their imterpretation is difficult. A small number of cases of active neurosyphilis are said to show negative serology. In many neurological diseases a small rise occurs in the CSF protein, but this is a very non-specific finding. Its main value is often to indicate that there is organic disease present. Straight radiology of the spine is useful and may show evidence of cervical or lumbar spondylosis, or of disseminated malignancy. Electromyographic and nerve conduction studies will help to distinguish between disease of the peripheral nerve and the muscle and will be pathognomonic in dystrophia myotonica.

CLINICAL PROBLEM

T	P	BP	R
37.2	90	190/100	20

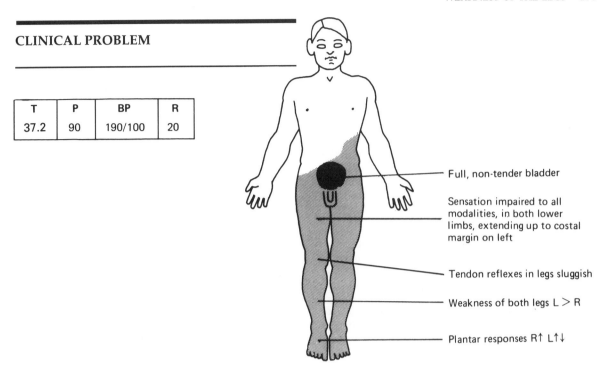

Full, non-tender bladder

Sensation impaired to all modalities, in both lower limbs, extending up to costal margin on left

Tendon reflexes in legs sluggish

Weakness of both legs L > R

Plantar responses R↑ L↑↓

A 49-year-old businessman consulted his general practitioner because of low lumbar pain which had come on gradually over the previous 10 days. The pain was dull and aching and had developed after a long car journey. It troubled him especially at night and also if he coughed or strained. He had continued working during this time, taking large amounts of aspirin. Initially this controlled the pain but had subsequently proved ineffective. Furthermore, over the preceding few days the pain had begun to spread into his right buttock and down the back of the right thigh.

In the past he had been generally well except for a previous epidsode of back pain 8 years ago which had responded to bed rest. He was known to be mildly hypertensive and had been taking a thiazide diuretic for several years. He smoked 20 cigarettes daily and drank fairly heavily, mainly in the context of his job. His father and one brother had both died from myocardial infarction.

Examination revealed an obese man, pulse 72 regular. Blood pressure 200/105. The fundi showed Grade I changes. There was loss of the normal lumbar lordosis and the lumbar spine was a little tender on percussion. Straight leg raising on the right was limited to 60 degrees and on the left to 80 degrees.

He was admitted to a private nursing home for bed rest and over the next 2 weeks his symptoms and signs improved rapidly.

Routine investigation showed: Hb 16.5 g/dl. WBC and differential normal. ESR 28 mm in 1 hour. Urea 4.8 mmol/l. MSU: normal. CXR showed slight cardiomegaly but was otherwise clear. X-ray of the spine showed early spondylitic changes, with narrowing of the disc spaces of L4/L5 and L5/S1.

He was being considered for discharge when he complained that for the previous 24 hours he felt his legs had become weak and that he had difficulty in walking to the toilet. He had also noticed some hesitancy in his micturition. He had not passed urine for 12 hours.

Examination (see diagram) revealed a full bladder which was not tender. The prostate appeared normal. There was weakness of both legs, more marked on the left, tone was not obviously abnormal, and the tendon reflexes in the legs were sluggish. The plantar response was thought to be extensor on the right and equivocal on the left. Sensory testing revealed some impairment of all modalities in both lower limbs, and this extended up to the costal margin on the left. No abnormality was found in the upper limbs.

QUESTIONS

1. What are the likely reasons for this patient's sudden deterioration?
2. What would be your immediate management?

DISCUSSION

Early in his illness the patient was thought to have a mechanical derangement of the lumbosacral region; probably a prolapsed disc with root pressure. The story he gave was completely compatible with such a diagnosis, both in the nature and site of his pain, its relationship to coughing and sneezing (manoeuvres which raise the CSF pressure) and its pattern of radiation. Prolapsed intervertebral disc (PID) is undoubtedly the commonest cause of such a syndrome, but it is important to remember that many other disease processes can produce nerve root compression and present in a similar manner.

His obesity and the fact that he had suffered an episode of back pain in the past supports the diagnosis of PID, while the findings of local tenderness, loss of the lumber lordosis, and limitation of straight leg raising are indicative of local pathology with root irritation. His investigations are also compatible with this diagnosis, except that the ESR is a little high. His initial management, therefore, with bed rest was reasonable. Usually this would be combined with a low-calorie reducing diet, sedation and analgesia.

His obesity, heavy cigarette smoking, hypertension, and bad family history also suggest that he is a candidate for vascular disease and that the rare condition of spinal artery occlusion must be considered.

The deterioration which occurred shortly before his discharge is obviously a very sinister event. The difficulty with micturition, the extensor plantar response, and the sensory level suggest a lesion involving the spinal cord rather than the nerve roots. This could obviously not occur with a disc lesion at the level of L5/S1. Higher disc lesions may occur but are very rare.

The common causes of a clinical picture of this type are very varied. Trauma is a frequent reason, but is self-evident and not relevant here. Demyelinating disease, either the common multiple sclerosis or the rare variant neuromyelitis optica may present in this way. However, there have been no previous episodes of neurological disease, there are no signs of lesions elsewhere in the nervous system, and he is a little old for this disease. Furthermore, it would not explain his initial presentation with back pain and root irritation.

A transverse myelitis can result from infection. This may occur as a result of local infections, either tuberculous or pyogenic, spreading to involve the cord and its blood supply, or it may be as a complication of one of the common exanthemata such as herpes zoster. There is no history of recent infection in this patient and such an interpretation is unlikely.

Neoplastic disease may involve the meninges either directly or by spread from the vertebral bodies. This can result from disseminated carcinoma, and may also be a complication of the lymphomas and leukaemias. Initial presentation of the disease with a neurological syndrome such as cord compression is well recognized, and must certainly be considered here. He is a heavy smoker and carcinoma of the bronchus is not excluded by a single normal chest X-ray. Primary tumours of the meninges and nerve roots such as meningioma and neurofibroma can cause spinal cord compression, but usually there is a longer story of progressive disability.

The most important investigation in this patient is further radiology. Myelography should be performed. In addition to showing any block, it may, by indicating the exact site of any pathological lesion, also suggest its nature.

Radioisotope scanning of the skeleton may show evidence of any disseminated malignancy and is more sensitive in showing metastases than conventional radiology early on. If leukaemia or lymphoma is suspected a marrow aspiration is indicated.

In this patient lumbar puncture showed the typical changes of spinal block and myelography showed that this was due to an extramedullary, extradural lesion at the level of D6. Emergency laminectomy at this level revealed extensive tumour tissue spreading from the vertebral bodies, and histology showed this to be probably anaplastic carcinoma of the bronchus. This was confirmed by the later progression of the disease.

26. Pruritus

Pruritus or itching can simply be defined as the desire to scratch. It is best regarded as a mild type of pain caused by tissue damage of a low order of magnitude. There is undoubtedly considerable variation between individuals in the threshold of stimulation at which the sensation is experienced. In the same way as one can describe one person as being more ticklish than another, so some are more susceptible to itching.

Itching is certainly the most important single dermatological symptom. It is usually a symptom of primary skin disease but diagnostic difficulty may occur when pruritus is the presenting symptom of a systemic disease. Although there may be an associated rash, this too may be a manifestation of an underlying disease.

An erroneous primary dermatological diagnosis may be made if the secondary effects of scratching on the skin are not appreciated. There may be obvious scratch marks. When over a period of time they leave depigmented scars surrounded by an area of hyperpigmentation, the skin changes are called prurigo. Persistent rubbing, gives rise to lichenification where the skin becomes thickened and raised in violet-brown lozenge-shaped patches between normal skin creases. This localized disorder is called neurodermatitis or lichen simplex. Other particularly troublesome localized forms are the closely related pruritus ani and pruritus vulvae. The diagnosis of general, senile or psychogenic (idiopathic) pruritus should not be made until all possible aetiological factors have been excluded.

GENERALIZED PRURITUS

Liver disease

Pruritus occurs commonly in all forms of obstructive jaundice. As such it is a helpful symptom in the differential diagnosis of jaundice, suggesting that it is due to cholestasis rather than hepatocellular damage or haemolysis. The cause of the pruritus is thought to be the retention of bile salts rather than the elevated bilirubin. This seems borne out by the success of symptomatic oral treatment with the bile salt binding resin cholestyramine, used when the obstruction is not complete. Methyl testosterone acts, by an unknown mechanism, as an effective antipruritic despite causing further elevation of the bilirubin.

Obstructive jaundice due to gallstones, pancreatic carcinoma or drugs such as chlorpromazine will usually be easily detected. Likewise most patients with biliary cirrhosis will have jaundice, but pruritus without jaundice may be the presenting symptom of primary biliary cirrhosis. Itching may occur in other forms of non-icteric cirrhosis so that one should always look for signs of liver disease – hepatosplenomegaly, spider naevi, palmar erythema, leuconychia – in a patient presenting with pruritus.

Pregnancy

Pruritus may occur in the last trimester and disappear 2 or 3 days post-partum. It frequently recurs in subsequent pregnancies and may also be precipitated in such women by the taking of the contraceptive pill. Most of these patients will have an obvious associated cholestatic jaundice. The syndrome is thought to be due to a disturbance of the liver metabolism of steroid hormones, with either a failure of degradation or an excess production of normal steroids, or the production of an abnormal steroid. Diagnostic difficulty may arise in some patients with pruritus who are not clinically jaundiced. There will, however, usually be biochemical abnormalities to suggest cholestasis such as a raised liver alkaline phosphatase.

Herpes gestationis is a rare condition occurring in pregnancy. There is a skin eruption resembling pemphigoid, which is accompanied by intense itching.

Renal failure

Pruritus may be an early feature of chronic renal failure from any cause but does not occur in acute renal failure. The mechanism by which pruritus occurs is not understood. In those patients who develop secondary hyperparathyroidism, and who have pruritus, rapid relief of itching may occur after parathyroidectomy, though the impairment of renal function remains unchanged. It is possible, in these cases, that the elevated calcium–phosphate product causes pruritus through its deposition in the skin. Pruritus does not occur with hypercalcaemia due to other causes which are not associated with a raised serum phosphate and where the calcium–phosphate product is not greatly elevated. Ultraviolet radiation (UVB) may also give relief by mechanisms which are not understood.

Diabetes mellitus

Hyperglycaemia and glycosuria predispose to infection, especially with yeasts. Candida infection, particularly of the anogenital region, is a common complication causing pruritus. There is also a form of generalized pruritus of unknown cause that may rarely occur particularly at the onset of diabetes. In these patients other paraesthesiae may also occur, suggesting that there is a metabolic disturbance of the peripheral nerves.

Malignant disease

The skin manifestations of internal malignancy are becoming increasingly recognized. Pruritus can be a presentation of a remote cancer on rare occasions. Pruritus is a feature of Hodgkin's disease in some patients. When it occurs it may antedate the diagnosis by years. The itching may be intense and is often worse at night, and often affects the palms of the hands and soles of the feet. It is a most distressing, intractable and untreatable symptom and is only relieved by treatment of the underlying disease. Curiously it is a very uncommon symptom in non-Hodgkin's lymphoma. A related but separate condition is the lymphoma directly involving the skin known as mycosis fungoides. The mycotic phase of ulcerating skin tumours is often preceded for many years by a variety of premycotic lesions. These may be erythrodermic (synonymous with exfoliative dermatitis), eczematous or psoriasiform and are all associated with intense pruritus.

Disorders of blood

Pruritus may be a presenting symptom of leukaemia. It occurs, in the form of erythroderma, in some patients with chronic lymphatic leukaemia. In the rare monocytic leukaemia pruritus and rash may be present for some time before blood abnormalities. At this early stage skin biopsy will show infiltration with monocytes.

Pruritus is a common symptom in primary polycythaemia and, as with some of the other causes of itching, it may be precipitated by taking a hot bath or shower. Using this 'provocative test' an incidence of 20–50% has been described. Usually, however, other symptoms of headache, dizziness, dyspnoea or thrombotic episodes in the heart or brain, will predominate. On rare occasions pruritus may be a symptom of a severe anaemia, especially pernicious anaemia, and is also said to occur with iron deficiency even in the absence of anaemia.

Malabsorption syndrome

In steatorrhoea, especially that associated with gluten sensitivity, a variety of non-specific skin disorders may occur. For example, pruritus may thus be associated with eczema-like lesions or pigmentation.

Collagen diseases

In systemic sclerosis, where there is scleroderma together with involvement of the oesophagus, gut, lungs and kidneys, pruritus may occur. Dermatomyositis is an uncommon condition in which pruritus may also rarely occur. There is proximal limb girdle muscle weakness, together with skin involvement often affecting the upper eyelids or knuckles.

Thyroid disorders

Pruritus can be a symptom of both thyrotoxicosis and myxoedema. It occurs so rarely as to be more of a curiosity than of diagnostic value, and in the latter, may be another manifestation of dryness of the skin.

Drugs

Drug eruptions frequently itch and do not cause too much diagnostic difficulty. Occasionally pruritus may be the only manifestation of an otherwise subclinical sensitivity reaction. Cocaine characteristically causes itching. Another agent whose effect on the skin is not clinically visible is fibreglass used for insulation purposes.

LOCALIZED PRURITUS

Itching is a feature of many skin disorders. In these cases a dermatological diagnosis can be made from the appearance and distribution of the lesion or the demonstration of the causative agent. Pruritus is prominent in scabies, pediculosis, urticaria and eczema and dermatitis herpetiformis, and the prodrome of shingles (Herpes zoster).

Proctologists and gynaecologists are frequently consulted because of pruritus. In pruritus ani and pruritus vulvae there are numerous local disorders which may be responsible, some being common to both conditions.

Pruritus vulvae

Perspiration and lack of hygiene predispose to pruritus vulvae, as may previous gynaecological operations. It may also complicate incorrect treatment with locally irritant or sensitizing preparations, such as topical antihistamines. Topical steroids or broad-spectrum antibiotics may cause monilial infection. The glycosuria of uncontrolled or undetected diabetes mellitus may give rise to moniliasis and thus present as pruritus vulvae. This complication has also been described in users of the contraceptive pill.

Pruritus ani

Pruritus may be confined to the anus in the diseases which can cause generalized pruritus mentioned above. Similarly, primary dermatological disorders such as psoriasis, contact dermatitis, lichen planus, lichen sclerosis, leucoplakia or local neoplasms may cause pruritus ani and pruritus vulvae.

Many local anorectal conditions have pruritus as a presenting symptom, along with soreness, bleeding and discharge. The commonest, of course, is haemorrhoids but fissure, fistula, condylomata, polyps and even carcinoma of the rectum can be responsible. Faecal soiling may be a factor common to these conditions. Treatment of the underlying disease should of course, cure the pruritus.

Infections are a common cause of pruritus ani. Moniliasis (candidiasis) due to the yeast, *Candida albicans*, is as important here as in pruritus vulvae and has the same predisposing causes. Fungal infection with epidermophyton is the cause of tinea cruris (Dhobi itch). This may spread from the groin to involve the anus. Another infection of intertriginous areas, which may involve the anus, is erythrasma due to *Corynebacterium minutissimum* which can be identified using fluorescence in ultraviolet light since the organism produces a porphyrin. The threadworm, *Oxyuris*, may cause nocturnal pruritus ani, especially in children, and when the worms are seen in the stool, there is great alarm in the parents. The diagnosis is best confirmed by applying Scotch tape to the perianal skin on waking and microscopically identifying the ova that adhere to it.

CLINICAL PROBLEM

T	P	BP	R
37·2	68	110/70	26

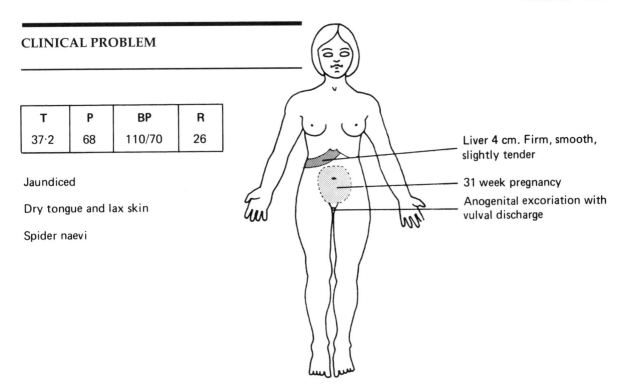

Jaundiced

Dry tongue and lax skin

Spider naevi

Liver 4 cm. Firm, smooth, slightly tender

31 week pregnancy

Anogenital excoriation with vulval discharge

A 25-year-old unmarried hairdresser was admitted to hospital because of jaundice. She was 31 weeks pregnant and had been well for the first 20 weeks of her pregnancy, without nausea, vomiting or heartburn. She had suffered from haemorrhoids for some years which had recently become worse. She had developed frequency of micturition at 24 weeks which, a week later, was associated with dysuria. Her own doctor initially advised her to drink more fluids but when her symptoms became worse gave her a 10-day course of sulphadimidine. This relieved the dysuria but her frequency persisted. Two weeks after admission the dysuria recurred, and associated with it, she developed intense pruritus of the perineum involving both the anus and vulva. Ten days before admission she was started on ampicillin 500 mg 6 hourly in an effort to control her presumed urinary infection. Again the dysuria improved within a few days, but her other symptoms persisted. Five days before admission she developed nausea and vomiting. She noticed her urine becoming darker followed by yellowness of her eyes and skin. Her pruritus and frequency continued.

There was no relevant past or family history. Apart from the drugs already mentioned she had been taking ferrous sulphate during pregnancy. Although she had been greatly upset when pregnancy had been confirmed, she had apparently accepted the fact but was planning to have her baby adopted. She strongly denied the suggestion that she might have been taking any other drugs.

On examination, she had a dry tongue and lax skin. She was moderately jaundiced but not anaemic and spider naevi were present on the arms, shoulders and face. In the abdomen, the uterus was enlarged corresponding to 31 weeks of pregnancy. The liver was palpable 4 cm below the costal margin; it was firm, smooth and slightly tender. The skin of the vulva and around the anus was excoriated and inflamed, and there was a whitish vulval discharge. On rectal examination and proctoscopy she had haemorrhoids which did not prolapse. The remainder of the examination was normal and she was afebrile.

QUESTIONS

1. What are the probable causes of her jaundice?
2. What are the probable causes of her pruritus?
3. What is the connection, if any, between these two symptoms?
4. What immediate investigations would be of value?

DISCUSSION

In addition to the various causes of jaundice in a young woman, certain causes specifically related to pregnancy will have to be considered.

Viral hepatitis occurs predominantly in young adults and carries a worse prognosis in pregnancy. The prodromal illness of 5 days in this patient would be unusually short, though it is somewhat difficult to separate from her symptoms of urinary tract infection. Hepatomegaly with some tenderness and spider naevi could both be features of hepatitis. However, spider naevi are also a common finding in pregnancy, and palmar erythema may also occur.

Although gallstones are also more common in pregnancy, no doubt related to the hypercholesterol-aemia that occurs, the absence of pain makes this an unlikely cause for her jaundice.

Drug-induced jaundice is an important cause to be considered. It may give rise to either a cholestatic or hepatocellular jaundice or to a mixed pattern. Drug jaundice may either be due to a hypersensitivity reaction or a direct toxic effect on the liver which is dose related. The only three drugs this patient has had are ferrous sulphate, sulphadimidine and ampicillin, and the first two can cause jaundice under certain circumstances. Ferrous sulphate has a toxic effect on the liver only if taken in considerable overdose, when abdominal pain, vomiting and diarrhoea would occur. Sulphonamides cause jaundice very rarely; when it occurs it may be purely cholestatic or of a mixed cholestatic–hepatocellular type.

Other causes of jaundice in pregnancy include acute yellow atrophy or acute fatty liver. The clinical picture is of vomiting, jaundice, bleeding and renal failure. Both conditions carry a bad prognosis and one would expect the patient to be more severely ill. In contrast, intrahepatic cholestasis of late pregnancy is a benign condition, and generalized pruritus is a very common feature in this disorder.

Pruritus confined to the vulva and anus is very unlikely to be due to a systemic disorder such as cholestasis and a local cause must be sought.

Although haemorrhoids may cause irritation of the anus, this would not explain pruritus vulvae. Broad-spectrum antibiotics predispose to moniliasis which is a common cause of pruritus ani and vulvae. However, the pruritus in this patient antedated the use of ampicillin.

The glycosuria of uncontrolled diabetes mellitus is another common cause of itching and pruritus may be the presenting symptom of this disease. This patient had frequency of micturition followed by dysuria; when the presumed infection was treated the dysuria improved but the frequency persisted. It is unlikely that the frequency was due to a high fluid intake alone as the patient showed signs of dehydration on admission. Diabetes beginning in mid-pregnancy, complicated by urinary infections and moniliasis, is very likely in this patient. It is therefore unlikely that there is any connection between the jaundice and the localized itching.

The investigations in this patient should be directed towards establishing the diagnosis of diabetes and the presence of moniliasis as both these conditions require treatment. Attempts to establish the cause of the jaundice from liver function tests are likely to be unrewarding, particularly as the advanced pregnancy precludes liver biopsy unless it is considered to be of vital importance.

The urine should therefore be tested for glucose, and a random and fasting blood sugar obtained, probably followed by a glucose tolerance test or measurement of glycosylated haemoglobin in case there is a lowered renal threshold for glucose, as may occur in pregnancy. The vulval discharge must be examined microscopically and cultured for *Candida albicans*, and the patient started on treatment with nystatin pessaries and ointment. A blood count may show a leucocytosis due to the recent urinary infection, and the presence of a lymphocytosis or viral lymphocytes might suggest hepatitis. Liver function tests would be performed to establish the pattern of jaundice but are unlikely to reveal the underlying cause. There may be a purely cholestatic pattern with bilirubinuria and urobilinogen absent from the urine, together with markedly raised alkaline phosphatase but moderate elevation of transaminase. This would favour a diagnosis of sulphonamide hypersensitivity or the cholestasis of pregnancy. Hepatocellular jaundice with bilirubinuria and excess urobilinogen in the urine, high transaminases and slight elevation of alkaline phosphatase would be more suggestive of infective hepatitis.

Glycosuria and an abnormal glucose tolerance test confirmed the presence of diabetes. *Candida* was easily seen on smear. The jaundice faded over the next 10 days and the investigations showed a mixed hepatocellular and obstructive jaundice for which no definite cause was established.

27. Polyarthritis

A common presenting complaint is swelling and pain in joints. One of the main problems is to try and establish whether or not one is dealing with a primary rheumatic disorder, or whether the symptom is part of another underlying disease. Early on precise diagnosis may be impossible, and only with the passage of time does the picture become clear. Nevertheless, every attempt must be made to reach a diagnosis quickly and here the clinical history and the pattern of joint involvement are the most valuable guides.

HISTORY

It is important to enquire very carefully about the true onset of the disorder. Often, when pressed, patients will remember having had recurrent attacks of transient swelling or discomfort in a joint over periods of months or years. Such a history is often found in rheumatoid arthritis. An acute onset over a few weeks, involving many joints, frequently occurs in other connective tissue disorders, such as systemic lupus erythematosus (SLE) or polyarteritis nodosa, as well as in rheumatoid arthritis. The important feature of rheumatoid arthritis is that the joint involvement is characteristically symmetrical, and the joints when involved, normally remain inflamed for a long period of time. This is in marked contrast to the flitting arthritis often seen in rheumatic fever, and sometimes in subacute bacterial endocarditis. A history of morning stiffness, improving with exercise, is typical of rheumatoid arthritis, and may occur early in the disease. In contrast, pain rather than stiffness is common in osteoarthritis, and is often made worse by use of the joints.

The pattern of joint involvement is of great importance. Gout, which often involves more than one joint, nevertheless has a strong predilection for the metatarsophalangeal joints. The small joints of the hands are often involved in rheumatoid arthritis, but the distal interphalangeal joints are characteristically spared. This is not the case with psoriatic arthritis in the hands, where the distal interphalangeal joints may be involved, often not symmetrically. The small joints of the hands may also be affected in systemic lupus erythematosus, which in the early stages, may be very difficult to distinguish from rheumatoid arthritis. Other characteristic sites of involvement in each disease will be discussed below. Arthralgia, which is pain in joints without swelling, may occur in any arthritic disorder and may herald the onset of true arthritis.

Of equal importance with the onset, site, and progression of the arthritis are details of any associated systemic symptoms. Fever, malaise and weight loss are found in many connective tissue diseases, and also occur with the arthropathy which may accompany malignant disease. Some systemic infections such as subacute bacterial endocarditis may be accompanied by polyarthritis even though the joints may not be directly invaded by the organism. On the other hand when there is direct infection of a joint, for example with gonococcal arthritis, a monoarthritis is more usual. In both situations fever and rigors may occur. The exclusion of an infective cause is particularly important in a patient with a short history.

A history of skin eruptions must be carefully sought. Transient rashes are common in many connective tissue disorders, especially SLE and polyarteritis nodosa. They may also occur in rheumatic fever. The distribution of the rash may be characteristic, for example the facial 'butterfly' rash of SLE, or the erythema nodosum over the shins which may accompany sarcoidosis or rheumatic fever. Arthritis may accompany psoriasis, even when the primary skin disorder is not severe.

Pain and redness of the eyes may be due to the conjunctivitis and iritis accompanying Reiter's syndrome, or to the iritis of ankylosing spondylitis. Diarrhoea and abdominal pain suggest ulcerative colitis or Crohn's disease, where arthritis may be prominent.

CAUSES OF POLYARTHRITIS

Rheumatoid arthritis

If a middle-aged woman complains of the gradual symmetrical involvement of joints, including the hands, with effusions and morning stiffness and without a great deal of constitutional disturbance, the diagnosis of rheumatoid arthritis is difficult to avoid. Any large joint may be involved, but the small joints of the hands and feet, and the cervical spine are characteristically affected. The temporomandibular, and cricoarytenoid joints can also be involved. When arthritis appears suddenly, involving several joints, other diagnoses such as SLE will also have to be considered. In the early phases of the disease, with involvement of only one or two joints, a firm diagnosis may not be possible, even with X-rays and serological tests.

The essential feature of the arthritis is the destruction of articular cartilage and bones. Consequently joint deformity, including subluxation, and lateral and anteroposterior instability is very common. Capsular thickening is normally prominent and large effusions can occur. In the knee, these may form large cystic swellings, which may sometimes rupture into the calf, simulating deep venous thrombosis. Subcutaneous nodules over extensor surfaces of limbs and flexor and extensor tendons are characteristic of the condition.

Systemic features sometimes occur, such as pleural effusion, peripheral neuropathy and splenomegaly. When these features are present there may be some difficulty in distinguishing the disease from SLE. This is not usually a problem if it is remembered that the arthritis in SLE is not nearly so destructive, and that glomerulonephritis, which is common in SLE, does not occur in rheumatoid arthritis. In rheumatoid arthritis, some degree of anaemia is common. Renal amyloidosis is not unusual in long-standing cases, occasionally giving rise to the nephrotic syndrome. Sjögren's syndrome is keratoconjunctivitis sicca and xerostoma in association with rheumatoid arthritis or another connective tissue disease.

Still's disease is a variant of rheumatoid arthritis occurring in children. Some cases have a severe systemic illness with fever, pericarditis, skin rash, peritonitis and anaemia. Glomerulonephritis does not occur. The joint disease is similar to the adult form, but tests for rheumatoid factor are negative and ankylosing spondylitis or rheumatoid arthritis may develop after many years.

Degenerative joint disease (osteoarthritis, osteoarthrosis)

The characteristic features of degenerative joint disease are the involvement of only one or two joints, often asymmetrically, the very slow progression of the disorder in most patients, the advanced age at which it most commonly appears, and the lack of systemic complications. It often arises in a single joint as a result of previous trauma, other joints being spared.

In some patients a history of trauma is lacking and the disease may affect several joints. In this form of the disorder the hands are often involved, especially distal interphalangeal joints and the metacarpo-

phalangeal joint of the thumb. Heberden's nodes are a characteristic finding, related to the affected distal interphalangeal joints. Some patients with the generalized form may have a family history of the disease. In this form of the disorder distinction from rheumatoid arthritis can be difficult. Degenerative joint disease is a frequent sequel to rheumatoid arthritis whether active or not.

There is usually crepitus on moving the affected joint, and joint effusions may be present which when aspirated show clear fluid with little cellular content.

Gout and pseudogout

This is a diagnosis which must always be considered, since specific treatment is available. Although the first metatarsophalangeal joint is usually involved, gout may affect any joint, and may occur in more than one joint at a time. Joint swelling may persist after the acute attack has subsided and this may create diagnostic difficulty. The onset of the attack is typically much more acute and painful than in any other form of polyarthritis, and often resembles pyogenic arthritis in the degree of inflammation present. Sometimes the onset is much milder and the disease may progress in a chronic fashion. The ears should be examined for tophi, which may also accumulate around the joints, especially in the hands. These may be confused with the synovial swelling commonly found in severely affected joints in rheumatoid arthritis. In primary gout there is often a family history of the disorder. Gout may be secondary to polycythaemia rubra vera and myeloid metaplasia in the elderly, and acute leukaemia in the young. An acute attack is sometimes provoked by treatment of these diseases and lymphoma by cytotoxic drugs. In primary gout trauma and operations may provoke an acute attack.

The serum urate is nearly always raised in gout. Aspiration of the joint fluid and its examination under polarized light for the presence of the negatively birefringent urate crystals in polymorphonuclear leucocytes is the definitive diagnostic test. Aspiration will also exclude pyogenic arthritis which is the main differential diagnosis.

A clinically similar monoarthritis, which is being increasingly recognized, is 'pseudogout' or calcium pyrophosphate gout. This condition primarily affects large joints in which there is often chondrocalcinosis. The onset is abrupt, often following trauma. Calcium pyrophosphate crystals which are weakly birefringent, can be seen in polymorphs in the joint fluid. The disease is sometimes a complication of hyperparathyroidism.

Ankylosing spondylitis

Peripheral arthritis occurs in about 20% of patients with ankylosing spondylitis, and when it occurs usually involves proximal large joints, knees and feet. The diagnosis should be suspected if the arthritis occurs in a young man, and if there is a history of lumbar backache. There may be associated iritis, and aortitis causing aortic incompetence.

Polyarthritis is more likely to occur in adolescents, when it is more frequently associated with iritis and aortitis. In women the disease is rare, and may occur in association with ulcerative colitis and Crohn's disease.

Systemic lupus erythematosus (SLE)

This disease, with its diversity of symptoms and signs, may present as a polyarthritis, whose distribution can be identical to rheumatoid arthritis. The onset of the disease is usually abrupt and constitutional upset is often severe. The disease may be precipitated by exposure to sunlight. A similar disease can be provoked by drugs such as hydrallazine, procainamide, phenytoin and propranolol. Abdominal pain, pleurisy, neuropathy, pericarditis, fever anaemia, psychosis, skin rashes of many types and glomerulonephritis are all common. Further distinction from rheumatoid arthritis lies in the important fact that renal disease occurs in approximately half of the patients with SLE while in rheumatoid arthritis the only major renal complications are due to amyloid disease and analgesic abuse, both of which are uncommon.

Polyarteritis nodosa

This disorder, like SLE, has numerous possible presentations apart from polyarthritis. These include asthma, skin rashes, mononeuritis multiplex, muscle pains, pericarditis, pulmonary infiltration, pleurisy, glomerulonephritis and hypertension. The widespread vascular disturbance may cause acute inflammation of the gallbladder and testes, while cerebral arteritis is not uncommon.

This is very unlike the clinical picture found in rheumatoid arthritis. The arthritis of polyarteritis may have a similar distribution to rheumatoid arthritis, but has a predilection for large joints, is usually abrupt in onset, may move from joint to joint, and deformity and erosion of joints are not common. Approximately 30% of patients have a positive test for hepatitis B surface antigen.

Rheumatic fever and Still's disease

The classical history of arthritis, developing rapidly in one joint, and then moving from joint to joint, without causing any permanent damage, is usually all that is required to distinguish this disease from other forms of polyarthritis. An antecedent sore throat or the finding of cardiac involvement further supports the diagnosis. The response to salicylates is not diagnostic, since many inflammatory polyarthritides will remit partially on large doses of aspirin. An interesting, albeit rare, sequel to rheumatic fever, especially if recurrent, is a form of chronic mild deformity of joints (often small joints of the hand) first described by Jaccoud, and further delineated by Bywaters. This is not likely to be a diagnostic problem since it occurs in the context of clearly established rheumatic fever.

Small nodules may appear over the elbows and knees. They are distinguished from those found in rheumatoid arthritis by their small size, their site over the joints rather than over the neighbouring bones and tendons, and by the fact that the nodules of rheumatoid arthritis accompany chronic joint deformity.

Reiter's syndrome

The triad of arthritis, urethritis and conjunctivitis, usually leads to early diagnosis. The onset is abrupt, often following sexual exposure, although bacillary dysentery may be a precipitating cause. Sometimes the urethritis can be so mild and the conjunctivitis so fleeting, that diagnostic difficulty can occur. Balanitis may be present and shallow painful ulcers can occur over the penis and in the mouth. A slit-lamp examination of the eyes is mandatory in all suspected cases, since iritis is often present and can lead to blindness. Keratodermia blenorrhagica occurs over the soles of the feet and palms. It is characterized by small vesicles and brown scaly papules, and the rash may be indistinguishable from psoriasis.

Sacroiliitis is not uncommon in this disorder and X-rays of the spine may show changes similar to those seen in ankylosing spondylitis, although they are more unevenly distributed. Plantar fasciitis and calcaneal spurs are characteristic of the syndrome. The arthritis is acute and destructive, often leading to deformity. It involves the hands, sometimes asymmetrically, and often only one or two fingers. Large joints in the legs are also affected, usually symmetrically. Aortitis has been described. The condition is relapsing and in some attacks symptoms of conjunctivitis and urethritis may be very mild or absent. A careful history will then reveal that these features were present in an earlier, initial episode (often with a long interval between attacks).

Ulcerative colitis and Crohn's disease

It is now clear that both these diseases may be complicated by a form of joint disease which is not due to coincidental rheumatoid arthritis.

The large joints are usually involved, and sometimes the arthritis may antedate the bowel symptoms. A most interesting feature in both diseases is that sacroiliitis can occur, and some patients show changes indistinguishable from ankylosing spondylitis in the lumbar spine. These individuals are often HLA-B27 positive. As in ankylosing spondylitis, aortitis and iritis are occasionally seen. The significance of the association between spondylitis, iritis, and aortitis seen in these disorders and in Reiter's syndrome is not understood.

Although it is not likely to present diagnostic difficulty, the polyarthritis associated with these disorders should always be kept in mind, especially if the patient is a woman with sacroiliitis or spondylitis.

Sarcoidosis

Two forms of arthritis are seen in this condition. The first is an acute arthritis, which usually occurs in the context of erythema nodosum and constitutional upset. The knees and ankles are usually involved, and the arthritis settles without deformity. The second form is a chronic disorder seen in long-standing sarcoidosis. Joints which are adjacent to underlying bone disease are often involved. Both large and small joints may swell, and sarcoid granulomata can be found on synovial biopsy. Although the arthritis usually occurs in the presence of obvious disease, it should be borne in mind in any patient with a puzzling chronic polyarthritis.

Psoriasis

Polyarthritis may complicate this disorder, and the skin eruption does not have to be severe for the joint complication to develop. There is usually a long history of psoriasis. The arthritis may involve the small joints of the hand. Here it may be asymmetrical, and involve distal interphalangeal joints, which help to distinguish it from rheumatoid arthritis.

When the hands are involved, a careful examination will often show pitting of the nails or subungual keratosis. Interestingly, this often occurs in the nail of the digit affected by arthritis. Any large joint may be involved and distinction from rheumatoid arthritis may be difficult unless a careful search for the skin lesions is made. The arthritis may be highly destructive, with erosion of bone and marked deformity. Further points of distinction from rheumatoid arthritis lie in the occasional occurrence of sacroiliitis (20% of cases) and the negative serological tests.

Subacute infective endocarditis

Polyarthritis may occur in this condition and can be acute, resembling a septic arthritis, or subacute. The large joints are particularly affected, although any joint may be involved. The arthritis may move from joint to joint as in rheumatic fever. However, haematuria, a cardiac murmur, fever, anaemia and Osler's nodes are often present. The diagnosis of infective endocarditis should be considered in a patient with systemic upset, polyarthritis and a cardiac murmur. Under such circumstances, blood cultures must always be taken. A disastrous mistake would be to treat such patients with corticosteroids on the presumption that they have a 'collagen' disease.

Other infective causes

Pyogenic arthritis usually affects one joint only. Staphylococci, gonococci, pneumococci, streptococci and pseudomonas are the commonest infecting organisms. It may, however, occur in a joint of a patient with rheumatoid arthritis, when it may be misdiagnosed as a relapse of the condition and treated with steroids. Such a joint should always be aspirated. Gonococcal infection may present with an arthritis which moves from joint to joint, and is often accompanied by a rash. It is especially likely to present in this way in women, as opposed to men in whom urethritis is a prominent symptom resulting in early treatment. After meningococcaemia a sterile polyarthritis may occur. Osteomyelitis may be accompanied by an effusion in an adjacent joint. Radiological changes in bone may occur late and antibiotic therapy must not be delayed if the diagnosis is likely.

Arthritis and sacroiliitis occur in brucellosis and this might be suggested by a history of drinking raw milk. Virus diseases are being increasingly recognized as a cause of transient polyarthritis with a good prognosis. Of these rubella is the commonest. The arthritis is not usually severe and is self-limiting. It may also follow rubella vaccine and vaccination against smallpox. Chickenpox, infective hepatitis, *Mycoplasma pneumoniae*, infectious mononucleosis and mumps are all recognized causes.

Malignant disease

A common accompaniment of carcinoma of the bronchus is hypertrophic pulmonary osteoarthropathy. Although this is not a true arthritis, it may occasionally be misdiagnosed as such. The presence of clubbing will point to the correct diagnosis, and the radiological appearance of symmetrical periosteal reaction at the ends of the long bones are characteristic.

Occasionally polyarthritis may be the first feature of an occult neoplasm. The association has been reported with a wide variety of malignant tumours. The arthritis may resemble rheumatoid arthritis and sometimes remits when the tumour is excised. Although rare, this form of polyarthritis should be borne in mind in a middle-aged or elderly person, especially if there is weight loss or anaemia.

Miscellaneous causes

Arthritis occurs as part of *Henoch–Schönlein purpura*, but the other features of this disorder will point to the correct diagnosis. Arthritis, similar to rheumatoid arthritis, may occur in *systemic sclerosis (scleroderma)*. Usually the skin changes are obvious, but occasionally only the visceral features of the disease are present. *Whipple's disease* may be accompanied by recurrent flitting polyarthritis. The association with steatorrhoea and skin pigmentation will suggest the diagnosis. *Alkaptonuria* (ochronosis) predisposes to the development of osteoarthritis involving the knee and spine. The intervertebral discs become calcified and are visible on X-ray. In *Behçet's syndrome* oral and genital ulceration are combined with skin rashes, encephalitis, iridocyclitis and arthritis of one or two joints; venous and arterial thromboses and vascular involvement of the eye are the most serious complications. Acute arthritis, especially of the ankles and knees, commonly occurs in *erythema nodosum*. Although sarcoidosis is the commonest cause, drugs, streptococcal infection, fungal and tuberculous infections can also give rise to the syndrome.

Systemic sclerosis may sometimes be associated with arthritis and arthralgia early in the disease before the other features (skin, lung and gut fibrosis, calcinosis, Raynaud's phenomenon and renal failure) occur.

RADIOLOGICAL INVESTIGATION

In the early stages of most of these disorders, X-rays of the affected joints often do not provide diagnostic information. In rheumatoid arthritis, for example, one of the earliest appearances is juxta-articular osteoporosis, and only later do the characteristic X-ray appearances develop.

Narrowing of the joint space signifies loss of articular cartilage; it occurs quite quickly in many inflammatory arthritides, especially in rheumatoid arthritis. It occurs after a longer period of time in degenerative joint disease, and by then the other signs of this disorder are usually present with sclerosis of underlying bone, and osteophyte formation at joint margins. Erosion of bone is typical of rheumatoid arthritis, and should be looked for carefully. The hands and feet, if involved, are good sites to observe these changes. The erosions appear as a ragged margin in the surface of the bone, usually seen first at the edge of the articular surface. The destruction extends and soon becomes obvious. In rheumatoid arthritis, if the wrists are involved clinically, X-ray often shows erosion of the ulnar styloid early on (Fig. 27.1).

In psoriasis, the destruction may be difficult to distinguish from rheumatoid arthritis. The heads of the metacarpals may be lost entirely and there is usually considerable deformity. Subluxation and gross deformity are typical of advanced rheumatoid arthritis, and secondary degenerative changes are usual.

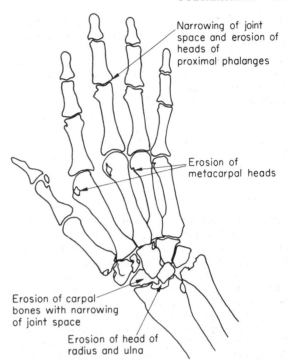

Narrowing of joint space and erosion of heads of proximal phalanges

Erosion of metacarpal heads

Erosion of carpal bones with narrowing of joint space

Erosion of head of radius and ulna

Fig. 27.1 Radiological changes in rheumatoid arthritis

The bones themselves may show lesions. In gout punched-out lytic areas are commonly seen, which are usually adjacent to the articular surface. Cystic areas in bone may also occur in rheumatoid arthritis, and sometimes in degenerative joint disease. In sarcoidosis granulomata may occur in bone, often in the metacarpals. The bone is often slightly expanded, and there are lytic areas.

Periostitis is the hallmark of hypertrophic pulmonary osteoarthropathy, and is usually best seen along the ends of long bones. Appearances of damage to the joint itself do not occur. Local periostitis also occurs in many other conditions where there is true arthritis. For example, it is often seen near involved joints in Reiter's syndrome and in juvenile rheumatoid arthritis.

The sacroiliac joints are involved in many disorders and views of these joints may be helpful. There is narrowing of the joint space, often with sclerosis of the adjacent bone, and erosions may be seen at the joint margins. Ultimately these changes result in fusion of the joint. X-rays of the spine in ankylosing spondylitis initially may show 'squaring' of the vertebral bodies, the characteristic calcification of intervertebral ligaments occurring only later.

SEROLOGICAL TESTS

Many doctors place too much trust in the diagnostic value of serological tests in arthritis. Clinical criteria usually give the diagnosis, and serology is often only of marginal help. The reasons for this are that the serum factors which are being looked for are often only byproducts of the basic disease process and may be produced under a variety of other circumstances.

Rheumatoid factor

This is a large molecular weight antibody which is directed against altered human gamma globulin. It probably arises wherever altered gamma globulin is present in the blood, for example as circulating immune complexes, or adherent to bacteria. The antibody is found most consistently and in the highest titre in rheumatoid arthritis. Interestingly, the antibody is nearly always present if the patient has rheumatoid nodules or vascular lesions, and many believe that patients with rheumatoid arthritis who have rheumatoid factor (about 75–85%) have a more destructive disease than those who do not.

Rheumatoid factor is also found in some patients with SLE, polyarteritis, sarcoidosis, leprosy, subacute infective endocarditis and in 5–10% of normal elderly people. It is absent in ankylosing spondylitis, psoriasis, and Reiter's syndrome. It is detected by the capacity of the patient's serum to agglutinate latex or bentonite particles coated with human gamma globulin, or to agglutinate sheep red cells coated with rabbit gamma globulin (the Rose–Waaler test). It can be discovered, by more complex techniques, in some patients with rheumatoid arthritis where conventional tests are negative.

Antinuclear factors (ANF)

In SLE a variety of antibodies directed against various nuclear constituents may be found in the bloods. They are usually detected by immunofluorescent techniques, although latex and bentonite agglutination tests have been developed. In active SLE especially with nephritis, ANF is almost always present, and its absence is strongly against the diagnosis. However, ANF is found in patients with rheumatoid arthritis and polyarteritis nodosa and is occasionally seen in sarcoidosis, lepromatous leprosy and subacute infective endocarditis. The pattern of fluorescence is of significance: a diffuse staining is seen with SLE and a speckled appearance with mixed connective tissue disease. It is possible that ANF has pathogenetic significance in SLE: the nephritis, for example, is probably due to combination of anti-DNA antibody with free circulating DNA and deposition of these circulating complexes in the glomeruli. Anti-DNA antibodies can now be measured by DNA binding, techniques and are present in highest titre in active SLE.

HLA typing

It is rarely necessary to tissue-type patients to make a diagnosis. A remarkably close association has been found between ankylosing spondylitis and the HLA-B27 type. Over 90% of patients have this histocompatibility antigen. A slightly less strong association exists between HLA-B27 and Reiter's syndrome although 10% of people who are HLA-B27 develop Reiter's syndrome after Shigella infection.

CLINICAL PROBLEM

T	P	BP	R
37·6	92	130/80	26

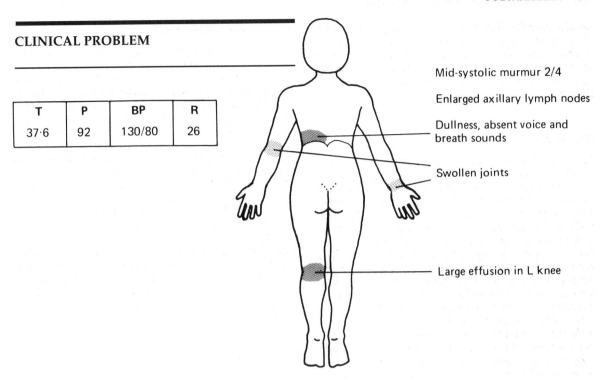

Mid-systolic murmur 2/4

Enlarged axillary lymph nodes

Dullness, absent voice and breath sounds

Swollen joints

Large effusion in L knee

A housewife of 54 was referred to the outpatient's clinic with the complaint that for the preceding 6 weeks she had had pain and swelling in the joints. She had noticed the rapid onset of arthritis in the left elbow, both knees, and right wrist, and in the second and third proximal interphalangeal joints of both hands. She had started to feel unwell 8 weeks before being seen, while on a camping holiday in Portugal with her family. She had felt feverish, and had a poor appetite. During the course of the illness she had lost 5 kg in weight. Two weeks before being seen she had developed a persistent unproductive cough.

In the past she had been well, apart from menopausal symptoms which had started at the age of 48 and had lasted 4 years.

On examination she was clinically anaemic and had a slight fever. There was no evidence of heart failure but a mid-systolic murmur was present, heard best at the apex and left sternal edge, but not conducted to the neck or axilla. In the chest there was dullness to percussion with absent breath sounds and voice sounds at the left base posteriorly and in the left axilla. There was swelling of the left elbow and knee and right wrist, with pain and limitation of movement. There was a large effusion in the left knee. The affected joints in the hands showed swelling and limitation of movement. There was considerable soft-tissue swelling in the fingers of both hands and pain on flexion of the fingers. There were enlarged axillary lymph glands.

QUESTIONS

1. In what way may the signs in the chest be related to the arthritis?
2. What investigations would be of value?
3. What should be the immediate management?

DISCUSSION

This patient has an acute onset of polyarthritis involving small and large joints. In addition she has signs of a pleural effusion, and there is a severe constitutional disturbance with weight loss, anaemia and fever. There is evidence of tendon sheath effusions in the fingers.

The pleural effusion may be part of the disease causing the arthritis or an unrelated finding. Pleural effusion is the commonest pulmonary manifestation of rheumatoid arthritis. It more commonly occurs in men who less commonly have rheumatoid arthritis. It may occur at the beginning of the illness or during its course. The effusion typically has a high protein content and low glucose concentration. A large pleural effusion without pleuritic pain is less common in systemic lupus erythematosus, and although this diagnosis should be considered, it is much less common than rheumatoid arthritis in post-menopausal women.

The pleural effusion may be caused by a coincidental disease. Primary or secondary cancer of the lung, or tuberculosis are possible diagnoses in this case. A pulmonary neoplasm, either primary or secondary, may cause a pleural effusion, and can rarely cause a polyarthritis. Although lymph node enlargement always suggests the possibility of malignancy, moderate local lymph node enlargement is very common in acute arthritis from any cause, and is a usual finding in rheumatoid arthritis. There is nothing in the history to suggest that the effusion is post-pneumonic, or that it follows pulmonary infarction.

The acute arthritis will have a wider differential diagnosis if the effusion is not part of the disorder. Brucellosis in particular must be considered, since she has recently been on a camping holiday and may have drunk infected milk. Subacute infective endocarditis is a possibility, but her cardiac murmur is equally well explained by anaemia and fever and there are no other signs to support such a diagnosis.

Investigation must include a chest X-ray, which will confirm the presence of a pleural effusion and may show signs of a neoplasm or of pulmonary tuberculosis. A full blood count will confirm the presence of anaemia. A neutrophil leucocytosis would be in favour of an infective cause of the arthritis, but may occur to some degree in any acute inflammatory polyarthritis. The sedimentation rate will be raised whatever the diagnosis. The centrifuged urine must be examined microscopically. Haematuria is usually present in infective endocarditis but is also seen in nephritis due to SLE. It does not occur in rheumatoid arthritis. Blood cultures should be taken as infective endocarditis is a possible diagnosis, and they may also be positive in brucellosis. Aspiration of the pleural effusion is essential together with biopsy of the pleura. A straw-coloured effusion with a low glucose content will be found in rheumatoid arthritis. Pleural biopsy may show tuberculosis or secondary carcinoma. In rheumatoid arthritis diagnostic histological features are not usually found. If the effusion is haemorrhagic, this will strongly suggest carcinoma (see Ch. 9).

There is little to suggest direct invasion of the joints by pyogenic bacteria, but aspiration and culture of the fluid in the knees may be worthwhile if the diagnosis is still unclear after other investigations. Tests for rheumatoid factor will probably be positive if the pleural effusion is due to rheumatoid arthritis. A negative test has little diagnostic significance. Tests for antinuclear factors, (especially anti-DNA antibodies) will be positive if there is active SLE, but may also be positive in rheumatoid arthritis. If negative, the tests make SLE highly unlikely.

Initial management must be with bed rest and salicylates. Steroids should be withheld until a diagnosis is reached. In particular an infective cause for the arthritis and pleural effusion must be firmly excluded.

The diagnosis was acute rheumatoid arthritis with pleural effusion. The patient was treated with steroids and the disease settled down for a period of 6 months. Two years later, she had widespread rheumatoid arthritis with subcutaneous nodules.

28. Anaemia

Many patients who are anaemic have become so from a cause which is easily discovered and treated. At the other extreme, the diagnosis of some anaemias can present a most difficult task.

Certain symptoms and physical signs are common to all patients with anaemia regardless of its cause. Many patients complain of tiredness, fatigue and dyspnoea on exertion. The level of haemoglobin at which symptoms appear depends on the individual, his age and occupation, and the rapidity with which the anaemia has developed.

Angina pectoris may be provoked, especially in the elderly population with ischaemic heart disease or left ventricular hypertrophy due to hypertension or aortic valve disease. If either heart disease or anaemia is severe, congestive cardiac failure may develop. In the elderly mental confusion is commonly exacerbated.

Specific features of history and physical examination will be dealt with later. Pallor of the nails and conjunctivae is the cardinal sign of anaemia, but is often not noticeable even with quite severe anaemia. The physical signs of congestive cardiac failure may be present, and there is often a tachycardia with bounding peripheral pulses and a systolic ejection murmur.

The confirmation of the clinical suspicion of anaemia is by measurement of the haemoglobin. The next step in diagnosis is the thorough examination of a blood film. The type of anaemia can then be divided into three broad categories: microcytic, normocytic, and macrocytic.

MICROCYTIC ANAEMIA

On the blood film, the red cells appear poorly haemoglobinized. The MCHC (mean corpuscular haemoglobin concentration) is reduced and this used to be the most reliable of the red cell indices. Nowadays blood samples are usually analysed automatically, and the red cell count has become more accurate. Indices based on the red cell count are therefore more reliable and the MCV (mean corpuscular volume) and the MCH (mean corpuscular haemoglobin) are now used as the indices indicating microcytosis and hypochromia.

By far the commonest cause of hypochromic microcytic anaemia is iron deficiency. Absorption and loss of iron are normally in balance (see Fig. 28.1). The body iron is in haemoglobin and the reticuloendothelial system, and bleeding gives rise to a negative iron balance. An iron deficiency blood picture

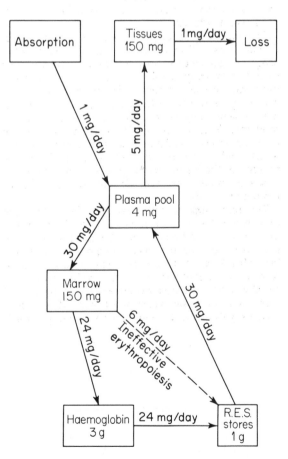

Fig 28.1 Pathways of iron metabolism
Figures on the arrowed pathways indicate the amount of iron passing daily in this direction. Other figures indicate the size of the various pools.

develops when the stores are exhausted. Before that time, normochromic anaemia will be present if the bleeding is rapid. The diagram shows how small the plasma pool is, and how rapidly it is turning over as iron is supplied to the marrow from reticulo-endothelial cells. When the iron stores are exhausted, the plasma iron falls and insufficient iron is available to the marrow for haemoglobin synthesis, resulting in anaemia. Iron deficiency anaemia with a low plasma iron may also occur if the reticuloendothelial cells are unable to relinquish their iron into the plasma. This occurs in chronic infection and malignancy (the 'anaemia of chronic disease'). In sideroblastic anaemia, on the other hand, a hypochromic microcytic anaemia arises because the bone marrow cannot incorporate iron into red cells properly. In this type of anaemia, however, the plasma iron level is not depressed. Finally, a hypochromic microcytic type of anaemia may occur even if the storage, release and uptake of iron are all normal. This situation occurs when synthesis of haemoglobin is impaired due to an inborn error of globin production, as in thalassaemia.

History and examination

The vast majority of patients with hypochromic microcytic anaemia have iron deficiency and the majority of these have blood loss as the cause. If the symptoms of anaemia have come on over a few weeks then gastrointestinal haemorrhage is likely and symptoms of melaena or haematemesis may be obvious. Occult bleeding from the gastrointestinal tract is common. In elderly women oesophagitis due to gastro-oesophageal reflux is a common cause and is often asymptomatic. A history of anorexia, nausea, dysphagia or altered bowel habit may point to an underlying neoplasm. Malabsorption syndrome may be suggested by the passage of bulky pale stools, but may be present even when the bowel habit is normal (see Ch. 13). Hookworm infestation usually presents with iron deficiency anaemia rather than with symptoms of the primary infestation.

Bruising and bleeding from sites such as gums and urinary tract are serious symptoms suggestive of leukaemia or malignancy besides providing a reason for iron deficiency. In premenopausal women iron deficiency is usually due to excess loss in menstruation, although a history of a great excess of bleeding may not be present because their iron balance is normally precarious. In all age groups, but especially in children and the elderly, dietary lack of iron may be important, and will only be discovered if a careful history is taken of what the patient actually eats.

The anaemia of chronic infection may be hypochromic, and tuberculosis or localized collections of pus will be suspected by the characteristic fever and the local symptoms of the infection. Rheumatoid arthritis and other connective tissue disorders may all cause hypochromic anaemia but other signs of the disease will be present. Malignant neoplasms at any site can cause hypochromic anaemia, and weight loss, anorexia and other specific localizing symptoms such as haematuria may all be pointers to the diagnosis.

On examination the signs of iron deficiency may be present, with smooth tongue, cheilitis and koilonychia. An abdominal mass may indicate a gastrointestinal carcinoma or hypernephroma. The liver and spleen may be enlarged in a patient with hepatic cirrhosis and bleeding varices and in patients with thalassaemia major. The latter condition should always be considered in patients who derive from the Mediterranean littoral, central Africa and certain parts of Asia. Splenomegaly may rarely occur in severe iron deficiency anaemia from any cause. An enlarged lymph node may indicate an unsuspected neoplasm, while more generalized lymphadenopathy occurs in lymphomas or tuberculosis. Rectal examination may reveal haemorrhoids, a melaena stool or a rectal carcinoma.

Investigation

Thrombocytopenia may be present and the cause may be suggested by the white count (e.g. leukaemia). Differential diagnosis is discussed in Ch. 29. The serum iron is an important investigation, since it will be low in iron deficiency anaemia with an increased iron binding capacity (transferrin). In the anaemia of chronic disease (which may be mildly hypochromic) the serum iron is also low but there is no rise in the transferrin (Total Iron Binding Capacity – TIBC). In sideroblastic anaemias and in thalassaemia the serum iron will be normal or raised. The serum ferritin is a guide to the body iron stores and is low in iron deficiency.

In most patients with hypochromic microcytic anaemia the cause of iron deficiency will be discovered easily. This will usually turn out to be occult gastrointestinal blood loss, dietary deficiency, or menstrual loss. If the serum iron is low and there is no stainable iron in the marrow, the problem is to find the cause of iron deficiency. Repeated examination of stools for occult blood, sigmoidoscopy, barium swallow and meal and barium enema examination may all be needed. In the elderly and in young children careful dietary assessment is necessary.

A bone marrow examination will be helpful in difficult cases. In iron deficiency there will be erythroid hyperplasia and no stainable iron in the marrow. Iron will be present in the anaemia of infection and in sideroblastic anaemia. In the latter condition the iron is arranged in clumps around the cell nucleus of erythroid precursors – so-called 'ring sideroblasts'. A marrow aspirate may also show evidence of a primary blood disorder such as leukaemia, or secondary carcinoma.

In some patients oral iron will have been given, without adequate response. The commonest reasons for a failure of response of anaemia to oral iron are: that iron deficiency is not present (in particular that the patient has the anaemia of chronic disease); that occult bleeding is continuing; that the patient has not taken the tablets; or that there is failure of absorption of iron such as occurs after gastrectomy and in malabsorption syndrome.

If the serum iron is normal the diagnosis may be sideroblastic anaemia or thalassaemia. Most cases of sideroblastic anaemia are acquired, and the disorder usually occurs in late middle age. Sideroblasts may be seen in the marrow in a variety of other conditions such as haemolytic anaemia, carcinoma, leukaemia, and in nutritional and megaloblastic anaemias. Many acquired sideroblastic anaemias are idiopathic. The blood film usually shows anisocytosis and poly-chromasia, and some red cells are normochromic. The bone marrow appearance, with ring sideroblasts, is typical. Some of the idiopathic cases respond to large doses of pyridoxine, and in some an element of folate deficiency is present.

Thalassaemia major is a severe and fatal disease readily distinguished from iron deficiency anaemia because of the clinical and haematological charac-teristics. Patients with the less obvious condition of thalassaemia minor are often erroneously and harmfully treated with iron. The blood film usually shows target cells and basophilic red cells due to immature red cells. Diagnosis is by haemoglobin electrophoresis, which shows a moderate increase in HbA$_2$, and by finding affected relatives.

NORMOCYTIC ANAEMIA

It is in this group of anaemias that some of the most difficult problems in diagnosis arise. A classification of the causes is shown in Table 28.1

History and examination

The diagnosis is usually indicated by the clinical details. Acute blood loss will be obvious, and occult bleeding has already been discussed. Malignancy is a common cause of normocytic anaemia in middleaged and elderly patients. Although the history may be typical, and signs of a tumour may be present, it is not uncommon for the tumour to be occult. General malaise, fever, weight loss and anaemia may be the only signs of the underlying disease. An abdominal mass and enlargement of lymph nodes must be sought.

Chronic renal failure will often be missed clini-cally, but must be excluded in any patient with a normocytic anaemia. A history of polyuria and noc-turia may be present, and the patient may show pig-mentation and be hypertensive.

Myxoedema may be accompanied by mild normo-cytic anaemia, as may pituitary and adrenal insuffi-ciency. There may be obvious features on history and examination to suggest these diagnoses, but the most important step is to consider these disorders in a patient with undiagnosed anaemia.

Table 28.1 Causes of normocytic anaemia

1. Blood loss
Acute or subacute before iron deficiency occurs

2. Inflammation
Pyogenic
Infective endocarditis
Tuberculous
Connective tissue diseases (e.g. rheumatoid arthritis, polymyalgia rheumatica)

3. Malignancy
Disseminated carcinoma
Bone marrow replacement: myeloma, leukaemia, metastatic carcinoma, myelofibrosis (these often cause a leucoerythroblastic anaemia)

4. Chronic renal failure

5. Aplastic anaemia

6. Endocrine disorders
Myxoedema
Hypopituitarism
Addison's disease

7. Malnutrition
Protein calorie malnutrition
Scurvy

8. Haemolytic anaemias
Due to intrinsic red cell defects:
    hereditary spherocytosis and elliptocytosis
    abnormal haemoglobins; thalassaemia; sickle-cell disease
    enzyme defects (e.g. pyruvate kinase deficiency)

Due to extrinsic factors:
    autoimmune haemolytic anaemias due to drugs (usually in G6PD deficient individuals)
    cold haemoglobinuria
    hypersplenism
    disseminated intravascular coagulation (e.g. due to septicaemia)

Conditions causing bone marrow infiltration, such as myeloma, will usually be accompanied by bone pain and perhaps by pathological fractures. If there is thrombocytopenia there may be bruising and pur-pura. Myelofibrosis is invariably accompanied by massive splenomegaly.

Haemolysis may be suspected by a history of jaundice without dark urine. The spleen will usual-ly be enlarged if the cause is hereditary sphero-cytosis or autoimmune haemolytic anaemia. Here-ditary spherocytosis will be suspected if there is a family history of anaemia. Jaundice is often present, and recurrent haemolytic crises with deepening jaundice occur. Pigment gallstones frequently deve-lop and may cause symptoms including obstructive jaundice.

In children, autoimmune haemolytic anaemia may follow viral infections, while in adults it may some-times be associated with diseases such as SLE, lymphomas, chronic lymphatic leukaemia, or drugs such as methyldopa. If there is long-standing splenomegaly from any cause this may be the cause of the anaemia as a result of hypersplenism.

If the haemolysis is acute and intravascular there will be haemoglobinuria. In paroxysmal nocturnal haemoglobinuria there is haemoglobinuria on waking which may be accompanied by abdominal or loin pain. In paroxysmal cold haemoglobinuria there is acute intravascular haemolysis after exposure to cold. There may be signs of syphilis, which is a common cause.

In glucose-6-phosphate dehydrogenase deficiency, the patient is usually black or Mediterranean. The disorder has a sex-linked inheritance of variable expression. The clinical picture is of acute haemolysis following exposure to a drug or broad beans (favism). There is jaundice and there may be haemoglobinuria. Occasionally acute infections may precipitate an attack. A wide variety of drugs can provoke haemolysis: antimalarials, sulphonamides, nitrofurantoin, analgesics, and sulphones.

In aplastic anaemia the patient may present with anaemia or symptoms of infection due to neutropenia. A history of exposure to drugs such as chloramphenicol or chemicals such as benzene should be sought.

Lead poisoning, although uncommon, is often accompanied by anaemia and may not be remembered as a possible cause of anaemia in young children. It may also occur in adults in the appropriate occupations.

Sickle-cell anaemia usually presents in early childhood. The symptoms of anaemia are present and sickling crises occur with bone and joint pain, abdominal pain, fever and cerebrovascular accidents. Although splenomegaly is common in children, in adults it is less so because of repeated splenic infarctions during sickling crises. There is commonly a mild degree of jaundice, which is more apparent during a crisis. Cardiomegaly is usually present, and a systolic murmur is often heard. Leg ulcers are common.

A variety of inherited red cell enzyme defects are described which are often accompanied by a haemolytic anaemia. The commonest is pyruvate kinase deficiency which is inherited as an autosomal recessive character. The presentation is usually in childhood, and the degree of haemolysis varies from mild to severe. Slight jaundice is often present, splenomegaly is common, and slight enlargement of the liver is not unusual. Inherited red cell enzyme defects should be thought of in any child or young adult with congenital haemolysis when spherocytosis is not present.

Investigation

Examination of the peripheral blood will often indicate the type of anaemia present. The red cells will show spherocytosis in hereditary spherocytosis, and some degree of spherocytosis is common in autoimmune haemolytic anaemias. Marked anisocytosis and poikilocytosis suggest bone marrow infiltration or disseminated carcinoma. In chronic renal failure there may be burr cells present, and target cells in liver disease. A reticulocytosis always suggests acute blood loss or haemolysis as a cause of the anaemia. Basophilic stippling is found in G6PD deficiency and in lead poisoning. Heinz bodies (haemoglobin precipitate) may be seen during haemolysis in G6PD deficiency and in some patients with inherited defects of haemoglobin which render the haemoglobin unstable (e.g. Hb Koln and Hb Zurich). Howell–Jolly bodies are found in hyposplenism, which is a feature of coeliac disease, where anaemia due to multiple deficiencies may be present. If there is bone marrow infiltration from myeloma, there is often marked rouleaux formation due to the paraprotein. Marrow replacement will also be suggested if a leucoerythroblastic blood picture is present with normoblasts, immature white cells and thrombocytopenia. A low white count may occur in aplastic anaemia or aleukaemic leukaemia, while a raised white count may occur in renal failure and disseminated malignancy as well as in infections.

The ESR may be helpful. It will not be raised in myxoedema or hypopituitarism or in blood loss from non-malignant causes. It will be raised in most other conditions, but very high values suggest myeloma or a connective tissue disease, especially polymyalgia rheumatica and polyarteritis.

Haemolysis will be suggested by spherocytosis, jaundice (indirect hyperbilirubinaemia), reticulocytosis, increased urinary urobilinogen and splenomegaly. Further investigation of the cause will be discussed later.

A chest X-ray is essential. It may show malignant deposits in the lungs, a primary bronchial carcinoma, and myeloma or secondary carcinoma in the ribs. Enlarged hilar or paratracheal nodes may be present, suggestive of lymphoma or tuberculosis. The lungs may also show tuberculosis, and a right-sided pleural effusion, perhaps with elevation of the hemidiaphragm, may point towards an underlying hepatic or subphrenic abscess although this will normally have been suspected on other grounds. Disseminated carcinoma and bone marrow infiltrations may be demonstrated by skeletal X-rays.

The urine may show red cells and white cells, suggesting renal infection or glomerulonephritis. Persistent microscopic haematuria is strongly suggestive of renal or bladder carcinoma. Proteinuria will usually be present in chronic renal disease. Culture of the urine is important, and a sterile urine with the presence of pus cells always suggests renal tuberculosis. Any of these findings will be an indication for further investigation, including blood urea and intravenous pyelography.

The gastrointestinal tract is a common site of hidden malignancy, and the stools may contain occult blood. Barium meal and enema examinations will be necessary to exclude this possibility. However the anaemia of blood loss is much more likely to be hypochromic.

A bone marrow aspiration will usually demonstrate leukaemia or myeloma if present, but a bone marrow biopsy may be needed in some cases of aplastic anaemia and myeloma, and in many cases of secondary carcinoma of bone and myelofibrosis.

Liver function tests, tests for SLE, myxoedema and hypopituitarism will be carried out where appropriate.

If haemolysis is suspected on clinical grounds or because of jaundice and reticulocytosis, a variety of further investigations are needed. If haemolysis is suspected but not definitely present, then a raised urinary and faecal urobilinogen and decreased plasma haptoglobin may indicate its presence. Haemolysis can be confirmed by finding a decreased red cell half-life after injecting the patient's chromium-labelled erythrocytes intravenously. This test is only of value if there is no bleeding.

An osmotic fragility test will show a decreased resistance to hypotonic solutions in hereditary spherocytosis, and to a lesser extent in autoimmune haemolytic anaemias. The indirect antiglobulin test will be positive in the vast majority of cases of chronic autoimmune haemolytic anaemia during a relapse. In acute autoimmune haemolytic anaemias, only half of the cases have a positive antiglobulin test.

Further investigation of haemolytic anaemias will depend on the clinical picture. In autoimmune haemolytic anaemia, a positive antinuclear antibody test will support a diagnosis of SLE and biopsy of an enlarged lymph node may reveal an underlying lymphoma or chronic lymphatic leukaemia of which the anaemia is a manifestation. Sickle-cell anaemia will be demonstrated by the sickling test and by haemoglobin electrophoresis, and the latter test will show other abnormal haemoglobins. Estimation of G6PD activity can be made, and other red cell enzymes such as pyruvate kinase can be estimated in cases of congenital non-spherocytic haemolytic anaemias. The Donath–Landsteiner antibody is detectable in paroxysmal cold haemoglobinuria, and the acid haemolysin and sucrose lysis tests are positive in paroxysmal nocturnal haemoglobinuria.

MACROCYTIC ANAEMIA

Macrocytes in the peripheral blood are usually the result of megaloblastic erythropoiesis in the bone marrow. Macrocytes are apparent to the skilled observer on a blood film, and increase in the MCV is a reliable guide to macrocytosis. However, it is not uncommon for a mixed iron deficiency and megaloblastic process to be present in the same patient and the automated red cell indices can then indicate normocytic cells, while examination of the blood film will show a dimorphic picture with microcytic hypochromic cells and macrocytic normochromic cells.

Although macrocytosis usually means that megaloblastic erythropoiesis is occurring, this is not always so, and normoblastic changes can be found under some circumstances. Some degree of macrocytosis is common in haemolytic anaemias and in post-haemorrhagic anaemia where larger more immature erythrocytes are released into the circulation.

Many of the conditions where normocytic anaemia occurs may occasionally cause macrocytosis. These include myxoedema, hypopituitarism, bone marrow infiltration, acute leukaemia, and aplastic anaemia. Macrocytosis is a frequent and sensitive accompaniment of alcohol excess, probably due to failure of folate utilization rather than folate deficiency. Liver disease from any cause may result in macrocytosis, part of which may be due to folate deficiency. The diagnosis of these conditions has been discussed. If there is any doubt as to the cause of a macrocytic blood picture, a bone marrow examination will be made. If normoblastic erythropoiesis is found then diagnosis will proceed along lines already discussed.

The main causes of megaloblastic erythropoiesis are summarized in Table 28.2

Table 28.2 The causes of megaloblastic erythropoiesis

1. Lack of vitamin B_{12}
Due to inadequate dietary intake:
  dietary deficiency in strict vegetarians
  fish tapeworm

Due to lack of intrinsic factor:
  pernicious anaemia
  total gastrectomy
  partial gastrectomy and gastric atrophy

Due to failure of intestinal absorption:
  disease or resection of terminal ileum
  stagnant loop syndrome
  tropical sprue

2. Lack of folic acid
Due to inadequate intake:
  dietary deficiency (especially in the elderly and in alcoholics)
  pregnancy (increased demand)
  chronic haemolytic anaemia (increased demand)

Due to failure of intestinal absorption:
  coeliac disease
  tropical sprue
  anticonvulsant drugs

History and examination

Pernicious anaemia occurs in the middle-aged and elderly, although a rare juvenile form occurs. The onset is insidious with symptoms of anaemia. Glossitis is common and may be present before anaemia. Central nervous system symptoms may also be the presenting feature, especially in men. The complaint is usually of paraesthesiae and numbness in the hands and feet due to neuropathy, and unsteadiness of gait with weakness of the legs. Mental disturbance is common, with confusion and dementia. Loss of control of rectum and bladder occurs late, and external ocular palsy and retrobulbar neuritis are rare manifestations. Anorexia, weight loss and fever are common. Symptoms identical with those of pernicious anaemia may occur in any of the conditions which lead to lack of vitamin B_{12} and a history of previous gastric or intestinal surgery may be present, or of terminal ileal disease such as Crohn's disease or tuberculosis. The fish tapeworm *Diphyllobothrium latum* does not usually cause symptoms other than those due to B_{12} deficiency. It lives for many years and only a small proportion of those infested develop anaemia.

Folic acid deficiency also causes glossitis and loss of appetite, but neurological symptoms do not develop. There may be a history of underlying disease causing malabsorption syndrome, or the patient may be epileptic on anticonvulsant drugs when folate deficiency may occur possibly due to interference with folate absorption. Superadded folic acid deficiency may occur in chronic haemolytic states.

On examination, the physical signs will be those of anaemia, together with glossitis. In the case of pernicious anaemia the patients are often prematurely grey, and a mild degree of jaundice is common. In the nervous system there may be mental confusion, peripheral neuropathy, upper motor neurone signs in the legs and also posterior column signs. In severe cases retinal haemorrhages occur.

In folate deficiency there may be other signs also related to an underlying cause such as gluten enteropathy, causing malabsorption (see Ch. 14).

Investigation

The blood film often shows hypersegmentation of neutrophils when there is megaloblastic erythropoiesis from any cause. There may be slight neutropenia and thrombocytopenia as well. Anisocytosis and poikilocytosis are marked in both B_{12} and folate deficiency. Where the cause is nutritional, iron deficiency may coexist and a dimorphic blood picture may be seen.

A marrow aspiration will establish whether there is megaloblastic erythropoiesis. Usually the cause will be clear, but serum B_{12} and folate estimations will be diagnostic. Assay of B_{12} is especially helpful if the diagnosis of subacute combined degeneration is suspected in a patient with little or no anaemia.

If the serum B_{12} is low, a Schilling test (in which the absorption of radioactive B_{12} is measured with and without intrinsic factor) will help to determine whether there is an intestinal defect of absorption or whether there is lack of intrinsic factor. Confirmatory evidence that pernicious anaemia is present will come from finding anti-intrinsic factor and anti-parietal cell antibodies in the serum. In juvenile pernicious anaemia, the antibody tests are negative. If intestinal malabsorption of B_{12} is demonstrated by the Schilling test, radiological investigation of the small bowel will be required.

If folic acid deficiency is shown, investigation for steatorrhoea will be needed (see Ch. 14), and an assessment of the patient's dietary intake will be necessary. The folic acid deficiency caused by anticonvulsants (phenytoin, primidone and phenobarbitone) responds rapidly to folic acid administration.

Finally, a possible cause of megaloblastic erythropoiesis, and an established cause of macrocytic anaemia is scurvy. The megaloblastic changes may be due to vitamin C lack itself or to a concomitant folic acid deficiency which is often present. The disease should be suspected in an anaemic patient with haemorrhagic manifestations and follicular hyperkeratosis in the skin. The white cell vitamin C content will be low.

CLINICAL PROBLEM

T	P	BP	R
37	106 reg.	200/80	28

Anaemia, mental confusion,
weight loss

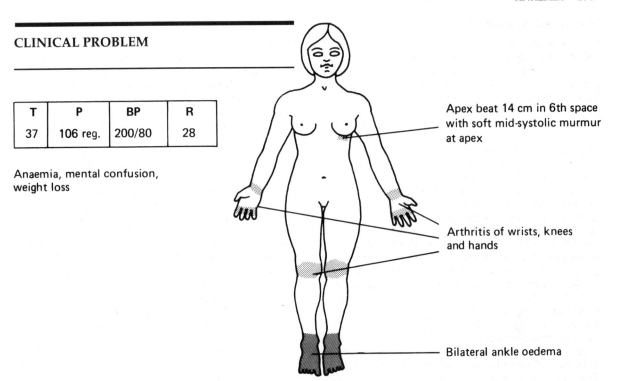

Apex beat 14 cm in 6th space
with soft mid-systolic murmur
at apex

Arthritis of wrists, knees
and hands

Bilateral ankle oedema

A woman of 82 was admitted to hospital having been found wandering in the street at night. She was confused and obstreperous and neighbours had called an ambulance when she refused to return to her own home. Her daughter said that following the death of the patient's husband 3 years previously she had become depressed and withdrawn. She had not gone out of the house much and had refused all offers of assistance. Her daughter had tried to help by bringing in food and cleaning her flat. She had noticed that her mother had been losing weight for 6 months previously, and 3 months before admission the patient consulted her family doctor because of ankle swelling, and shortness of breath on exertion and at night-time in bed. These symptoms had responded to diuretic treatment. For 2 months she had been irritable and uncooperative, and her daughter had noticed that she had become untidy and forgetful.

She had had a hysterectomy 30 years previously for post-menopausal bleeding. For 20 years she had suffered from rheumatoid arthritis with deformity in the small joints of the hands and swelling and pain intermittently in the knees, wrists and elbows. She had taken a variety of anti-inflammatory drugs for several years, and for the preceding 2 years her joints had not been troublesome and had not imposed any limitation on her activities.

On examination she was rather dirty and was clearly confused. Apart from absent ankle jerks there were no other abnormal signs in the nervous system. Temperature 37°C. Pulse 106 regular. Blood pressure 200/80. R 28/min. She was clinically anaemic, and her tongue was smooth and depapillated. The nails were cracked. The jugular venous pressure was not raised, but there was some ankle oedema bilaterally. The heart was enlarged with the apex beat 14 cm out in the 6th space (in the anterior axillary line). A soft mid-systolic murmur was present at the apex. She had clearly lost some weight, but there were no other abnormal physical signs in the lungs and abdomen. Rectal examination was normal. She had rheumatoid arthritis involving the hands, knees and wrists, with some deformity but little pain on movement.

Investigations: Hb. 8.2g/dl. ESR 86 mm/h. MCH 29 pg. MCV 80 fl. WBC 4.2 × 10^9/1 with normal differential count. Platelets 259 × 10^9/1. Chest X-ray showed cardiac enlargement with distension of upper lobe veins.

QUESTIONS

1. Which aspects of the history and physical signs might be related to the cause of her anaemia?
2. How would you interpret the red cell indices?
3. How would you investigate her further?

DISCUSSION

Elderly people are prone to nutritional deficiencies and social isolation increases the likelihood of this occurring. The patient had been depressed and isolated since the death of her husband 3 years earlier. From the point of view of causing anaemia, dietary deficiency of iron and folic acid are the likeliest causes, since dietary B_{12} deficiency is very uncommon, unless very strict vegetarian diets are adhered to for a long time, as the liver stores are long lasting. Dietary iron deficiency will quickly cause anaemia if there is blood loss as well. The possible causes of blood loss in this patient are occult malignancy which is suggested by her weight loss over the preceding 6 months, and analgesic ingestion as treatment of her chronic rheumatoid arthritis although this had been inactive for some time.

The onset of congestive cardiac failure can be attributed to her anaemia. The physical signs of a wide pulse pressure, a large heart and a mid-systolic murmur, supports this, as does the radiographic finding of cardiomegaly and distension of upper lobe veins. A cardiac murmur in an anaemic patient with a raised ESR raises the possibility of subacute infective endocarditis which must be excluded by blood cultures as other classical symptoms and signs may be absent.

The mental confusion may have several causes. Any severe anaemia in elderly people, who are likely to have some degree of cerebral arteriosclerosis, may provoke mental confusion and disorientation, especially in those who are socially isolated. The combination of mental confusion and anaemia raises the possibility of B_{12} deficiency, and although there is nothing in the history to suggest a cause of B_{12} deficiency in this patient, this must be excluded. Her confusional state may also be caused by cerebral secondaries from an occult malignancy, or by cerebrovascular disease alone.

Physical examination in this patient does not give much information as to the cause of the anaemia. The smooth depapillated tongue might be due to iron or B_{12} deficiency. Absent ankle reflexes are common in old age and do not necessarily indicate peripheral neuropathy associated with B_{12} deficiency or underlying carcinoma. There is no bruising or follicular hyperkeratosis suggestive of scurvy.

The red cell indices indicate a normochromic normocytic anaemia. This is unlike the findings in iron, folate or B_{12} deficiency. Normochromic, normocytic anaemia suggests disseminated malignancy as a more likely diagnosis in this patient. Rheumatoid arthritis may also cause this type of anaemia and a raised sedimentation rate. The fact that the arthritis is quiescent at present is strongly against this as a cause.

The red cell indices may however be misleading if taken in isolation. Indices indicating normochromic normocytic anaemia may be found if there is microcytosis and macrocytosis present at the same time. Such a situation often arises if iron deficiency is combined with deficiency of folate or B_{12}. This combination of events is especially likely in the elderly. The meaning of these indices cannot be assessed unless a blood film is examined, when hypochromic cells may be seen, and macrocytes, with anisocytosis and poikilocytosis. There may be hypersegmentation of the nucleus of polymorphonuclear leucocytes in folate and B_{12} deficiency. If the blood film suggests that a 'dimorphic' blood picture is present, then serum iron, folate and B_{12} should be estimated. If these are normal then the likelihood of occult malignancy is strengthened. However chronic renal failure should also be excluded, especially in view of the history of analgesic treatment for years, which might have caused analgesic nephropathy. Thyroid function should be checked.

If investigations show that there is a deficiency of iron, folate or B_{12} then most physicians would simply treat the anaemia appropriately, without a sternal marrow examination, in a patient of this age. Iron deficiency however should be investigated further in view of her weight loss, since a remediable condition may be found, such as giant gastric ulcer, or a slow-growing carcinoma of the colon, or chronic aspirin ingestion. Careful dietary assessment and barium studies will be needed.

If no deficiency is found, or if the result of treatment is only a small rise in haemoglobin, then barium studies may show the site of an underlying cancer. A CT brain scan and an ultrasound liver scan, both of which are non-distressing investigations, may be very suggestive of secondary deposits rendering further investigation and treatment inadvisable. Cerebral atrophy may be present.

> This patient had combined iron and folate deficiency. The latter was thought to be dietary in origin. The iron deficiency was attributed to gastrointestinal bleeding as a result of analgesic ingestion.

29. Bruising and bleeding

Many patients say that they bruise easily, but only a minority turn out to have an underlying blood disorder. The diagnosis of the cause of a bleeding tendency covers a wide range of medicine, but clinical evidence alone will often provide the answer without the necessity for complicated laboratory tests.

Purpura is due to bleeding into the skin. The appearance is of numerous small haemorrhages in the skin, clearly defined, not raised, and distinguished from telangiectases by the fact that they do not blanch on pressure. Ecchymoses are larger purpuric areas. Both ecchymoses and purpura are a result of increased capillary fragility, by far the commonest cause of which is thrombocytopenia. Bruises are larger areas of bleeding, usually occurring subcutaneously. They may be found in thrombocytopenic patients, who may also have purpura. On the other hand, when there is a deficiency of a clotting factor, the capillaries are not unduly fragile and significant bruising may be found without purpura.

HISTORY

When taking the history one should enquire closely into the length of time the patient has noticed the tendency to bleed, and ask about operations and tooth extractions, and about past attacks of joint swelling. Haemophiliacs usually begin to notice their symptoms when they are old enough to run about and hurt themselves. The onset of symptoms, in thrombocytopenic purpura may be very abrupt, especially in children.

The extent of the bleeding should be ascertained. One should enquire whether the patient has noticed blood in the urine or stools. Visceral bleeding is of especial importance since, although it may occur in any patient with a bleeding tendency, it may equally well indicate underlying disease of the gut or urinary tract which the bleeding tendency has brought into light. Conversely, although localized bleeding, as from the gastrointestinal tract, will usually indicate a local disorder, one should always consider the additional possibility that this may be the only sign of a generalized bleeding disorder.

Joint symptoms are of great importance for two reasons. Firstly, haemarthrosis is a very common feature of many bleeding disorders, especially haemophilia and Christmas disease. Secondly, polyarthritis may accompany diseases in which bleeding is a feature, such as allergic purpura, systemic lupus erythematosus and drug sensitivity.

Constitutional symptoms may be present. Fever is a common symptom in leukaemia, and may also occur as a result of infection in any condition where there is bone marrow depression. A febrile illness, sometimes viral, commonly precedes acute thrombocytopenia in children. Weight loss is an important symptom, often indicating an underlying neoplasm or lymphoma.

Drugs may cause thrombocytopenia alone, or a general bone marrow aplasia. The commonest are phenylbutazone, gold, chloramphenicol, thioureas, chlorothiazide and carbamazepine. Sedormid, now seldom prescribed, and quinidine cause a selective thrombocytopenia due to an immune destruction of platelets. It is obvious that severe bleeding may result from anticoagulant therapy, particularly if inadequately controlled. Similarly, most cytotoxic drugs will produce marrow depression as a direct toxic effect rather than due to idiosyncrasy.

Finally, a family history of any tendency to bruise or bleed should be sought. In haemophilia not only is there a family history, but the severity of the disorder tends to be similar in different members of the same family.

PHYSICAL EXAMINATION

Examination of the skin is very important. Purpura always suggests thrombocytopenia, although it also occurs in capillary disorders such as scurvy and von Willebrand's disease. 'Senile' purpura is often seen over the hands, forearms and shins of the elderly. The skin is usually smooth, atrophic and hairless, and there is no other abnormality.

The distribution and nature of the rash is characteristic in Henoch–Schönlein purpura. It is usually present over the legs and buttocks and around the elbows. The lesions are unusual because the bleeding is due to local capillaritis. They are often raised and accompanied by erythema, quite unlike thrombocytopenic purpura. While examining the skin, one should look for the facial and buccal lesions of hereditary haemorrhagic telangiectasia, and the thickened lax skin of pseudoxanthoma elasticum which is often best seen around the neck. In scurvy, purpura mainly affects the legs, and is associated with a rough skin due to follicular keratosis and corkscrew hairs.

A number of important signs may be seen in the mouth. Loose teeth and bleeding gums suggest scurvy, while palatal and faucial ulceration are serious signs suggesting the neutropenia of aplastic anaemia or leukaemia. Palatal ulceration also occurs in infectious mononucleosis, in which thrombocytopenia may sometimes occur. Oral thrush commonly complicates aplastic anaemia and leukaemia. Gum hypertrophy occurs in monocytic leukaemia, and palatal haemorrhages in thrombocytopenia from any cause.

The musculoskeletal system is important in both diagnosis and management. Recurrent haemarthroses often occur in haemophilia and Christmas disease. As a result, there may be loss of range of joint movement, fibrous ankylosis of joints, wasting of surrounding muscle groups and entrapment neuropathies. Sternal tenderness and pain in the bones are signs suggestive of acute leukaemia, or some other malignant process causing bone marrow infiltration. Subperiosteal haemorrhages may occur in a variety of bleeding disorders, especially scurvy, and may occasionally be misdiagnosed as bone tumours.

Enlargement of the spleen suggests lymphoma, leukaemia, or myeloproliferative disorders. However, splenomegaly due for example to portal hypertension, may itself give rise to hypersplenism and pancytopenia.

In the central nervous system, any acute neurological disturbance in a patient on anticoagulants should raise the possibility of localized bleeding as a cause. The optic fundi may show retinal haemorrhages, especially in thrombocytopenia. They also occur in systemic infections such as subacute infective endocarditis. Retinal exudates may occur in systemic lupus erythematosus which is sometimes accompanied by thrombocytopenia. Occasionally the retinae may be infiltrated with leukaemic or lymphomatous deposits.

Generalized lymph node enlargement occurs in acute leukaemia, lymphoma and in chronic lymphatic leukaemia. Enlargement of cervical lymph nodes as a result of oral and pharyngeal inflammation is common in aplastic anaemia, acute leukaemia, and infectious mononucleosis.

SIMPLE INVESTIGATIONS

In the majority of cases one will have been able to decide, on clinical grounds, whether the bleeding tendency is due to disturbance of clotting or of platelet function, and the cause which might underlie

either. The following simple tests will usually confirm the diagnosis.

Full blood count. An automated blood count (haemoglobin white cell count and platelet count) must always be supplemented by examination of the peripheral blood film. The diagnosis of thrombocytopenia is confirmed by the platelet count. It is a curious fact that although, in general, the lower the platelet count the greater the risk and extent of bleeding, this relationship does not always hold true, and in some diseases other factors have been postulated which affect the capillaries independently of the platelets. The presence of immature white cells with blast forms suggests an acute leukaemia, while the appearance of both immature red and white cells – a leucoerythroblastic blood picture – always suggests marrow infiltration, by carcinoma, lymphoma or myelofibrosis. Chronic myeloid leukaemia and chronic lymphatic leukaemia are easily recognized on a peripheral blood film. The atypical mononuclear cells of infectious mononucleosis may be seen.

Bleeding and clotting times. The cessation of capillary bleeding depends on the formation of a platelet thrombus at the site of the wound, and on the ability of the small vessels to contract. It does not depend to any great extent on coagulation factors. The bleeding time is therefore prolonged in thrombocytopenia, scurvy, hereditary capillary fragility and von Willerbrand's disease. The test gives useful information, but technique is important and false positives and negatives occur.

The whole blood clotting time measures the function of all the blood clotting factors apart from those in the 'extrinsic' system. It is prolonged in haemophilia and Christmas disease as well as in fibrinogen deficiency. It should be stressed that the test is a crude one and considerable deficiency of a factor, such as factor VIII (AHG) can be present without the test being abnormal.

THE CAUSES OF THROMBOCYTOPENIA
(see Table 29.1)

Bone marrow infiltration. Acute leukaemia must always be excluded in a thrombocytopenic patient. The peripheral white cell count may confirm the diagnosis, but in aleukaemic leukaemia it may be normal or show a neutropenia. Chronic myeloid and lymphatic leukaemia, on the other hand, are accompanied by a characteristic white count and usually obvious physical signs. Secondary carcinoma, lymphoma, and myeloma must be considered as possible causes.

The major physical sign in myelofibrosis is splenomegaly, which is usually gross. The disease may complicate polycythaemia rubra vera and myeloid metaplasia. It is usually accompanied by a leucoerythroblastic blood picture, and the platelet count is often reduced later in the disease. Occasionally the

Table 29.1 Causes of thrombocytopenia

1. Bone marrow infiltration
Leukaemias
Lymphomas
Myeloma
Secondary carcinoma
Myelofibrosis
Infections such as tuberculosis
Rare hereditary disorders (marble bone disease,
    Gaucher's disease)

2. Bone marrow depression
Drugs
Metabolic (e.g. uraemia)
Infection (severe systemic infection, e.g. septicaemia,
    typhoid)
Megaloblastic anaemia
Rare inherited disorders of platelet production (e.g.
    Wiskott–Aldrich syndrome)

3. Increased platelet destruction
Antibody mediated:
    idiopathic thrombocytopenic purpura
    drugs
    post-transfusion
    viral infections (e.g. infectious mononucleosis,
        measles)
Hypersplenism
Disseminated intravascular coagulation
Thrombotic thrombocytopenic purpura

4. Intrinsic platelet defects
Myeloproliferative disorders (including
    thrombocythaemia)
Hereditary disorders (e.g. Glanzmann's disease)

platelet count may be raised with large abnormal forms present.

Bone marrow depression. Aplastic anaemia is almost always accompanied by thrombocytopenia, and leucopenia is commonly present. Some drugs such as phenylbutazone may primarily affect platelet formation. Toxic depression of the marrow occurs as a direct effect of cytotoxic drugs and ionizing radiation. It may also occur in uraemia and in any severe systemic infection.

Increased platelet destruction. In some patients who have thrombocytopenia as a result of drugs, circulating antibodies can be found which are directed against the platelet–drug combination. In most cases of idiopathic thrombocytopenic purpura, antibodies against platelets can be demonstrated, but the techniques are difficult and the results variable.

In patients with a big spleen from any cause – lymphoma, tropical disease, portal hypertension – platelets may be destroyed excessively in the spleen. Often there is an accompanying neutropenia and anaemia. This is called hypersplenism.

Intrinsic platelet defects. In the myeloproliferative syndromes, although platelets may be produced in excessive quantities they do not function normally,

and the effect is as though there is thrombocytopenia. The platelets often assume bizarre and giant forms. This may occur in the myeloproliferative disorders such as polycythaemia vera, chronic myeloid leukaemia and haemorrhagic thrombocythaemia. There is a rare congenital condition called Glanzmann's disease (or thromboasthenia) in which the platelets are normal in number but do not aggregate properly in response to various agents including ADP.

Other causes of thrombocytopenia. There are many other causes of thrombocytopenia (see Table 29.1), in some of which the mechanism of production of the disorder is unclear.

FURTHER INVESTIGATION OF PLATELET DISORDERS

It is clear that a wide variety of further investigations may be needed in order to define the cause of thrombocytopenia. The most important is examination of the marrow, since this may show leukaemia or cancer cells. The presence or absence of megakaryocytes in normal numbers will provide information as to whether there is defective production of platelets. If bone marrow aspiration is normal or a dry tap is obtained, a trephine biopsy should be done. It may show infiltration by carcinoma or lymphoma, or the appearances of myelofibrosis. It can also confirm the presence of aplasia.

Other investigations which may be indicated are blood urea, radiological skeletal survey, urine examination, protein electrophoresis, ANF tests.

CLOTTING DEFECTS

A simple but workable scheme of clotting is seen in Fig. 29.1. The simplest initial tests in determining the cause of a coagulation defect are as follows.

The prothrombin time. Tissue thromboplastin, in the form of brain extract, and calcium is added to the patient's plasma. The extrinsic system is activated and clotting will normally occur within 15 seconds. The intrinsic system is also activated, but takes longer to produce clotting, making the prothrombin time a test of the extrinsic system (Factor VII) and the common pathway. If Factors X, V, prothrombin and fibrinogen are reduced, then the prothrombin time will also be prolonged, but in this case tests of the intrinsic system will also be abnormal. Although it is called the prothrombin time and used to control anticoagulant therapy, in practice prothrombin reduction is not the most important effect of these drugs.

The partial thromboplastin time and the kaolin cephalin clotting time. These tests eliminate some of the variability of the whole blood clotting time. They provide a reliable surface for activation and an essential phospholipid. The intrinsic system (essentially Factors VIII and IX) is measured, since tissue juices are

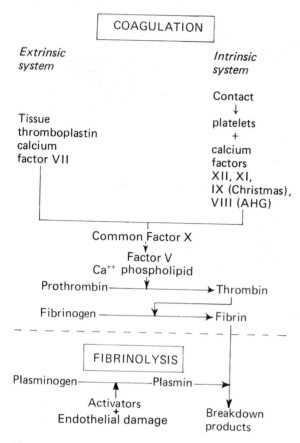

Fig. 29.1 A simplified scheme of coagulation

not added to the test system. The test normally produces clotting in about one minute. It will also be prolonged if the common factors X, V, prothrombin and fibrinogen are deficient.

These tests will give a good idea of what kind of clotting defect is present. The thromboplastin generation test will define whether Factor VIII or IX is missing from the intrinsic system but specific assays are now available.

The thrombin time. A solution of thrombin is added to plasma and the time taken to clot is measured. Prolongation is seen in hypofibrinogenaemia and during heparin therapy.

CAUSES OF CLOTTING DEFECTS

A widely accepted current view is that coagulation is proceeding all the time, with fibrin deposition in blood vessels preserving the integrity of the vascular endothelium. Fibrinolytic mechanisms are also active, continuously removing excess fibrin and ensuring the patency of the vascular channels. Defects in coagulation can be considered under the following headings.

Inherited defects of specific clotting factors. The

commonest deficiency states are haemophilia A, inherited as a sex-linked recessive, in which there is a deficiency of Factor VIII activity (AHG) and haemophilia B (Christmas disease, also a sex-linked recessive) where the deficiency is of Factor IX activity. (In some cases of haemophilia a form of Factor VIII is present which has no biological activity.) Many haemophiliacs know when they are bleeding even though there are no clinical signs of haemorrhage. Bleeding from any site may occur in either disease. The diagnosis is made on the history and nowadays by assay of the activity of the specific factor. The thromboplastin generation test is also used in the diagnosis of these two disorders.

In von Willebrand's disease (autosomal dominant) there is a deficiency of Factor VIII activity and an abnormality of platelet function in which the platelets do not aggregate in the presence of ristocetin. Factor VIII activity is dependent on von Willebrand's factor (VWF) for prolongation of its half-life, and VWF also binds platelets to the exposed endothelium. Absence of VWF thus causes deficient clotting and prolongation of the bleeding time.

Acquired defects in thrombin formation. The commonest cause by far is the use of anticoagulants, but deficiency of vitamin K and liver disease both produce very similar effects. Production of Factor VII is mainly affected, but IX and X are also reduced in amount, as is prothrombin itself.

Disorders due to circulating coagulation inhibitors. Occasionally a bleeding tendency occurs due to the formation of inhibitors of coagulation factors. These substances can occur in connective tissue diseases, in patients with malignancy, and in pemphigus. Occasionally they develop in elderly men without a predisposing cause. Usually the inhibitor is an antibody to AHG, but in systemic lupus erythematosus the inhibitors affect thrombin formation. Antifactor VIII antibodies may be produced in haemophiliacs undergoing prolonged treatment with cryoprecipitate or Factor VIII.

Disseminated intravascular coagulation. As a result of septicaemia, particularly Gram-negative septicaemia, a widespread intravascular coagulation can occur with generalized fibrin deposition. The whole clotting mechanism is activated and thus clotting factors and platelets are greatly reduced in amount. This acute defibrination is often called 'consumption coagulopathy'. There is a severe haemorrhagic disorder and often circulatory collapse. A similar state of affairs may occur as a result of antepartum haemorrhage or amniotic fluid embolism, probably as a result of autoinfusion of tissue thromboplastin. The disorder may also be found in association with some carcinomas, particularly of the prostate, although it is often less acute. A diagram of the sequence of events is shown (Fig. 29.2). A similar process occurs in the haemolytic uraemic syndrome. The haemolysis in this condition is caused by damage

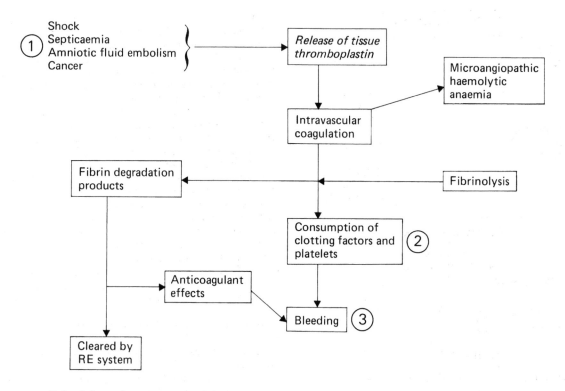

Shock
Septicaemia
Amniotic fluid embolism
Cancer

Release of tissue thromboplastin

Microangiopathic haemolytic anaemia

Intravascular coagulation

Fibrin degradation products

Fibrinolysis

Consumption of clotting factors and platelets

Anticoagulant effects

Bleeding

Cleared by RE system

Principles of management
1. Treatment of cause
2. Replacement of clotting factors
3. Transfusion of blood

Fig. 29.2 Disseminated intravascular coagulation

to erythrocytes in the fibrin mesh deposited in small vessels. In these cases treatment with fibrinogen may be harmful.

Release of plasminogen activator and excess fibrinolysis occurs in situations of tissue trauma and intravascular coagulation. Thus in all the disorders outlined as a cause of acquired fibrinogen deficiency, excess fibrinolysis is occurring too, and may aggravate the bleeding tendency. In addition, after prostatectomy, urokinase, which is an activator of fibrinolysis, may be liberated, and this may account for some cases of excessive bleeding after this operation. Tests of fibrinolysis are not well standardized. In general they involve measurement of the time taken to lyse blood clot, and the detection of fibrin breakdown products.

CLINICAL PROBLEM

T	P	BP	R
37·4	92	150/80	24

Anaemic

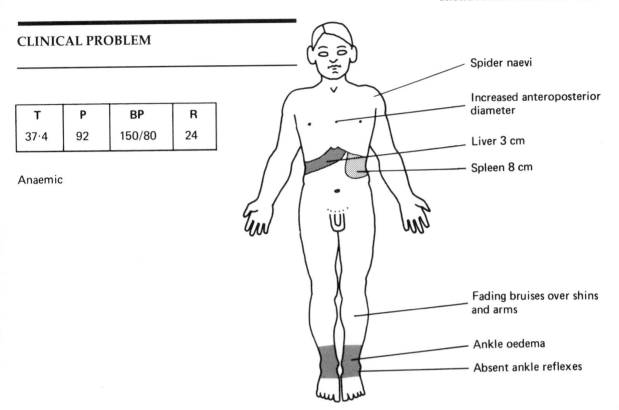

Spider naevi

Increased anteroposterior diameter

Liver 3 cm

Spleen 8 cm

Fading bruises over shins and arms

Ankle oedema

Absent ankle reflexes

An oil company executive aged 55 returned home to England from Nigeria, having been dismissed from his job. He had been abroad for 15 years after demobilization from the army. He had been ill for the past year with weight loss and loss of appetite. There had been no alteration in bowel habit. For 2 months he had noticed moderate ankle oedema, and over the same period of time he had noticed that he was bruising easily. There had not been bleeding from other sites. He was a heavy smoker, having smoked 40 cigarettes a day for 35 years, and had a cough productive of mucoid sputum. He drank spirits regularly.

He had lived a solitary life abroad, in rural Nigeria. He had never married. There was no family history of any bleeding tendency.

On examination he looked unwell. He was clinically anaemic, but not jaundiced or cyanosed. There was moderate ankle oedema, but no other evidence of congestive cardiac failure. The heart was not enlarged. BP 150/80. Pulse 92 regular. In the chest there was an increased anteroposterior diameter, and occasional rales in both lungs which cleared on coughing. In the abdomen the liver was palpable 3 cm below the costal margin, and was smooth. There was enlargement of the spleen, 8 cm below the costal margin. There were no abnormal abdominal wall veins and no ascites. The skin showed occasional purpuric areas over the backs of the hands, and fading bruises over the shins and arms. There were a few spider naevi over the shoulders. The central nervous system was normal apart from loss of both ankle reflexes.

Investigation. Hb 8.1 g/dl. MCV 96 fl. WBC 2.4 × 10^9/l Neutrophils 1.0 × 10^9/l. Lymphocytes 1.2 × 10^9/l. Eosinophils 0.2 × 10^9/l. Platelets 48 × 10^9/l. Prothrombin time 17 s (control 13 s).

QUESTIONS

1. What are the most likely diagnoses?
2. What further investigations should be undertaken?
3. What is the likely explanation of his bleeding tendency?

DISCUSSION

This patient has chronic ill-health, enlargement of the liver and spleen, ankle oedema and absent ankle reflexes. Cirrhosis of the liver is a strong possibility, the ankle oedema being due to hypoalbuminaemia. The possibility of an alcoholic aetiology should be borne in mind because of the social circumstances, and because the ankle reflexes are absent which may indicate alcoholic peripheral neuropathy.

Lymphomas can cause hepatosplenomegaly, and the differential diagnosis from cirrhosis of the liver can sometimes be difficult. There is often lymph node enlargement, but this is not always the case. Lymphosarcoma confined to the spleen can be especially difficult in this respect. Signs of hepatocellular failure such as spider naevi, palmar erythema, and leuconychia are common in cirrhosis but are not found in lymphomas.

Massive splenomegaly is usual in myelofibrosis, but the absence of a leucoerythroblastic blood picture is against this diagnosis. Thrombocytopenia, neutropenia and anaemia can occur in splenomegaly from any cause due to 'hypersplenism', and these findings do not help in the differential diagnosis of the cause of a very large spleen.

Secondary carcinoma is rarely associated with splenomegaly although it may occur if there is portal vein thrombosis. Thrombocytopenia may also be caused by carcinoma if it invades the bone marrow although again a leucoerythroblastic blood picture might be expected.

Great enlargement of the spleen due to chronic malaria is uncommon in European adults in Africa. Kala-azar causes hepatosplenomegaly, and this is a possible diagnosis. It is however an uncommon disorder among Europeans in West Africa, and there is usually marked fever.

Further investigation will include liver function tests including transaminase, γGT and alkaline phosphatase estimations, serum protein determination and serum electrophoresis. An active cirrhosis will be suggested by raised transaminases and hypoalbuminaemia, and a raised gamma globulin. However, any diffuse infiltrative disorders involving the liver may lower the serum albumin and cause a rise in alkaline phosphatase.

A barium swallow is an important investigation, since the presence of varices would greatly strengthen the diagnosis of portal hypertension due to cirrhosis. Their absence would not exclude it. In cirrhosis a liver scan would show a patchy hepatic uptake of isotope and an increased uptake in the spleen. A similar patchy uptake can be observed in any diffuse infiltrative process in the liver.

Liver biopsy is contraindicated because of the bleeding tendency. A bone marrow aspiration may show infiltration with lymphoma and is also of value in the diagnosis of Kala-azar. A marrow biopsy may be needed to exclude myelofibrosis, but this is not a probable diagnosis.

The likely explanation of the bleeding tendency is a combination of thrombocytopenia due to hypersplenism, and hypoprothrombinaemia due to liver disease. Further studies of clotting are not appropriate, since the object of investigation is to establish the primary diagnosis.

This man was dismissed from his post because of alcoholism. It transpired that he had been a heavy drinker for many years and recently his work had begun to suffer. He had portal cirrhosis.

30. Pyrexia of undetermined origin

PUO can be defined as a fever the cause of which is not clear after taking a history and performing a clinical examination. Unskilled or hurried clinical examination will mean that many patients are labelled as having a PUO. Such patients may be subjected to needlessly elaborate diagnostic investigations, often as part of a ritual, rather than with any clear idea in mind. It cannot be stressed too strongly that a meticulous history and examination is the most valuable means of achieving a diagnosis.

The causes of PUO are changing and vary greatly from place to place. For example, typhoid fever is now an uncommon disease in the UK, while this was not the case 75 years ago. Improved standards of hygiene and nutrition have made tuberculosis less common than formerly and rheumatic fever has also declined greatly in incidence. With modern air travel, knowledge of diseases common in the tropics is essential. This must include infections such as tuberculosis and typhoid as well as diseases conventionally associated with the tropics. The AIDS epidemic has led to a considerable change in the variety of infectious diseases which are now routinely encountered.

A brief classification of some causes of PUO which may be found in the United Kingdom at the present time is shown in Table 30.1. Viral infections are

Table 30.1 Some causes of PUO

1. *Bacterial infections*
Subacute infective endocarditis
Collections of pus: subphrenic, renal, intrahepatic, pelvic, empyema
Chronic septicaemia (e.g. meningococcal)
Tuberculosis*: miliary, pulmonary, gastrointestinal, spinal, renal, uterine
Brucellosis
Typhoid
Leptospirosis

2. *Malignant diseases*
Carcinomata:
 hypernephroma
 hepatoma
 secondary carcinoma in liver
 widespread metastases
Lymphoma
Acute leukaemia

3. *Granulomatous diseases of unknown cause*
Crohn's disease
Sarcoidosis

4. *Connective tissue disorders*
Systemic lupus erythematosus
Polyarteritis nodosa
Drug fever
Srill's disease
Giant cell arteritis/polymyalgia rheumatica

5. *Viral and rickettsia diseases*
Influenza
Infectious mononucleosis
Q fever (endocarditis especially)
Prodrome of acute exanthemata
Scratch fevers
HIV infection at ARC stage
Cytomegalovirus*

6. *Protozoal and fungal diseases*
Malaria
Amoebic abscess
Kala-azar
Trypanosomiasis
Histoplasmosis*
Toxoplasmosis*
Pneumocystis carinii*

7. *Unknown cause*
Mediterranean fever
Aetiocholanolone fever

8. *Drug fever*

9. *Factitious*

*Especially common in AIDS

placed last, although these are probably now the commonest cause of PUO. The diagnosis of viral illness is often based on insecure grounds, specific tests being unavailable or retrospective.

THE HISTORY

It is important to understand what the patient's occupation involves, since this may point to the diagnosis: for example, brucellosis in veterinary surgeons and farm workers. As previously mentioned, a careful history of the patient's recent travels is of great importance. A history of malaise and weight loss over a period of time, especially in the middle-aged person, always raises the possibility of cancer, while pruritus points towards the diagnosis of a lymphoma. Joint pains and arthritis are common in subacute infective endocarditis, in chronic gonococcal and meningococcal infections, and in connective tissue diseases.

Skin rashes, which are often transient, may occur in immunological diseases of many kinds, especially in systemic lupus erythematosus, where they may follow exposure to sunlight, and drug allergy. They also occur in chronic bacterial infections such as subacute infective endocarditis and meningococcaemia.

The Acquired Immune Deficiency Syndrome (AIDS) is now so widespread that it must be considered in any patient with PUO. After infection with HIV there is a transient febrile illness followed by a prolonged latent period. Subsequently persistent generalized lymphadenopathy (PGL) develops, followed by a constitutional illness of sweats, fevers and weight loss (AIDS-related complex – ARC). Later, neurological symptoms, due to CNS infection with HIV, and opportunistic infection, may occur. At this stage fever may be the main sign and the diagnosis only becomes apparent when clinical or radiological signs develop. Patients may pass through some or all of these stages at varying rates. While HIV is especially common in male homosexuals, i.v. drug abusers and haemophiliacs, heterosexual transmission is accounting for an increasing number of cases, especially in patients from Africa.

Factitious fever is suggested by the fact that the fever disappears when measured under careful supervision. Occasionally the fever may be genuine but induced by the patient (usually female and often associated with medical work). The patient infects herself deliberately (e.g. by self-catheterization).

PHYSICAL EXAMINATION

An essential point about the physical examination is that it should be repeated regularly. The tendency is all too often to examine the patient once and then to await the results of laboratory tests. Physical signs may develop while the patient is under observation and frequently indicate the diagnosis. Examples of this are obvious: the development of a cardiac murmur,

fundal haemorrhages, skin lesions, or haematuria in subacute infective endocarditis; the development of choroidal tubercles in miliary tuberculosis, or the appearance of a cervical lymph node as the first sign of a lymphoma or carcinoma.

Enlargement of the spleen occurs in many disorders but usually indicates a generalized disease such as septicaemia, connective tissue disease, lymphoma, sarcoidosis, leukaemia or tropical disease. Splenomegaly makes local collections of pus or primary and secondary carcinoma less likely diagnoses.

The presence of signs of disease in many systems makes connective tissue diseases and diffuse infiltrative disease more likely. For example, a patient with polyarteritis nodosa may have mononeuritis, arthritis, skin rash and renal disease; while in sarcoidosis there may be involvement of lymph nodes, lungs, liver, spleen and skin.

Careful examination of the eye with an ophthalmoscope, and, if indicated, with a slit lamp is essential. Retinal haemorrhages or infiltrates may develop in leukaemia or lymphoma as well as in subacute infective endocarditis. Uveitis may occur in sarcoidosis, tuberculosis and toxoplasmosis.

Careful examination of the lymph nodes is of great importance. Enlargement of a single node suggests a secondary spread of carcinoma, or tuberculosis, while generalized lymph node enlargement points to a diagnosis of lymphoma, leukaemia or sarcoidosis. The testes may be the site of a seminoma, which has metastasized to the retroperitoneal lymph nodes.

THE TEMPERATURE CHART

The pattern of the fever may be of diagnostic help (examples are shown in Fig. 30.1).

An intermittent fever is one in which the temperature rises for a few hours and then returns to normal for varying periods. Malaria is the classic intermittent fever, but a similar pattern may be seen in many pyogenic infections, for example ascending cholangitis.

Remittent fever, in which the temperature returns towards normal for a variable period, but is always elevated, is often seen in collections of pus (empyema, etc.) and in carcinoma. It is also a common feature of lymphoma and may occur in abdominal tuberculosis.

In brucellosis, in subacute infective endocarditis and in Hodgkin's disease there may be periods of fever lasting for several days, followed by periods with very little fever (undulant fever).

The temperature chart may, however, show an irregular or continuous fever with no special distinguishing features. Furthermore in many illnesses, pyogenic or malignant, the pattern of fever may vary from one time to another. So many patients have been given broad-spectrum antibiotics before being

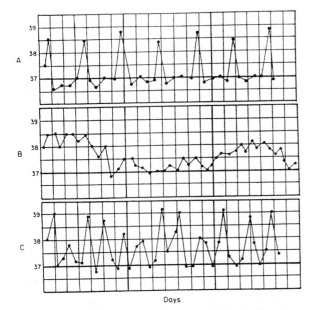

Fig. 30.1 Examples of various patterns of fever **A.** Quartan malaria **B.** Undulant fever (due to Hodgkin's disease) **C.** Empyema of gallbladder

seen in hospital that the patterns of fever from infective causes are no longer typical.

BASIC SCREENING INVESTIGATIONS

Certain simple investigations are performed as a routine in any patient with a fever, because they often indicate the type of disease process which may be present, and which of the many possible more complex investigations are likely to be helpful in diagnosis.

The haemoglobin, red cell indices and blood film. Anaemia is a common concomitant of many diseases but severe anaemia always suggests malignancy. If the blood film and indices show iron deficiency, then occult blood loss and gastrointestinal malignancy are again highly probable. Normochromic normocytic anaemia is a common finding and not of great diagnostic help. Anaemia makes a viral infection less likely.

The white blood count. The hallmark of pyogenic infection is neutrophil leucocytosis, with immature granulocytes and toxic granulation. However there may not be a leucocytosis, especially if the infection has been partially treated by the indiscriminate use of antibiotics. A rise in the neutrophil count can also occur in diseases such as Hodgkin's lymphoma.

Some patients may have a neutrophil leucocytosis of great degree, and this, with the presence of immature white cells, may lead to a mistaken diagnosis of leukaemia. Leukaemoid reactions of this type may be seen in any pyogenic infection. The

differentiation from acute leukaemia may at times be difficult, but in acute leukaemia there is usually a high proportion of blast cells, together with thrombocytopenia and anaemia.

Neutropenia is suggestive of viral infection although it is by no means always present and also occurs in typhoid fever and SLE. In many viral infections, but especially in infectious mononucleosis, atypical mononuclear cells may be seen.

A lymphocytosis sometimes occurs in tuberculosis and can occasionally be of such a degree as to be confused with lymphatic leukaemia. The presence of immature red and white cells in the blood – a leucoerythroblastic blood picture – must always suggest marrow replacement especially by disseminated malignancy.

The erythrocyte sedimentation rate (ESR). Although the ESR is raised in most causes of PUO, levels of 100 mm/h, or more are suggestive of a connective tissue disease or malignancy.

The chest X-ray. Pyogenic infection in the lung, such as an abscess, pneumonia, bronchiectasis or empyema are usually symptomatic and the diagnosis can be made without difficulty. Pulmonary infiltrates occur in connective tissue disease, although they are often transient. In AIDS, pneumocystis carinii pneumonia typically presents with breathlessness and pulmonary infiltrates, although the X-ray may be normal. If suspected, bronchial lavage may be necessary for diagnosis. Secondary deposits may be seen in both the lung fields and as osteolytic or osteosclerotic lesions in ribs. Miliary mottling suggests tuberculosis (especially in HIV-positive patients), sarcoidosis or histoplasmosis. The hilar lymph nodes may be enlarged and if so, tuberculosis, lymphoma, sarcoidosis and secondary carcinoma are probable diagnoses.

Examination of the urine. Proteinuria is a nonspecific finding in a febrile patient, but heavy proteinuria must suggest renal disease, either inflammatory or neoplastic. All kidney infections including tuberculosis are commoner in diabetics, and glycosuria must be excluded. A fresh centrifuged urine must always be examined. Numerous white cells suggest infection, while granular or red cell casts suggest renal inflammation of any cause such as connective tissue diseases and especially subacute infective endocarditis. The haematuria accompanying a hypernephroma may only be detectable on microscopy.

FURTHER LABORATORY INVESTIGATION

A common and most difficult problem is when there are no features in the history of physical examination to suggest the diagnosis and where no evidence is forthcoming in spite of repeated careful examination in hospital.

The problem is the distinction between infection either pyogenic or tuberculous, malignancy including lymphoma, and a connective tissue disease. The diagnosis of a connective tissue disease presenting as a PUO depends on histological evidence or on the later development of the distinguishing features of the disorder. The diagnosis is difficult to make but becomes more likely the longer the patient remains undiagnosed.

Repeated and careful bacteriological investigations are essential. Urine must be cultured in every case. A sterile pyuria suggests tuberculosis and is an indication for culture of the urine for *Mycobacterium tuberculosis*. It also occurs in inadequately treated pyelonephritis. Sputum, if present, must be cultured for *Mycobacterium tuberculosis* as well as pyogenic organisms. Blood cultures are an essential part of the examination and every attempt should be made to culture the blood on at least three occasions before treatment is started. The technique is important, care being taken to prevent skin contamination, and if possible to take the culture as the temperature begins to rise.

In addition to the standard cultures of urine and sputum in the search for tubercle bacilli, culture and inoculation of marrow aspirate, and lymph node and liver biopsy material may also be of value.

Serological tests are a useful adjunct to bacteriological investigation. If AIDS is suspected, the patient should be asked if an HIV test can be performed. Agglutination tests for the detection of *Salmonella* are an essential part of investigation, while brucellosis and Q fever endocarditis can often only be diagnosed in this way. An important point is that a rising titre is of great value in demonstrating active infection, and so the initial serology must always be done as early as possible in the investigation. In rheumatic fever, although a very high ASO titre is diagnostic of recent streptococcal infection, a rising titre is equally valuable. A Paul–Bunnell test for infectious mononucleosis should be performed if the diagnosis is at all likely. Cytomegalovirus infection and toxoplasmosis may closely resemble infectious mononucleosis, but the Paul–Bunnell test remains persistently negative.

Further investigations are undertaken as appropriate. The serum alkaline phosphatase and the SGOT are often elevated in liver disease, and may suggest the need for more tests such as an ultrasound liver scan when abscess or carcinoma is suspected, or a liver biopsy when diffuse infiltration or carcinoma is a possibility. If the scan suggests a space-occupying lesion, more precise knowledge of its nature and site may be gained from a CT scan. If doubt persists then a fine-needle aspiration with culture and cytological examination of the specimen may be diagnostic. Low-grade fever may occur due to cirrhosis itself, or as a result of a complication such as hepatoma, Gram-negative septicaemia, or tuberculosis. If there is a suspicion of disease in the bowel such as tuberculous enteritis, Crohn's disease or lymphosarcoma, then a barium follow-through may be helpful. Often, the nature of the intestinal lesion can only be decided at laparotomy. Pyogenic abscesses and Crohn's disease can sometimes be demonstrated by scanning with [111]Indium-labelled leucocytes (from the patient) which localize at the infection.

Connective tissue diseases may cause great diagnostic difficulty. The DNA antibody test is nearly always positive in active SLE, as are tests for anti-nuclear factor, although the latter are of less diagnostic value. The tests for rheumatoid factor may also be positive in any of the connective tissue diseases, while subacute infective endocarditis, chronic suppuration, and sarcoidosis may all be associated with positive latex fixation tests for rheumatoid factor. In the case of polyarteritis the diagnosis is best established when necrotizing arteritis has been found in tissue such as muscle, skin, kidney or testis. Blind biopsies of these organs are seldom rewarding but a biopsy should be undertaken if there is reason to suspect arteritis in a particular site. Coeliac angiography may reveal characteristic appearances of small vessel disease in polyarteritis. In an elderly patient with PUO and a high ESR a biopsy of the temporal artery, whether tender or not, may show giant-cell arteritis. The response to steroids is characteristically swift.

Ultrasound and CT scanning are of great value in the diagnosis of intra-abdominal tumours. If the disease remains a mystery after exhaustive investigation, or if the patient's condition is deteriorating, then a laparotomy should be seriously considered, since occult cancers, especially lymphomas may defy all attempts at preoperative diagnosis.

Ideally, treatment should never be started until the diagnosis is established. If this proves impossible, then a trial of a broad-spectrum antibiotic is a logical first step. Steroids are never given alone unless tubercle or pyogenic infection can be confidently excluded as a cause of the PUO and this is not often the case. If the probability of tuberculosis seems high, then a therapeutic trial of specific antituberculous drugs – ethambutol and INAH – must be seriously considered.

CLINICAL PROBLEM

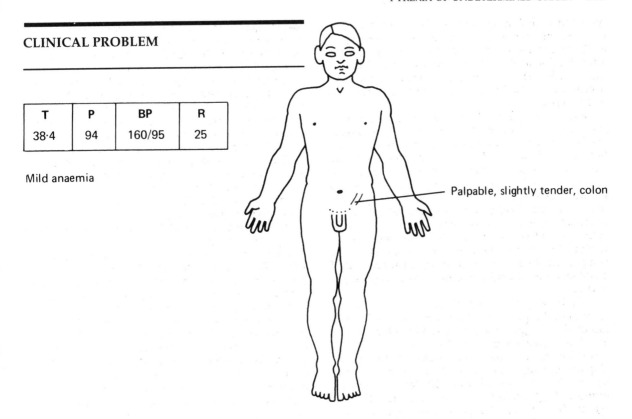

T	P	BP	R
38·4	94	160/95	25

Mild anaemia

Palpable, slightly tender, colon

A 65-year-old businessman presented with a 6-week history of rigors, weight loss and malaise. His wife had died 5 years earlier, and he had been very depressed and had been drinking heavily since that time. He had suffered from constipation for many years, for which he had regularly taken laxatives. On the advice of his family doctor he had gone on a recuperative holiday to southern Italy, and while there had had an episode of left iliac fossa pain and diarrhoea with some blood in the stool. He had received a 5-day course of a broad-spectrum antibiotic and the illness had subsided after 3 days. He had not had any recurrence of diarrhoea. Two weeks after his return he had begun to feel unwell with fevers, and vague upper abdominal discomfort.

On examination he was mildly anaemic. Temperature 38.4°C. There were no other abnormal physical signs except that the descending colon was palpable and slightly tender. Rectal examination was normal. Over the next few days in hospital he had an irregular continuous fever with temperatures varying between 37.5°C and 39.5°C.

Investigation. Hb 10.2 g/dl. MCV 100 fl. MCH 31 pg. WBC 10.4 × 10^9/l (80% neutrophils, 17% lymphocytes, 3% eosinophils). ESR 72 mm/h. Chest X-ray showed a small right pleural effusion and fibrosis at the left apex. MSU – trace of protein, no other abnormality. Serological tests for Salmonella were negative with the exception of *Salmonella typhi* H antigen, which was positive at 1/10 on two occasions 10 days apart.

QUESTIONS

1. What do you consider to be the most likely diagnosis?
2. Which investigations would be most helpful in diagnosis?
3. What would be your immediate management?

DISCUSSION

This patient had an episode of diarrhoea treated with broad-spectrum antibiotics before his present illness began. There is a strong possibility that his illness is related to this. There are no physical signs to suggest a local collection of pus in the abdomen or pelvis, but an hepatic or subphrenic abscess might well be present. The former is more likely, since his previous illness settled down quickly and it is unlikely that he perforated a viscus at that time. A liver abscess is more likely to occur in debilitated elderly patients, and when it does so it often produces few localizing signs. The small right pleural effusion would be compatible with either diagnosis. The slight neutrophil leucocytosis might occur in a partially treated infection of this kind.

An occult carcinoma is a possibility and the stomach, liver and intestine would be the likely primary sites. In Europeans hepatoma nearly always arises in a cirrhotic liver. It is difficult to explain his previous illness on this basis; the duration of his symptoms is only 6 weeks, and there is no evidence of metastases.

His chest X-ray shows apical fibrosis but there is little to suggest pulmonary tuberculosis in this patient. Abdominal tuberculosis causing diarrhoea would not resolve with broad-spectrum antibiotics. Involvement of retroperitoneal nodes is possible, but would not account for his previous episode of diarrhoea.

The course of the illness is too prolonged for typhoid fever. The serology is compatible with TAB immunization but not with infection. The high intermittent fever and rigors are not typical of brucellosis. A lymphoma involving retroperitoneal nodes can produce fever, but the illness is of short duration and the previous episode of diarrhoea would not be accounted for by this diagnosis. Despite the absence of signs of hepatic disease, this patient could have cirrhosis due to his heavy drinking which may cause low-grade fever, or be complicated by Gram-negative septicaemia.

On investigation, an ultrasound liver scan would be very valuable since it may show a filling defect if an hepatic abscess is present. If a filling defect was found, a CT scan might help to differentiate an abscess from a tumour. Blood cultures should be taken. A barium meal and follow-through and barium enema would be helpful, if the liver scan is normal, to look for a carcinoma of the stomach or intestine. A high alkaline phosphatase of liver origin with a low serum albumin would suggest an expanding intrahepatic lesion. If an intrahepatic lesion is found, a fine-needle aspirate should be considered for bacteriological and cytological examination.

If these investigations are normal, laparotomy should be considered. Before diagnosis, no treatment should be given. Immediate management is symptomatic.

> This patient had a pyogenic liver abscess following an attack of diverticulitis. A liver scan showed a filling defect, and treatment with aspiration and antibiotics resulted in cure.

31. Polyuria

Thirst and drinking habits are greatly influenced by social factors, and therefore the daily urine output varies greatly from one individual to another. Polyuria as a symptom means that the patient considers he is passing more urine than he should. There may or may not be associated frequency of micturition, or nocturia. Frequency, a common symptom of urinary tract infection, is not the same as polyuria, although the two symptoms may be confused by the patient. If the patient who has noticed polyuria has not also developed an increased thirst, then with a few important exceptions the complaint is unlikely to have an organic basis. The cause of polyuria can often be determined by the history and physical examination alone.

HISTORY

The age of the patient is important. In children, diabetes insipidus may follow exanthemata, a fracture of the base of skull, or be due to eosinophilic granuloma. Diabetes mellitus may occur at any age, and associated infection and weight loss will strongly suggest this disease. Chronic renal failure is notoriously difficult to diagnose clinically, and polyuria, often with nocturia, may be the presenting symptom of a patient whose kidney disease is already well advanced. Failure to concentrate the urine is particularly characteristic of the renal lesion found in sickle-cell anaemia, and other features suggesting this disorder may be present.

Compulsive water-drinking can provide difficult diagnostic problem, and a careful enquiry must be made into the patient's past and present mental state. Of particular importance is a history of great fluctuation in the severity of symptoms, with periods of remission and relapse. Both these features are unlike diabetes insipidus, but are frequent in compulsive water-drinking.

Hypokalaemia causes impaired renal concentrating ability with resulting polyuria. Long-standing diuretic therapy, ACTH secreting small-cell carcinoma of the bronchus, and prolonged diarrhoea may all be causes of potassium deficiency. A history of the drugs the patient is taking must therefore be obtained, together with details of any respiratory or alimentary disturbances. Hypercalcaemia may cause polyuria, and the associated abdominal pain, constipation and vomiting may suggest that the serum calcium is elevated, as may a history of renal stones. Hypothalamic tumours may present with headache and failing vision together with diabetes insipidus. Polyuria may also accompany the early stages of pregnancy, and occasionally occurs in thyrotoxicosis, but there will usually be other features suggesting these possibilities.

THE PHYSICAL EXAMINATION

Rapid weight loss in a young adult suggests diabetes mellitus. Chronic renal failure is often accompanied by anaemia, and acidotic respiration may be present. A lot of information may be obtained by looking at the eyes. Exophthalmos may occur in eosinophilic granuloma and may be unilateral or bilateral. The cornea may show calcification, which may accompany hypercalcaemia from any cause. It is best seen at the lateral aspects of the corneo-scleral junction. The visual fields may reveal bitemporal hemianopia if a pituitary tumour is present, although in hypothalamic tumours the field defect is often less characteristic. On ophthalmoscopic examination, there may be dot-shaped haemorrhages and exudates in patients with diabetes mellitus, or the changes due to hypertension which often accompanies chronic renal diseases.

Signs of peripheral vascular disease and of motor and sensory neuropathy can occur in diabetes mellitus. Tendon reflexes are often lost in hypokalaemia from any cause, and there is commonly profound muscular weakness and abdominal distension. In the abdomen, the presence of masses in the loins will suggest polycystic disease of the kidneys.

INVESTIGATION

Many of the diseases discussed above are easily diagnosed clinically and by a few simple laboratory tests. More complicated investigations need to be carried out in hospital since accurate estimation of fluid intake and output is necessary.

Examination of the urine is an essential preliminary. If the polyuria is due to diabetes mellitus, this will be obvious, while the presence of proteinuria suggests renal disease. The specific gravity of the urine gives some information since it is low in compulsive water-drinking and diabetes insipidus and often 'fixed' at about 1010 in chronic renal failure.

A chest X-ray may show a carcinoma of the bronchus, pulmonary sarcoidosis as a cause of hypercalcaemia, or the deposits of eosinophilic granuloma in the bones. Measurement of the blood urea and electrolytes are obviously required as a test of renal function and to detect hypokalaemia. If hypokalaemia is present, estimation of the urinary electrolytes in a 24-hour collection will help to show whether or not it is due to a renal loss of potassium. If the hypokalaemia is due to diarrhoea for example, then there will be renal conservation of potassium. If it is due to hyperaldosteronism or a renal tubular defect, then the urinary excretion will be disproportionately high. The serum calcium should be measured. If it is high, then this may be due to a variety of causes such as hyperparathyroidism, metastatic carcinoma, sarcoidosis or vitamin D intoxication.

If an abnormality is discovered by these investigations, then clearly further investigation will follow a variety of different paths.

There remains the most difficult problem, which is the diagnosis of pituitary diabetes insipidus, nephrogenic diabetes insipidus and the distinction between these conditions and compulsive water drinking. Even with the most refined investigations it may be difficult to say with certainty which disorder is present.

THE REGULATION OF PLASMA OSMOLALITY

Before considering more complicated tests, an understanding of the function of antidiuretic hormone (ADH) in the maintenance of normal water balance is necessary.

The normal person's intake of water, as mentioned earlier, is greatly dependent on social and cultural habits. The sensation of thirst does not relate precisely therefore to any single physiological event. It is of course true that dehydration will give rise to thirst, but the strength of the response will vary greatly from one individual to another. There is no sensation which restrains a fully hydrated person from continuing to drink.

If there is excessive loss of water from any cause, the osmotic pressure of the plasma rises (this is measured in milliosmoles/kg and is termed osmolality). This rise in osmolality causes a sensation of thirst and the release of ADH. ADH acts on the distal tubule and collecting ducts, and increases reabsorption of water through a cyclic AMP mechanism, the urine becoming concentrated with a high osmolality. Conversely, if more water is drunk than is needed to replace obligatory losses, plasma osmolality falls. ADH release is inhibited, and a dilute urine (with low osmolality) is passed (Fig. 31.1).

Diabetes insipidus

Diabetes insipidus can arise if there is either no effective ADH formation or release – such as occurs in pituitary tumours – or if the formation and release of ADH is normal but the kidneys are unresponsive to its action – 'nephrogenic' diabetes insipidus. Both these conditions result in the formation of large amounts of dilute urine and result in polydipsia. In the case of nephrogenic diabetes insipidus, there will be no response to injected ADH, while in pituitary diabetes insipidus the kidney should respond by producing a concentrated urine when ADH is given.

The hypothalamic–pituitary system in which the antidiuretic hormone is produced may be damaged by tumours, both hypothalamic and pituitary. Exam-

Table 31.1   Causes of polyuria

1. Polydipsia
Psychogenic

2. Lack of ADH
Idiopathic
Post-surgical
Pituitary tumours
  Craniopharyngioma
  Secondary carcinoma, e.g. breast, bronchus
  Histiocytosis X
Pituitary granulomas
  Sarcoid
  Tuberculosis
Hypothalamic or pineal germ cell tumours
Familial
  Autosomal dominant
  Autosomal recessive
Vascular
  Post-partum pituitary
  Infarction
Infective
  Viral meningitis and encephalitis

3. Failure of renal response to ADH
Primary nephrogenic diabetes insipidus
Renal tubular diseases: chronic renal failure,
  Fanconi syndrome, sickle cell anaemia,
  amyloidosis, myeloma, obstructive myopathy,
  Sjogren's syndrome
Metabolic abnormalities affecting renal tubule:
  hypokalaemia, hypercalcaemia
Drugs affecting renal tubule: lithium,
  demethylchlortetracycline

4. Osmotic diuresis
Diabetes mellitus
Chronic renal failure
Mannitol

ples are pinealomas, gliomas, chromophobe adenomas and craniopharyngiomas. Granulomatous diseases such as sarcoidosis and eosinophilic granuloma may involve the pituitary fossa and the hypothalamic region. Acute viral infections in childhood may be followed by diabetes insipidus. If the cause of the diabetes insipidus is a tumour, then treatment must be directed to the cause of the disorder as well as the resulting hormonal disturbance. It is important to note that some hypothalamic tumours may destroy the 'thirst centre' in addition to the posterior pituitary. These patients are in serious difficulty because they pass large amounts of dilute urine (due to ADH lack) but feel no thirst. They are therefore liable to great increase in plasma osmolality, with marked hypernatraemia. This can lead to irreversible brain damage and death. In contrast, if the posterior pituitary is destroyed by a tumour, the diabetes insipidus tends to improve when there is subsequent destruction of the anterior part of the gland. This may be due to lack of adrenocortical hormones which are necessary for the excretion of a water load. The commonest causes are post-surgical and 'idiopathic' cases which are usually on the basis of autoimmune destruction of the posterior pituitary.

Nephrogenic diabetes insipidus may similarly arise from many causes (see Table 31.1). It can be inherited as a familial sex-linked condition without evidence of other renal disease. The condition appears to be due to a failure of ADH to activate the receptor on the renal tubule. The female carrier may have impaired urine concentrating ability. It may be part of amyloidosis, Fanconi syndrome or myelomatosis, and can follow the relief of chronic obstruction to the urinary tract. A most important cause of failure of concentration ability of the kidney is hypokalaemia, for example due to purgative addiction, or diuretic therapy. This may be accompanied by a total unresponsiveness to administered ADH. The polyuria caused by hypokalaemia, however, may in part be due to increased thirst the reason for which is not known.

Compulsive water-drinking, or psychogenic polydipsia, is characterized by the passage of large amounts of dilute urine due to the high fluid intake. The patient says that he has great thirst, but this has no basis in organic disease. Although a history of hysterical symptoms is common, there may be no other psychiatric abnormality and the true nature of the polyuria may be difficult to uncover. Sometimes the patient gives himself away by having periods when the urine output is normal, or by not having thirst or polyuria at night.

Further investigation

The basic techniques of investigation of these patients are simple. There have to be accurate fluid balance measurements and careful estimations of plasma and urine osmolality. The following is a scheme of investigation (Fig. 31.2).

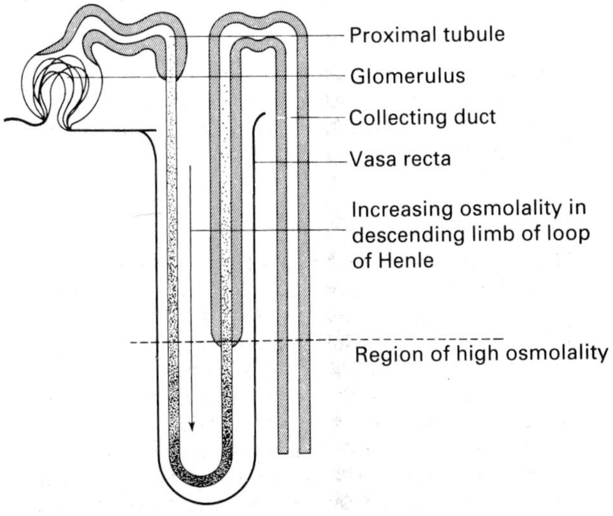

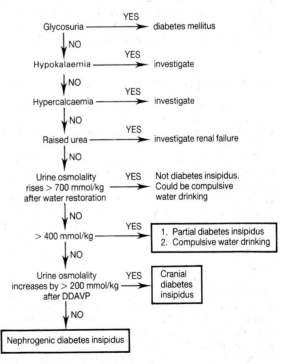

Fig. 31.1 Mechanism of concentration and dilution of the urine.
In the region of high osmolality ADH increases the passage of water out of the collecting duct

Fig 31.2 Investigation of polyuria

(a) Measurement of fluid intake and output, and plasma and urine osmolality. This will give an estimation of the degree of polyuria and polydipsia and forms a useful baseline for assessing treatment.

Wide daily fluctuations of intake and output are suggestive of compulsive water-drinking. The urine osmolality should be low constantly in pituitary and nephrogenic diabetes insipidus (usually below 170 mmol/kg). The plasma osmolality, on the other hand, is normal (270–290 mmol/kg) or high (290–310 mmol/kg) in these two disorders, because a slight degree of dehydration is usually present. In compulsive water-drinking the urine osmolality is also low, but values are often variable while the plasma osmolality is normal or low (250–270 mmol/kg) because there is often some degree of overhydration.

(b) Water-deprivation test. In this test, fluid is withheld until 3% of the body weight is lost. In a patient with pituitary diabetes insipidus or nephrogenic diabetes insipidus there is only a small rise in urine osmolality, and large volumes continue to be passed. The patient feels ill and thirsty and plasma osmolality rises above normal levels. It might be thought that this test will clearly differentiate compulsive water-drinking from the other two types of disorder. This is often the case, but unfortunately any patient who has been passing large amounts of dilute urine for long periods of time develops a partial unresponsiveness to the action of ADH and so fluid restriction in a patient with compulsive water-drinking may not always lead to the production of a normally concentrated urine. In addition patients with familial nephrogenic diabetes insipidus are sometimes able to concentrate their urine after a pro-

longed period of fluid restriction. The test can cause considerable distress and the information obtained from it can often be gained in other ways.

(c) The response to ADH. If the diabetes insipidus is 'nephrogenic' then there will be little or no response to administered ADH (usually administered as its analogue DDAVP – desmopressin). If the patient has pituitary diabetes insipidus or psychogenic polydipsia, there should be a response to ADH with the production of a concentrated urine and a fall in plasma osmolality. The hormone is given and the urine and plasma osmolality are measured over a 6-hour period. Because there may be an acquired resistance to the action of ADH in patients with pituitary diabetes insipidus and compulsive water drinking (due to a fall in osmolality in the renal medulla after a long period of polydipsia), this test may have to be carried out over several days, careful watch being kept on plasma osmolality to avoid overhydration, which is particularly likely to occur in patients with psychogenic polydipsia. Patients with polyuria due to hypokalaemia or hypercalcaemia also fail to concentrate their urine when ADH is administered.

(d) Assay of plasma ADH. Although the previous tests will usually differentiate between pituitary and renal diabetes insipidus and psychogenic polydipsia, they do not always do so. Reliable assays for ADH are not generally available. In renal diabetes insipidus the plasma levels of ADH are raised, while in pituitary diabetes insipidus or compulsive water-drinking the levels are low. In pituitary diabetes insipidus ADH levels do not rise normally after fluid restriction and a rise in plasma osmolality.

CLINICAL PROBLEM

T	P	BP	R
37·2	90	110/70	22

Depressed and withdrawn

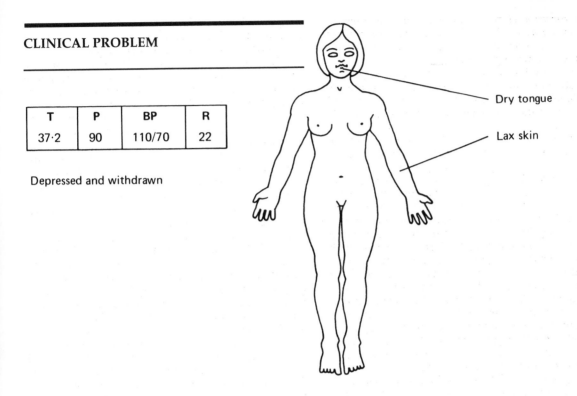

Dry tongue

Lax skin

A woman lawyer aged 35 presented with gradual alteration of mood, lethargy, depression and amenorrhoea of 6 months' duration. She had always been well apart from two attacks of frequency and dysuria 4 years previously, which had been treated successfully with antibiotics. During the previous 6 months she had lost all interest in her family, and her work had suffered greatly. Friends and colleagues had noticed that she had become forgetful, and that she had become prone to bouts of crying for no clear reason. There were no other specific symptoms. She had two children aged 10 and 8 years.

On examination she seemed depressed and withdrawn. She had impairment of recent memory and had difficulty in doing simple arithmetic. There were no localized neurological signs. The tongue was dry and the skin was lax. While in hospital it was noticed that she was getting up at night to pass large quantities of urine. Her family then reported that she had complained of passing more urine than usual for several weeks previously. Urine analysis was normal; specific gravity 1.006.

QUESTIONS

1. How would you account for the change in her personality?
2. What investigations would you perform?
3. What is the probable cause of her illness?

DISCUSSION

The history suggests organic brain disease, for it is unlikely that depression alone would account for the intellectual impairment. The combination of this with polyuria is in favour of a hypothalamic tumour, or an electrolyte disturbance. Hypercalcaemia may cause mental changes and polyuria. Hypernatraemia can be caused by excess water loss if the patient does not drink enough to maintain water balance, and may also cause dementia. This latter situation can occur in any process where there is destruction of the hypothalamus such as in granulomas, craniopharyngiomas or gliomas. A pituitary–hypothalamic disturbance is also suggested by the amenorrhoea. There is nothing to suggest nephrogenic diabetes insipidus, diabetes mellitus, or chronic renal failure. Compulsive water drinking would not account for the memory loss and amenorrhoea. Furthermore the patient did not herself complain of thirst and polyuria, as do patients with compulsive water-drinking. The most valuable initial investigation would be chest and skull X-ray, which might show evidence of a granulomatous disease or tumour in the pituitary region. Serum calcium must be estimated, and blood urea and electrolytes measured. Measurement of urine and plasma osmolality will be useful further investigations. Examination of the visual fields by perimetry may provide additional evidence of a field defect due to a tumour.

The most probable cause of her illness is a lesion in the hypothalamic and pituitary region causing failure of ADH release and dementia. The tumour may well have damaged the hypothalamic thirst centre, resulting in a failure to drink in response to the dehydration caused by progressive urinary water loss. The dementia may be due in part to hypernatraemia. There is no evidence from the history or examination to suggest hypercalcaemia, but this remains a possibility.

> This patient had histiocytosis X involving the pituitary – hypothalamic region with a diabetes insipidus-like picture but without any sensation of thirst. The resultant hypernatraemia had led to dementia which reversed when she was rehydrated (the serum sodium was 175 mmol/l).

32. The routine examination of urine

In a busy outpatient's clinic it is not usually possible for doctors to examine each patient's urine. Usually a simple test for sugar and protein is made. Even this limited investigation reveals unsuspected disease in many patients. In the ward, full analysis of the urine, including examination of the centrifuged deposit, should always be undertaken, and a great deal of useful information may be obtained.

In some cases the finding of an abnormality such as the presence of glucose or protein will be unexpected, and the underlying disease not immediately obvious. The problem may then be how far to investigate an apparently well patient in whom a routine urine examination has shown such an abnormality. The chemical analysis of the urine should always include tests for sugar and protein, and where indicated, tests for ketones and bile pigments. The fresh urine should be centrifuged and the deposit examined. Random measurements of specific gravity or acidity are seldom helpful.

The following account will consider the significance of the presence of glucose, ketones, protein or abnormal sediment in the urine. Tests for bile pigments are discussed in Ch. 15.

SUGAR

There are two standard ways of testing for sugar in the urine. The first is a modification of Benedict's test in which cuprous oxide is formed from copper sulphate and imparts a reddish colour, the intensity of which corresponds to the concentration of glucose present. The Clinitest tablet is the form of test most widely used, and the colour generated is compared with the manufacturer's colour chart. The tablets deteriorate unless they are dry. The second method of testing depends on the oxidation of glucose, by glucose oxidase, to gluconic acid. The enzyme is incorporated into a testing paper ('Clinistix' or 'Testape'). The hydrogen peroxide formed during the oxidation acts on an indicator dye (orthotolidine) to give a blue colour. This latter reaction requires an additional enzyme (peroxidase) which is also present on the paper. The paper is dipped into the urine and the colour develops within 1 minute after exposure to the air.

Benedict's test will give positive reactions with other sugars such as lactose and fructose, and with salicylate derivatives. Glucose oxidase is specific for glucose. Specimens should be tested for sugar within a few hours of collection, unless a preservative is added.

Normal young people excrete about 4 mmol glucose per day, but in later life the 'renal threshold' for sugar rises and this excretion diminishes. Generally speaking any concentration greater than 5.5 mmol/l is highly significant. This is well above the level of sensitivity of the glucose oxidase method, and a positive result with this technique should be checked with Clinitest. On the other hand, a positive Clinitest reaction may be due to substances other than glucose, in which case the glucose oxidase test will be negative.

Assuming that significant glycosuria has been confirmed, what may be its cause? Some patients will have such symptoms as thirst and polyuria which suggest diabetes mellitus, and an elevated blood sugar will confirm the diagnosis. If there is any doubt an oral glucose tolerance test may be needed. However, in elderly and obese patients glycosuria due to diabetes is often symptomless.

A large number of young people have glycosuria without a raised blood sugar. This is termed renal glycosuria, and is found in young men especially, and in about 25% of pregnant women, depending on the sensitivity of the test used. The renal glycosuria of pregnancy disappears within 1 week of delivery. In some patients there is a familial tendency to renal glycosuria usually appearing at about the time of puberty and inherited as an autosomal recessive. Renal glycosuria is due to defective reabsorption of glucose in the proximal tubule, but the nature of the defect is uncertain. The disorder is asymptomatic and affects 2–6 per 1000. There is no associated amino aciduria.

Some patients have a 'lag storage' response to a glucose load. This is a rapid rise in blood sugar, to above normal levels, followed by a rapid return to normal or subnormal levels. Glycosuria may occur transiently at the height of the response. This type of response often occurs after partial gastrectomy and is said to be due to excessive absorption of sugar from the intestine. It also occurs in thyrotoxicosis and in anxious people.

If the glucose oxidase test is negative but there is a positive Clinitest reaction, the patient may have been taking salicylates, or may have lactosuria, fructosuria, pentosuria or galactosuria. Lactosuria is common during pregnancy, and is in fact twice as common as glycosuria. A positive Clinitest is common, and the defect persists into the puerperium at a time when glycosuria has gone. Galactosuria occurs in infants with galactosaemia and is important in early recognition of the disorder. Fructosuria is a very rare condition inherited as an autosomal recessive. Fructose cannot be metabolized and fructosuria occurs after an oral fructose load. Pentosuria is a benign condition in which xylulose is excreted in the urine instead of being metabolized. Pentosuria may also occur after eating large quantities of fruit, and occasionally in morphine addicts.

The finding of a sugar which is not glucose will lead to further analysis of the urine to find out which of the alternative sugars is present.

KETONES

The Rothera test and Acetest tablets are both sensitive tests for acetone. The ferric chloride test for acetoacetate is less sensitive. None of these tests measure β-hydroxybutyric acid. The normal person excretes up to 100 mg of ketones per day, but in diabetic ketosis the excretion may be increased 1000-fold. A false positive ferric chloride test may be caused if salicylates are present in the urine, but the colour is more purple than with acetoacetate and does not disappear if the urine is boiled before performing the test.

Ketosis, as shown by a positive Acetest reaction, occurs in a wide variety of acute illnesses such as pneumonia, myocardial infarction, dehydration and starvation. In diabetes mellitus it is related to the degree of control of the disorder. Patients who are on phenformin often exhibit ketonuria, even though their blood sugar is well controlled. This ketonuria appears to have no harmful effect, but these patients also seem susceptible to the development of lactic acidosis.

PROTEIN

A small amount of protein is present in the urine of healthy people, and levels of up to 100 mg/day are probably within normal limits. This normal protein consists of plasma proteins which have crossed the glomerular basement membrane, tubular proteins probably derived from tubular cells and of small molecular weight. A major component of the tubular protein is a microprotein probably derived from the renal tubules known as the Tamm–Horsfall protein. The latter is a major constituent of the normal urinary protein. Its function is unknown but it is precipitated by albumin and forms a major constituent of urinary casts. Other proteins are derived from the lower urinary tract and seminal fluid.

In glomerular disease, increased quantities of protein may leak across the damaged glomerular basement membrane, in which case the urinary protein will be mainly derived from the plasma, and the size of the molecules passed in the urine will be related to the 'pore size' of the damaged membrane. Protein may also be passed into the urine by damaged tubules either as part of a generalized kidney disease such as chronic pyelonephritis or in diseases where the tubules are the main site of damage such as Fanconi's syndrome, or chronic cadmium poisoning. These proteins are of low molecular weight. Protein may also be derived from the lower urinary tract in acute cystitis or carcinoma of the bladder. These proteins will be normal plasma constituents.

The traditional, but now almost discarded, test for the presence of protein is to boil the urine. A considerable amount of protein has to be present for a visible precipitate to form. The test is still useful because it enables Bence–Jones protein to be detected. This protein consists of the light chains of immunoglobulins formed in patients with myelomatosis. The light chains have a molecular weight of 20 000 and readily cross the glomerular basement membrane. They are reabsorbed and catabolized in the proximal tubule, but some pass into the urine. They have the property of precipitating between 45°C and 55°C and redissolving at 95°C. The failure of the protein precipitate to redissolve, does not exclude the presence of Bence–Jones protein, since in some patients with myelomatosis, renal glomerular damage occurs (due to amyloid infiltration or to infiltration with myeloma) and this additional proteinuria will mask the presence of Bence–Jones protein.

A false positive precipitation may be caused by inorganic phosphates on boiling the urine. Acidification of the urine dissolves this precipitate but not coagulated protein.

A more widely used test is the addition of equal volumes of 25% salicylsulphonic acid to the urine when a cloudy precipitate forms. The degree of turbidity corresponds roughly to the concentration of protein present. False positives are given with radio-opaque diagnostic agents and with tolbutamide. Uric acid also precipitates when present in high concentration but the precipitate dissolves on heating. A positive salicylsulphonic acid test indicates clinically significant proteinuria, since normal concentrations of protein are not detected.

Albustix is a widely used method of testing for protein. A dye, tetrabromophenol blue, changes colour when the local pH is changed by presence of protein. The test is sensitive above 10 mg/dl and therefore also detects clinically significant protein concentrations. A major drawback is that it does not reliably detect low molecular weight proteins such as Bence–Jones protein or tubular proteins. In any patient where myelomatosis is suspected the urine should be heated, as described previously and tested with salicylsulphonic acid. The urine should be concentrated and electrophoresed if the suspicion that the patient has myelomatosis is strong.

There may be a clear reason why the patient has proteinuria, for example a history and physical signs suggestive of acute glomerulonephritis or acute pyelonephritis. Glycosuria or history of diabetes will suggest that the proteinuria is due to diabetic nephropathy (microalbuminuria). A common problem however, is the patient in whom proteinuria is discovered accidentally in outpatients or at an insurance examination when the significance of the finding may then be hard to assess. In particular, in young men postural and exercise proteinuria may present difficulty in diagnosis.

A thorough history and physical examination must be made. The history should include careful questioning about enuresis, nocturia and polyuria as indications of underlying renal disease with failure of ability to concentrate the urine. Illnesses suggestive of urinary infection may have occurred. Patients who have had several attacks do not always experience dysuria but frequency of micturition is a common symptom. In childhood failure to grow and bone pains may be due to chronic renal failure and osteodystrophy, and symptoms due to anaemia caused by chronic renal failure may be present at any age.

On examination the patient may have signs of chronic renal failure such as pigmentation, anaemia, acidotic respiration and peripheral neuropathy. The finding of hypertension in any patient with proteinuria suggests that the latter is due to renal damage.

Many patients with proteinuria have no symptoms or signs of underlying renal disease.

Investigation

The further investigation consists of a careful examination of the centrifuged deposit which may point to an underlying renal disease. This investigation is discussed fully below. The patient should be asked to provide a 24 hour urine collection for a precise estimation of the degree of proteinuria.

Massive proteinuria (more than 5 g daily) is characteristic of the nephrotic syndrome, and other features of this disorder may be present clinically and biochemically with oedema, hypoalbuminaemia, and hypercholesterolaemia. Oedema is likely to occur whenever the protein loss exceeds 0.1 g/kg body weight per day. In the nephrotic syndrome some information regarding the nature of the underlying glomerular damage can be determined by studying the relative clearances of high and low molecular weight proteins. In different types of nephrotic syndrome, the 'pore size' in the glomerular basement membrane differs. This results in protein molecules of different sizes leaking into the glomerular filtrate. Estimation of the concentration of these various sized molecules in a urine and plasma sample enables the clearance of each to be compared. A highly selective protein clearance, where lower molecular weight proteins such as albumin are found in the urine and the clearance of large molecules is very low, is suggestive of minimal change glomerulonephritis. Membranous glomerulonephritis is associated with an unselective clearance pattern and high molecular weight proteins are cleared to nearly the same extent as those of low molecular weight. The presence of renal failure imposes limitations on the conclusions that can be drawn from these tests.

If the nephrotic syndrome is confirmed then many physicians would advocate renal biopsy provided that renal failure was not present. A biopsy may show evidence of an underlying disease such as amyloidosis and may help to influence treatment depending on the histological appearances. In the nephrotic syndrome an intravenous pyelogram may be normal or show slightly enlarged kidneys.

Proteinuria which is not great enough in quantity to cause nephrotic syndrome may none the less be an important sign of renal disease. Chronic glomerulonephritis and chronic pyelonephritis are usually accompanied by proteinuria. Following an attack of post-streptococcal glomerulonephritis proteinuria may persist for weeks or months. Chronic analgesic ingestion may lead to chronic renal failure with proteinuria. If there are no clinical features to suggest these disorders, then the chief difficulty lies in distinguishing these conditions from postural and exercise proteinuria in a young patient.

In a patient with postural proteinuria the diagnosis can be confirmed by the patient lying down for 2 hours. After he has been lying for half an hour he collects a urine sample while recumbent, and again at the end of the 2-hour period. He then gets up and collects another specimen at the end of a 2-hour period. The first and third urine samples will contain protein, the second will not. A test such as this, combined with a normal centrifuged deposit and blood urea in a fit young man, would be regarded as adequate confirmation of the diagnosis of postural proteinuria.

However, in chronic renal disease of many types, the proteinuria is worse when erect and lessens when supine, and some studies have shown that a small number of patients who initially have only postural proteinuria subsequently develop evidence of renal damage.

Many forms of glomerular disease may be associated with asymptomatic proteinuria in an otherwise healthy person. These include focal segmental glomerulonephritis, membranous, proliferative and mesangiocapillary glomerulonephritis. Tubulo-interstitial renal disease and cystic disease of the kidney are other causes. If there is a low level of proteinuria, normal GFR and IVP and no urinary sediment, a 'wait and see' policy is justified.

If the patient is a woman, in whom chronic pyelonephritis is much more likely, or is middle aged, or has proteinuria both erect and supine, or has other evidence suggestive of renal disease such as nocturia or hypertension, then further investigation is always necessary. Examination of a centrifuged specimen is essential and white cells and casts, if present, will strongly suggest primary renal disease. Repeated culture of the urine, for tuberculosis as well as pyogenic organisms, is essential. Estimation of the blood urea is necessary and intravenous pyelography will usually be indicated. This may show small contracted kidneys suggestive of chronic glomerulonephritis or irregular scarring suggestive of chronic pyelonephritis. Changes suggestive of tuberculosis may be present. Clubbing of the calyces and hydronephrosis suggest lower urinary tract obstruction and a micturating cystogram may then be necessary to shown ureteric reflux.

Persistent proteinuria in the absence of definite evidence of structural damage to the kidneys is regarded by some physicians as an indication for renal biopsy. Changes of chronic glomerulonephritis, chronic pyelonephritis and focal glomerulonephritis may be found.

URINE MICROSCOPY

Examination of a centrifuged specimen of urine is a most important investigation and attention to technique is essential.

It is best to collect a sterile mid-stream specimen of urine. Approximately 15 ml are centrifuged for five minutes at 3000 r/min. The supernatant is decanted, but a few drops are left behind to resuspend the sediment, which is then examined.

Normal urine contains no more than two red cells, and two white cells in a 1/6th objective field, and occasional epithelial cells and hyaline casts.

Excessive numbers of epithelial cells occur in acute glomerulonephritis, when the cells are mainly derived from the renal tubule, and in acute cystitis when the cells are derived from the bladder mucosa. In heavy proteinuria due to the nephrotic syndrome tubular epithelial cells are often found which are laden with fat.

Microscopic haematuria may be found in any inflammatory lesion such as acute glomerulonephritis, subacute infective endocarditis, pyelonephritis, or cystitis. Red cells in the urine are an important indication of malignancy especially occult hypernephroma. Renal papillary carcinoma, and bladder papillomata and carcinomata may all bleed. Red cell casts nearly always mean glomerular damage due to acute glomerulonephritis or malignant hypertension.

White cells in excessive numbers can occur due to pyogenic inflammation anywhere in the urinary tract. In chronic pyelonephritis the rate of excretion of white cells commonly exceeds 200 000 in 1 hour, and this may be of diagnostic value. White cells are also found in sterile inflammation as in acute glomerulonephritis, and in general their presence indicates a renal parenchymal lesion. Granular casts may represent degraded white cell casts (or tubular casts) and can also occur with glomerular disease. Epithelial cells trapped in casts suggest glomerulonephritis. A few hyaline casts are a normal finding. Occasionally, in heavy proteinuria, refractive casts containing lipoprotein are found. The absence of casts in the specimen does not allow exclusion of any disease.

Many crystals form in normal urine, and on the whole, give little diagnostic information. In acid urine, uric acid, urates, oxalates and cystine crystals are formed, while in alkali urine crystals of phosphate, ammonium urate and carbonates may be seen.

CLINICAL PROBLEM

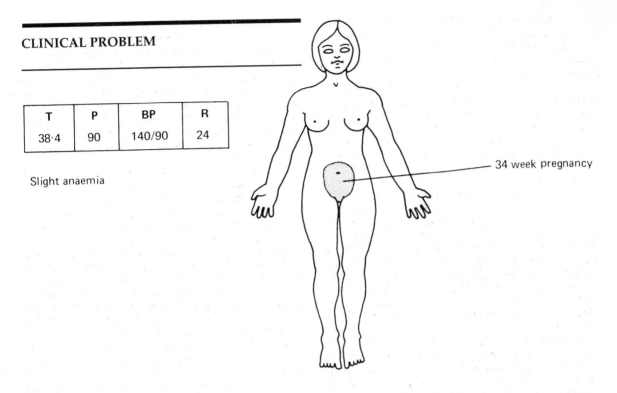

T	P	BP	R
38·4	90	140/90	24

Slight anaemia

34 week pregnancy

A 32-year-old store manageress from Sri Lanka became pregnant for the first time. She had been advised against becoming pregnant by a doctor in Colombo on account of moderately severe asthma which she had had since childhood, and which had been treated for 10 years with prednisone. On this treatment she had felt well and had little trouble from dyspnoea provided her dosage was not reduced below 10 mg/day.

During the first trimester she had a little urinary frequency which had not persisted and which was not associated with dysuria. Shortly afterwards her asthma worsened and she had to increase her prednisone to 25 mg/day, with good effect. At 30 weeks she began to feel rather tired and listless, but attributed this to the pregnancy. At about this time she noticed a return of her urinary frequency. On attending the antenatal clinic at 34 weeks a trace of protein was noted in her urine. She had no ankle swelling or swelling of the hands, but her blood pressure was slightly elevated at 140/95. She was admitted to hospital for rest.

On admission she seemed rather tired. Blood pressure 140/90. Temperature 38.4°C. There was a normal 34 week pregnancy and no other abnormality.

Further investigation revealed Hb 10.4 g/dl. MCV 80 fl. ESR 76 mm/h. Urine showed 2% glucose on Clinitest and was strongly positive with Clinistix, and moderate positive reaction with acetest. The Albustix test showed a 2+ positive reaction and there was a moderate precipitate of protein with salicylsulphonic acid. Examination of the centrifuged deposit showed 16 white cells per 1/6th field, 3–4 red cells, occasional white cell casts and epithelial cells. The urine was sterile on culture on three occasions.

QUESTIONS

1. What might be the cause of her glycosuria?
2. How would you account for the other urinary findings?
3. What further investigations would you do?

DISCUSSION

This patient has been on prednisone for asthma for several years. Asthma may be exacerbated by pregnancy, as in this case, and she had to increase her prednisone dosage. The glycosuria she subsequently developed might be due to the pregnancy itself although the degree of glycosuria is greater than one would expect from this cause alone. The glucose oxidase test confirms that this is glucosuria and not lactosuria. The moderate ketonuria is also not uncommon in pregnancy. Diabetes mellitus is a possibility in this patient and may well have been provoked by both the prednisone in increased dosage and the pregnancy itself. A blood sugar estimation is essential therefore and, if this is equivocal, a glucose tolerance test must be done. The proteinuria may of course be caused by toxaemia, and this is suggested by the rise in blood pressure which was the reason for her admission. However there are other features which suggest that this is not the case. There are numerous white cells in her urine with red and white cell casts. These cannot be accounted for by a very mild toxaemia of pregnancy. In addition she has felt unwell and has a slight fever and a raised ESR. Although the latter may be elevated during pregnancy, this degree of elevation would be unusual.

The illness suggests an underlying infective disorder and the urinary findings strongly point towards a renal cause. The urine has been cultured on several occasions and has been sterile. This, and the absence of urinary symptoms, makes acute pyelonephritis unlikely. Chronic pyelonephritis would account for the urinary findings, and sterile cultures are not infrequently found. This does not seem a likely diagnosis, since she was well before the pregnancy, and it does not account for her vague ill-health, fever and raised sedimentation rate. Pyogenic infection may occur above the site of a blockage to a ureter, for example by a stone, and the signs of inflammation might be masked by prednisone. One would expect some pain and local tenderness over the obstructed kidney and a history of an acute infection which had not settled down completely.

Renal tuberculosis is a strong possibility. A persistent sterile pyuria should always suggest this in any patient. There are several other reasons why the diagnosis should be suspected in this patient. Firstly she comes from Asia and tuberculosis is a common disease in immigrants from the tropical countries. She has been on steroids for several years, recently having had to increase the dose. Tuberculosis is frequently reignited by steroid treatment. Tuberculosis is more common in diabetics and there are grounds for suspecting that this patient may have diabetes; it is also sometimes exacerbated by pregnancy. Lastly, it would account for the urinary findings as well as her ill-health, fever, and raised sedimentation rate.

Further investigation should include examination of early morning urine specimens repeatedly for acid-fast bacilli, together with culture for mycotuberculosis. A Mantoux reaction at 1 in 10 000 will usually be positive if the patient has tuberculosis, and is not affected by steroid treatment in this dosage. A negative reaction would make the diagnosis very unlikely. A chest X-ray may show pulmonary tuberculosis or hilar lymph node enlargement. An IVP cannot be performed on a pregnant patient.

The blood urea should be measured, and the plasma electrolytes also estimated to exclude systemic acidosis. A ferric chloride test should be done as it is of more significance in the assessment of ketonuria than acetest tablets. If her fever persists blood cultures should be performed on several occasions to attempt to isolate a pyogenic organism.

This patient had a positive Mantoux and a normal chest X-ray. Although no acid-fast bacilli were found on microscopy, she was started on treatment with rifampicin, isoniazid and pyrazinamide. Labour was induced at 38 weeks, and a normal male infant was born. One week later the cultures of her urine grew *Mycobacterium tuberculosis* sensitive to all three drugs.

Index